D1216724

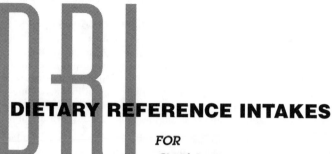

DIETARY REFERENCE INTAKES

FOR
Calcium,
Phosphorus,
Magnesium,
Vitamin D,
and
Fluoride

Standing Committee on the Scientific
Evaluation of Dietary Reference Intakes
Food and Nutrition Board
Institute of Medicine

NATIONAL ACADEMY PRESS
Washington, D.C.

NATIONAL ACADEMY PRESS • 2101 Constitution Avenue, N.W. • Washington, DC 20418

NOTICE: The project that is the subject of this report was approved by the Governing Board of the National Research Council, whose members are drawn from the councils of the National Academy of Sciences, the National Academy of Engineering, and the Institute of Medicine. The members of the committee responsible for the report were chosen for their special competences and with regard for appropriate balance. This report has been reviewed by a group other than the authors according to procedures approved by a Report Review Committee consisting of members of the National Academy of Sciences, the National Academy of Engineering, and the Institute of Medicine.

The Institute of Medicine was established in 1970 by the National Academy of Sciences to enlist distinguished members of the appropriate professions in the examination of policy matters pertaining to the health of the public. In this, the Institute acts under both the Academy's 1863 congressional charter responsibility to be an adviser to the federal government and its own initiative in identifying issues of medical care, research, and education. Dr. Kenneth I. Shine is president of the Institute of Medicine.

This project was funded by the U.S. Department of Agriculture (Grant No. 59-0700-6-061), the National Institutes of Health (Grant No. N01-OD-4-2139, TO 19), the Food and Drug Administration (Grant No. 223-90-2223), and with assistance from Health Canada. The opinions or conclusions expressed herein do not necessarily reflect those of the funders.

Library of Congress Cataloging-in-Publication Data

Dietary reference intakes for calcium, phosphorus, magnesium, vitamin D, and fluoride / Standing Committee on the Scientific Evaluation of Dietary Reference Intakes, Food and Nutrition Board, Institute of Medicine.
   p. cm.
  Includes bibliographical references and index.
  ISBN 0-309-06350-7 (cloth). — ISBN 0-309-06403-1 (pbk.)
  1. Diet. 2. Nutrition. I. Institute of Medicine (U.S.).
Standing Committee on the Scientific Evaluation of Dietary Reference
Intakes.
TX551.D466 1997
613.2′85—dc21   97-33777

Additional copies of this report are available from the National Academy Press, 2101 Constitution Avenue, NW, Lock Box 285, Washington, DC 20055. Call (800) 624-6242 or (202) 334-3313 (in the Washington Metropolitan Area). Order electronically via Internet at http://www.nap.edu.

For more information about the Institute of Medicine, visit the IOM home page at http://www.nap.edu/iom.

Printed in the United States of America

The serpent has been a symbol of long life, healing, and knowledge among almost all cultures and religions since the beginning of recorded history. The image adopted as a logotype by the Institute of Medicine is based on a relief carving from ancient Greece, now held by the Staatliche Museen in Berlin.

STANDING COMMITTEE ON THE SCIENTIFIC
EVALUATION OF DIETARY REFERENCE INTAKES

VERNON R. YOUNG (*Chair*),*† Laboratory of Human Nutrition, School of Science, Massachusetts Institute of Technology, Cambridge

JOHN W. ERDMAN, JR. (*Vice Chair*), Division of Nutritional Sciences, College of Agricultural, Consumer and Environmental Sciences, University of Illinois, Urbana-Champaign

JANET C. KING (*Vice-Chair*),* U.S. Department of Agriculture Western Human Nutrition Research Center, Presidio of San Francisco

LINDSAY H. ALLEN, Department of Nutrition, University of California, Davis

STEPHANIE A. ATKINSON, Department of Pediatrics, Faculty of Health Sciences, McMaster University, Hamilton, Canada

JOHANNA T. DWYER, Frances Stern Nutrition Center, New England Medical Center and Tufts University, Boston, Massachusetts

JOHN D. FERNSTROM, University of Pittsburgh School of Medicine, Western Psychiatric Institute and Clinic, Pittsburgh, Pennsylvania

SCOTT M. GRUNDY,* Center for Human Nutrition, University of Texas Southwestern Medical Center, Dallas

CHARLES H. HENNEKENS, Division of Preventive Medicine, Brigham and Women's Hospital, Boston, Massachusetts

SANFORD A. MILLER, Graduate School of Biomedical Sciences, University of Texas Health Science Center, San Antonio

U.S. Government Liaison

LINDA MEYERS, Office of Disease Prevention and Health Promotion, U.S. Department of Health and Human Services, Washington, D.C.

Canadian Government Liaison

PETER W.F. FISCHER, Nutrition Research Division, Health Protection Branch, Health Canada, Ottawa, Canada

Staff

ALLISON A. YATES, Study Director

CAROL W. SUITOR, Senior Program Officer, Study Director (April 1997–July 1997)

SANDRA A. SCHLICKER, Senior Program Officer

SHEILA A. MOATS, Research Associate (April 1996–November 1996)

---

* Member, Institute of Medicine.
† Member, National Academy of Sciences.

PANEL ON CALCIUM AND RELATED NUTRIENTS

STEPHANIE A. ATKINSON (*Chair*), Department of Pediatrics, Faculty of Health Sciences, McMaster University, Hamilton, Canada

STEVEN A. ABRAMS, Department of Pediatrics, Baylor College of Medicine, USDA Children's Nutrition Research Center, Houston, Texas

BESS DAWSON-HUGHES, Calcium and Bone Metabolism Laboratory, Jean Mayer USDA Human Nutrition Research Center on Aging, Tufts University, Boston, Massachusetts

ROBERT P. HEANEY, John A. Creighton University Professor, Creighton University, Omaha, Nebraska

MICHAEL F. HOLICK, Endocrinology, Nutrition and Diabetes Section and Vitamin D, Skin, and Bone Research Laboratory, Boston University School of Medicine and Boston Medical Center, Boston, Massachusetts

SUZANNE P. MURPHY, Department of Nutritional Sciences, University of California, Berkeley

ROBERT K. RUDE, Department of Medicine, University of Southern California, Los Angeles

BONNY L. SPECKER, Department of Pediatrics, University of Cincinnati and Children's Hospital Medical Center, Ohio

CONNIE M. WEAVER, Department of Food and Nutrition, Purdue University, West Lafayette, Indiana

GARY M. WHITFORD, Department of Oral Biology and Physiology, School of Dentistry, Medical College of Georgia, Augusta

Staff

SANDRA A. SCHLICKER, Study Director
SHEILA A. MOATS, Research Associate (April 1996–November 1996)
ELISABETH A. REESE, Research Associate
KIMBERLY A. BREWER, Research Assistant
ALICE L. KULIK, Research Assistant
DONNA M. LIVINGSTON, Project Assistant (April 1996–January 1997)
GERALDINE KENNEDO, Project Assistant
GAIL E. SPEARS, Administrative Assistant

v

SUBCOMMITTEE ON UPPER REFERENCE LEVELS OF NUTRIENTS

IAN C. MUNRO (*Chair*), CanTox, Incorporated, Mississauga, Canada
STEVEN A. ABRAMS, Baylor College of Medicine, USDA Children's Nutrition Research Center, Houston, Texas
ROBERT P. HEANEY, John A. Creighton University Professor, Creighton University, Omaha, Nebraska
WALTER MERTZ, Retired, Human Nutrition Research Center, Rockville, Maryland
RITA B. MESSING, Minnesota Department of Health, Division of Environmental Health, St. Paul
SANFORD A. MILLER, Graduate School of Biomedical Sciences, University of Texas Health Sciences Center, San Antonio
SUZANNE P. MURPHY, Department of Nutritional Sciences, University of California, Berkeley
JOSEPH V. RODRICKS, ENVIRON Corporation, Arlington, Virginia
IRWIN H. ROSENBERG,* Clinical Nutrition Division, USDA Human Nutrition Research Center on Aging, Tufts University and New England Medical Center, Boston, Massachusetts
STEVE L. TAYLOR, Department of Food Science and Technology, University of Nebraska, Lincoln
ROBERT H. WASSERMAN,† Department of Physiology, College of Veterinary Medicine, Cornell University, Ithaca, New York

Consultants

SHEILA DUBOIS, Food Directorate, Health Canada, Ottawa, Canada
HERBERT BLUMENTHAL, Retired, Food and Drug Administration, Washington, D.C.

Staff

SANDRA A. SCHLICKER, Study Director
SHEILA A. MOATS, Research Associate (April 1996–November 1996)
ELISABETH A. REESE, Research Associate
KIMBERLY A. BREWER, Research Assistant
ALICE L. KULIK, Research Assistant
DONNA M. LIVINGSTON, Project Assistant (April 1996–January 1997)
GERALDINE KENNEDO, Project Assistant
GAIL E. SPEARS, Administrative Assistant

---

* Member, Institute of Medicine.
† Member, National Academy of Sciences.

FOOD AND NUTRITION BOARD

vii

Ex-Officio Member

STEVE L. TAYLOR, Department of Food Science and Technology and Food Processing Center, University of Nebraska, Lincoln

Institute of Medicine Council Liaison

HARVEY R. COLTEN,* Northwestern University School of Medicine, Chicago, Illinois

Staff

ALLISON A. YATES, Director
GAIL E. SPEARS, Administrative Assistant
CARLOS GABRIEL, Financial Associate

Preface

This report represents the initial report of a major new activity of the Food and Nutrition Board (FNB): the development of a comprehensive set of reference values for dietary nutrient intakes for the healthy population in the United States and Canada. Hallmarks of the new activity include (1) the establishment of a set of reference values to replace the Recommended Dietary Allowances (RDAs) for the United States published previously by the FNB; (2) for the first time, a single set of reference values for the United States and Canada; (3) the clear documentation of the derivation of the reference values; (4) the promotion of nutrient function and biologic-physical well-being; (5) the consideration of evidence concerning the prevention of disease and developmental disorders in addition to more traditional evidence of sufficient nutrient intake (for example, prevention of deficiency); (6) the examination of data about selected food components that have not been considered essential nutrients; and (7) recommendations for future research directions based on the knowledge gaps identified.

Since the publication of the last version of the U.S. *Recommended Dietary Allowances* (NRC, 1989a) and of the Canadian *Recommended Nutrient Intakes* (Health Canada, 1990), there has been a significant expansion of the research base, an increased understanding of nutrient requirements and food constituents, and a better appreciation for the different types of nutrient data needed to address the applications of dietary reference values for individuals and population groups. There are now convincing reasons to conclude that past approaches to establishing and applying the RDAs can be improved.

Thus, the FNB considered it essential to reassess the nutrient requirement estimates that are needed for various purposes, how estimates of nutrient requirements should be developed, and how these values could be used in various settings of clinical and public health importance. To this end, the FNB's Standing Committee on the Scientific Evaluation of Dietary Reference Intakes (DRI Committee) is taking steps that should help eliminate some of the limitations, misinterpretations, and misuses of the 1989 RDAs and their predecessors. Indeed, the DRI Committee has already concluded that the 1989 edition of the *Recommended Dietary Allowances* should now be replaced in its entirety, rather than merely updated, by a new series of publications.

The DRI Committee aims to achieve a consistent and coherent definition of requirements and of reference intakes for all essential nutrients and food components evaluated. (A brief description of the process is given in Appendix A.) In this context, the reference intake values presented in this and subsequent reports should have a broad, enduring, and useful application.

This report defines requirements and other reference intake values for calcium, phosphorus, magnesium, vitamin D, and fluoride and represents the first in a series of reports providing both dietary reference intakes and guidance related to how to use them. Changes in the prepublication version (which was released in August, 1997) have been made to increase the readability and clarity of the information provided. Improvements in format and descriptions have been made consistent with the second report released in the series (which covers B vitamins and choline, the prepublication version of which was released in April, 1998). The DRI Committee deeply appreciates the comments received from many reviewers and individuals following the release of the prepublication version.

Because of the limitations of present scientific knowledge, there are differences of opinion among scientists about some of the matters covered in this report. Reaching agreement on the interpretation of the evidence relating to calcium requirements has been a challenge, both because of the compelling conceptual argument to use *maximal* calcium retention as an indicator of adequacy as was presented in the prepublication version of this report, and subsequent statistical questions raised in the methodology used to estimate it after that version was released. In order to address these statistical issues, the DRI Committee chose in this final printed version of the report to refer to the indicator of adequacy used to establish recommended intakes for calcium as *desirable* calcium retention. The balance data originally used in assessing maximal calcium retention were then recalculated (see Appendix E) to establish the estimates for adequacy of dietary calcium based on achieving the estimated desirable amount of calcium retention. In either case, consistent achievement of either *maximal* or *desirable* calcium intakes as the indicator of adequacy is presumed to reduce the risk of fracture secondary to osteopenia or osteoporosis.

After much careful weighing of the evidence, the DRI Committee determined that, because reducing risk of chronic disease was the intended endpoint and there were many uncertainties about the epidemiologic and experimental data, the setting of Estimated Average Requirements and Recommended Dietary Allowances for calcium could not be justified. Thus, as described in the report, Adequate Intake values were set instead.

It is not the function of this report, given the scope of work (see Appendix A, "Charge to the Panel on Calcium and Related Nutrients and Subcommittee on Upper Reference Levels"), to address applications of the DRIs. However, some uses for the different types of DRIs are described briefly in Chapter 9. The DRI Committee intends to issue a subsequent report that will focus on the uses of DRIs in various settings.

It is hoped that the critical, comprehensive analyses of available information and of knowledge gaps will greatly assist the private sector, foundations, universities, government laboratories, and other institutions with their research interests and with the development of an exciting and realistic research agenda for the next decade.

The support of Canada and Canadian scientists in this initiative for DRIs represents a pioneering first step toward the standardization of nutrient reference intakes at least within one continent.

This report reflects the work of the FNB's DRI Committee, an expert Panel on Calcium and Related Nutrients, and the Subcommittee on Upper Reference Levels of Nutrients. The committee, the panel, and the subcommittee owe a considerable debt of gratitude to the many experts who have assisted with this report. Many, but far from all, of these people are named in Appendix B. Thanks also go to the many experts who devoted so much time to discussing these issues and to Burton Altura, Chor San Khoo, and Charles Pak, initial members of the Panel on Calcium and Related Nutrients and/or the Subcommittee on Upper Reference Levels of Nutrients. The respective chairs and members of the panel and subcommittee have performed their work under great time pressure. It is because of their dedication that this report has come into being. All gave of their time willingly and without financial reward; both the science and practice of nutrition are major beneficiaries.

The DRI Committee wishes to acknowledge the tireless efforts of the former and present FNB chairs, Janet King and Cutberto Garza, who began the initiative and played a key role in securing the funding that has been received to date. Similarly, thanks go to Allison Yates who has been instrumental in guiding this complex activity, and to Stephanie Atkinson and Ian Munro, who gave generously of their time and effort in chairing the Panel on Calcium and Related Nutrients and the Subcommittee on Upper Reference Levels of Nutrients, respectively. Finally, it is the staff of FNB who get the work completed. Special gratitude is expressed to Sandra Schlicker, study director for both the calcium panel and subcommittee, and Carol Suitor, who assumed the added responsibility of acting director of the FNB during the last few months of this project. The committee also recognizes the contributions of Elisabeth Reese, Kimberly Brewer, Alice Kulik, Sheila Moats, Gail Spears, Donna Livingston, and Geraldine Kennedo. We also thank Judith Grumstrup-Scott for editing the manuscript and Mike Edington and Claudia Carl for assistance with publication.

Vernon Young
Chair, Standing Committee on the Scientific
Evaluation of Dietary Reference Intakes

Cutberto Garza
Chair, Food and Nutrition Board

Contents

xiii

Summary

BACKGROUND AND HISTORY

This report on calcium and related nutrients[1] is the first in a series of reports that presents dietary reference values for the intake of nutrients by Americans and Canadians. The overall project is a comprehensive effort undertaken by the Standing Committee on the Scientific Evaluation of Dietary Reference Intakes (DRI Committee) of the Food and Nutrition Board, Institute of Medicine, National Academy of Sciences, with the involvement of Health Canada. (See Appendix A for a description of the overall process and its origins.) This initial study was requested by the National Institute of Health's National Heart, Lung and Blood Institute; the U.S. Food and Drug Administration; and the Agricultural Research Service of the U.S. Department of Agriculture. Additional support was received by the U. S. Army Medical Research and Materiel Command,

---

[1]As this report was the first in the series intended to provide both quantitative recommendations for dietary reference intakes and guidance in how they should be used, changes in the prepublication version of this report have been made to increase the readability and clarity of the information provided. Improvements in format and descriptions are included in order to be consistent with the second report released in the series (DRIs for B vitamins and choline). Additionally, due to concerns raised about the statistical approach used in determining maximal calcium retention (see Appendix E), changes have been made with regard to the methodology for estimating calcium retention which were subsequently used in determining recommended intakes for calcium. See calcium discussion which follows in this summary.

Department of Defense and the Office of Disease Prevention and Health Promotion, U.S. Department of Health and Human Services.

WHAT ARE DIETARY REFERENCE INTAKES?

Dietary Reference Intakes (DRIs) are reference values that can be used for planning and assessing diets for healthy populations and for many other purposes. The DRIs replace the periodic revisions of the Recommended Dietary Allowances (RDAs), which have been published since 1941 by the National Academy of Sciences. DRIs encompass the Estimated Average Requirement (EAR), the Recommended Dietary Allowance (RDA), the Adequate Intake (AI), and the Tolerable Upper Intake Level (UL).

As has been the practice with dietary recommendations in the past from the Food and Nutrition Board (NRC, 1980, 1989a, 1989b) and Health Canada (1990), the DRIs included in this report apply to the healthy general population. In the case of RDAs and AIs, they are nutrient levels that should decrease the risk of developing a condition related to a nutrient and associated with a negative functional outcome. Intake at the level of the RDA or AI would not necessarily be expected to replete individuals previously undernourished, nor would it be adequate for disease states marked by increased requirements. Although at times these reference intakes may serve as the basis for recommendations for these other purposes, each situation calls for adaptation by qualified professionals.

For this report, consideration of the dietary practices associated with intakes of calcium and related nutrients has been limited to observations within U.S. and Canadian populations. The recommendations for the DRIs may not be generalizable globally, especially where food intake and indigent dietary practices may result in very different bioavailability of mineral elements from sources not considered in traditional diets of Canadians and Americans.

Estimated Average[2] Requirement

The *Estimated Average Requirement (EAR)* is the nutrient intake value that is estimated to meet the requirement defined by a specified indicator of adequacy in 50 percent of the individuals in a life stage

---

[2] It is recognized that the definition of EAR implies a median as opposed to a mean or average. The median and average would be the same if the distribution of requirements followed a symmetrical distribution, and would diverge as a distribution became skewed. Three considerations prompted the choice of the term

and gender group. At this level of intake, the remaining 50 percent of the specified group would not meet their nutrient needs. For some life stage or gender groups, data had to be extrapolated to estimate this value. In deriving the EARs, contemporary concepts of the reduction of disease risk were among the factors considered, rather than basing reference values solely upon the prevention of nutrient deficiencies.

The EAR is expressed as a daily value averaged over time, for most nutrients at least one week. Because the EAR is a dietary intake value, it includes an adjustment for an assumed bioavailability of the nutrient. The EAR is used in setting the RDA, and it may be used as one factor for assessing the adequacy of intake of groups and for planning adequate intakes by groups.

Recommended Dietary Allowances

The *Recommended Dietary Allowance (RDA)* is the average daily dietary intake level that is sufficient to meet the nutrient requirements of nearly all (97 to 98 percent) individuals in a life stage and gender group. The RDA applies to individuals, not to groups. The EAR serves as the foundation for setting the RDA. If the standard deviation (SD) of the EAR is available and the requirement for the nutrient is normally distributed, the RDA is set at 2 SDs above the EAR:

$$RDA = EAR + 2\ SD_{EAR}.$$

If data about variability in requirements are insufficient to calculate a standard deviation, a coefficient of variation (CV_{EAR}) of 10 percent is assumed in this report, and the resulting equation for the RDA is

$$RDA = EAR + 2\ (EAR \times 0.1)$$
$$RDA = EAR\ (1.2).$$

If the estimated CV is 15 percent, the formula would be

$$RDA = EAR\ (1.3).$$

---

estimated average requirement: (1) data are rarely adequate to determine the distribution of requirements, (2) precedent has been set by other countries that have used the same term for reference values similarly derived (COMA, 1991), and (3) the impreciseness of the data evaluated makes the determination of a statistically reliable median extremely unlikely.

If the nutrient requirement is known to be skewed for a population, other approaches are used to find the ninety-seventh to ninety-eighth percentile to set the RDA.

If data are insufficient for a specific life stage group to set an EAR, then no RDA will be set. An AI will be developed based on the data available (see below).

The RDA for a nutrient is a value to be used as a goal for dietary intake by healthy *individuals*. It is not intended to be used for *assessing* the diets of either individuals or groups or to *plan* diets for groups.

Adequate Intakes

The *Adequate Intake (AI)* is set instead of an RDA if sufficient scientific evidence is not available to calculate an EAR. The AI is based on observed or experimentally determined estimates of average nutrient intake by a group (or groups) of healthy people. For example, the AI for young infants, for whom human milk is the recommended sole source of food for the first 4 to 6 months, is based on the estimated daily mean nutrient intake supplied by human milk for healthy, full-term infants who are exclusively breastfed. The main intended use of the AI is as a goal for the nutrient intake of individuals. Other possible uses of the AIs will be considered by another expert group.

Tolerable Upper Intake Levels

The *Tolerable Upper Intake Level* (UL) is the highest level of daily nutrient intake that is likely to pose no risks of adverse health effects to almost all individuals in the general population. As intake increases above the UL, the risk of adverse effects increases. The term *tolerable intake* was chosen to avoid implying a possible beneficial effect. Instead, the term is intended to connote a level of intake that can, with high probability, be tolerated biologically. The UL is not intended to be a recommended level of intake. There is no established benefit for healthy individuals associated with nutrient intakes above the RDA or AI.

ULs are useful because of the increased interest in and availability of fortified foods and the increased use of dietary supplements. ULs are based on total intake of a nutrient from food, water, and supplements if adverse effects have been associated with total intake. However, if adverse effects have been associated with intake from supplements or food fortificants only, the UL is based on nutrient intake from those sources only, not on total intake. The UL applies to chronic daily use.

For some nutrients, there may be insufficient data on which to develop a UL. This does not mean that there is no potential for adverse effects resulting from high intake. When data about adverse effects are extremely limited, extra caution may be warranted.

COMPARISON OF RECOMMENDED DIETARY ALLOWANCES AND ADEQUATE INTAKES

Although the RDA and AI are used for the same purpose—setting goals for intake by individuals—the RDA differs from the AI. Intake of the RDA for a nutrient is expected to meet the needs of 97 to 98 percent of the individuals in a life stage and gender group. If the EAR is not known, as is the case when an AI is set, it is not known what percentage of individuals are covered by the AI. The AI for a nutrient is expected to exceed the average requirement for that nutrient, and it should cover the needs of more than 98 percent of the individuals, but it might cover the needs of far fewer (see Figure S-1). The degree to which an AI exceeds the average requirement is likely to differ among nutrients and population groups.

For people with diseases that increase requirements or who have other special health needs, the RDA and AI may each serve as the basis for adjusting individual recommendations; qualified health professionals should adapt the recommended intake to cover higher or lower needs.

In this report, AIs rather than EARs and RDAs are being proposed for all nutrients for infants to age 1 year, and for calcium, vitamin D, and fluoride for all life stages. The method used to derive the AI differs for each nutrient and for infants as follows.

Infants: Ages 0 through 6 Months

The AI is the intake by healthy breastfed infants as obtained from average human milk nutrient composition and average milk volume. Since infants self-regulate milk intake from the breast, it is presumed that larger infants, who may require more milk than the average population intake, will achieve this by increasing milk intake volume.

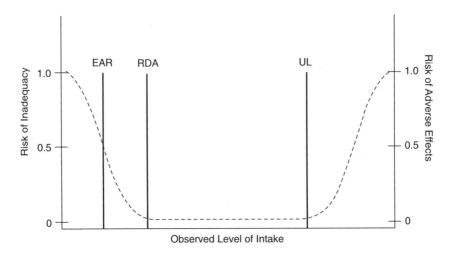

FIGURE S-1 Dietary reference intakes. This figure shows that the Estimated Average Requirement (EAR) is the intake at which the risk of inadequacy is 0.5 (50%) to an individual. The Recommended Dietary Allowance (RDA) is the intake at which the risk of inadequacy is very small—only 0.02 to 0.03 (2 to 3%). The Adequate Intake (AI) does not bear a consistent relationship to the EAR or the RDA because it is set without being able to estimate the average requirement. It is assumed that the AI is at or above the RDA if one could be calculated. At intakes between the RDA and the Tolerable Upper Intake Level (UL), the risks of inadequacy and of excess are both close to 0. At intakes above the UL, the risk of adverse effect may increase.

Calcium

In this report, three major approaches were considered in deriving the AIs for calcium—calcium balance studies of subjects consuming variable amounts of calcium, a factorial model using calcium accretion based on bone mineral accretion data, and clinical trials which investigated the response of change in bone mineral content/density or fracture rate to varying calcium intakes. The prepublication version of this report estimated per cent maximal calcium retention derived from calcium balance data as one of the three major approaches considered to develop the recommended intakes for calcium. Subsequent comments received following the report's release in prepublication form indicated concerns with the statistical methodology used to obtain such estimates from the available balance data. In response to the technical issues raised, the DRI Committee determined for this final printed version that it would estimate *desirable* calcium retention in place of estimating the per cent of maximal retention, using the same data and statistical methodology as was included in the prepublication version (see Appendix E).

Where sufficient data were available, values from balance studies for individual subjects within specific age groups were applied to a nonlinear mathematical model recently used by Jackman et al. (1997) which describes the relationship between varying calcium intakes and retention. The equation derived from this model was then solved to determine the calcium intake required to achieve retention of the desirable amount of calcium. The *desirable* retention varied by age group but for the most part reflected accretion of calcium in bone based on bone mineral accretion data available for some of the age groups.

Another major approach considered by the DRI Committee to estimate intake needed to maintain calcium adequacy was the factorial method. This is based on combining estimates of losses of calcium via various routes by apparently healthy individuals and then assuming that these represent the degree to which calcium intake, as corrected by estimated absorption, will balance these losses. The weakness of using this approach alone is that the data come from different studies, in different subjects, and the variation in absorption, particularly depending on previous intake, may be significant. The third approach derives calcium requirements from the few available clinical trials in which additional calcium was given and changes in bone mineral content or density or in fracture rate were measured over time.

Comparison of the intakes needed to achieve desirable calcium retention or maintain minimal calcium loss using each of these three methods gave reasonable confidence and concordance to the levels of intake recommended as AIs.

The decision to set AIs rather than EARs for calcium was based on the following concerns: (1) uncertainties in the methods inherent in and the precise nutritional significance of values obtained from the balance studies that form the basis of the desirable retention model described in the previous paragraph, (2) the lack of concordance between observational and experimental data (mean calcium intakes in the United States and Canada are much lower than are the experimentally derived values required to achieve desirable calcium retention), and (3) the lack of longitudinal data that could be used to verify the association of the experimentally derived calcium intakes for achieving a pre-determining calcium retention with the rate and extent of long-term bone loss and its clinical sequelae, such as fracture. Taking all of these factors into consideration it was determined that an EAR for calcium could not be established at the present time. The recommended AI represents an approximation of the calcium intake that, in the opinion of the DRI Committee and its Panel on Calcium and Related Nutrients, would appear to be sufficient to maintain calcium nutriture while recognizing that lower intakes may be adequate for many; however, this evaluation will have to await additional studies on calcium balance over broad ranges of intakes and/or of long-term measures of calcium sufficiency.

Vitamin D

The AI is the intake value that appears to be needed to maintain, in a defined group of individuals with limited but uncertain sun exposure and stores, serum 25-hydroxyvitamin D concentrations above a defined amount. The latter is that concentration below which vitamin D deficiency rickets or osteomalacia occurs. The intake value was rounded to the nearest 50 IU, and then doubled as a safety factor to cover the needs of all, regardless of exposure to the sun.

Fluoride

The AI is the intake value that reduces the occurrence of dental caries maximally in a group of individuals without causing unwanted side effects. With fluoride, the data are strong on risk reduction, but the evidence upon which to base an actual requirement is scant, thus driving the decision to adopt an AI as the reference value.

INDICATOR OF NUTRIENT ADEQUACY

The DRIs represent a new paradigm for the nutrition community: three of the reference values are defined by a specific indicator of nutrient adequacy, which may relate to the reduction of the risk of chronic disease or disorders; the fourth is defined by a specific indicator of excess where one is available. In the previous paradigm, the indicator of adequacy was usually limited to a classical deficiency state. Since the publication of the last revision of the *Recommended Dietary Allowances* in the United States (NRC, 1989a), the Canadian Recommended Nutrient Intakes (Health Canada, 1990), and the report on *Diet and Health* (NRC, 1989b), the research base related to the role of diet in chronic disease has expanded sufficiently to permit moving beyond deficiency indicators to other indicators with broader significance. Examples of such indicators are those related to decreasing the risk of chronic diseases such as osteoporosis, heart disease, or hypertension. However, there is insufficient scientific evidence to relate every nutrient to chronic disease. This is the case for phosphorus and magnesium. Thus, EARs and RDAs for these two nutrients are based on traditional indicators (for example, balance studies or circulating nutrient concentrations).

For calcium, it was initially planned to estimate calcium intakes which are thought to lead to the fewest diet-related osteoporotic fractures late in life; unfortunately, the available evidence does not presently exist to establish the precise relationship. Observational data linking calcium intake to fracture risk were considered, although the role of calcium intake at any single life stage in the etiology of osteoporosis is still unclear. Moreover, the long latency period for the development of osteoporosis complicates interpretation of both the epidemiological and experimental data. Epidemiological data are of limited use until more is known about the relationships between calcium intakes by individuals and the phenotypic expression of a specific risk of osteoporosis.

The approach taken was to consider information obtained from several types of studies, that could serve as a basis for setting an AI for each age group. The information reviewed came primarily from published calcium balance studies and calcium accretion data. These data were combined with information on bone mineral content and density using the new dual-energy x-ray absorptiometry technology adding new insights into calcium needs at various stages of the lifespan.

CRITERIA FOR DIETARY REFERENCE INTAKES

The scientific data for developing DRIs were obtained from clinical trials; dose-response, balance, depletion/repletion, prospective observational, and case-control studies; and clinical observations in humans. Studies that measured actual dietary and supplement intake were given more weight than studies that depended on self-reported food and supplement intake. Studies published in peer-reviewed journals were the principal source of data. The data were considered by life stage and gender to the extent possible. This allowed examination of possible physiologic differences in nutrient requirements and utilization. For some nutrients, the available data did not provide a basis for proposing different requirements for various life stage and gender groups. After careful review and analysis of the evidence, scientific judgment was used to determine what indicator of function or other criterion would be used as the basis of the requirement in establishing the EAR, AI, or UL.

For each nutrient, the strengths and weaknesses of relevant studies were assessed. The rationale for the inclusion or exclusion of evidence is given in Chapters 4 through 8. Where applicable, the strength, consistency, and preponderance of the data and the degree of concordance in epidemiological, clinical, and laboratory evidence influenced the selection of the indicators and the derivation of the EARs, AIs, or ULs.

USES OF DIETARY REFERENCE INTAKES

Uses of the DRIs are summarized in the following Box S–1:

For statistical reasons that will be addressed in a future report, the EAR is greatly preferred over the RDA for use in assessing the nutrient intake of groups.

International Uses of Dietary Reference Intakes

Until more is known about the prevalence of chronic disease risk and habitual nutrient intakes in other countries, the implications of these DRIs should be used with caution outside the United States and Canada. When requirements are estimated to decrease risk of disease, particularly chronic disease, associations may not be easily identified in short-term studies. Further, the AIs developed in this report may be at the upper range of intakes typically found in nationwide surveys if the criterion or outcome chosen involves chronic disease. The implication would be that it might be desirable to achieve an increase in the mean intake of the population in order to lower risk. However, the quantitative aspect is uncertain because of the approximate nature of the AI and limitations of the epidemiological and experimental data.

How to Meet Recommended Dietary Allowances or Adequate Intakes

A primary question that must be answered is "How can individuals consume the RDA or AI if surveys indicate that typical diets contain lower amounts?" This becomes a policy issue with regard to choosing methods to increase consumption of that nutrient in order to decrease the number of individuals at risk due to inadequate dietary intakes. Such methods include educating consumers to change their food consumption behavior, fortifying foodstuffs with

---

BOX S-1 Uses of Dietary Reference Intakes for Healthy Individuals and Groups

Type of Use	For the Individual	For a Group
Planning	**RDA:** aim for this intake.	**EAR:** use in conjunction with a measure of variability of the group's intake to set goals for the mean intake of a specific population.
	AI: aim for this intake. **UL:** use as a guide to limit intake; chronic intake of higher amounts may increase risk of adverse effects.	
Assessment[a]	**EAR:** use to examine the possibility of inadequacy; evaluation of true status requires clinical, biochemical, and/or anthropometric data.	**EAR:** use in the assessment of the prevalence of inadequate intakes within a group.
	UL: use to examine the possibility of overconsumption; evaluation of true status requires clinical, biochemical, and/or anthropometric data.	

EAR = Estimated Average Requirement
RDA = Recommended Dietary Allowance
AI = Adequate Intake
UL = Tolerable Upper Intake Level

[a]Requires statistically valid approximation of usual intake.

---

the nutrient, providing dietary supplements, or a combination of the three methods. It is not the function of this report, given the scope of work outlined, to provide an analysis of the impact of using these three methods.

Obtaining recommended intakes from unfortified foodstuffs has the advantage of providing intakes of other beneficial nutrients and of food components for which RDAs and AIs may not be determined, and of the potential enhancement of nutrient utilization through interactions with other nutrients simultaneously. It is recognized, however, that the low energy intakes reported in recent national surveys may mean that it would be unusual to see changes in food habits to the extent necessary to maintain intakes by all individuals at levels recommended in this report. Eating fortified food products represents one method by which individuals can increase or maintain intakes without major changes in food habits. For some individuals at higher risk, use of nutrient supplements may be desirable in order to meet recommended intakes.

It is not the function of this report, given the scope of work (see Appendix A, Origin and Framework of the Development of Dietary Reference Intakes), to address in detail applications of the DRIs, including considerations necessary for the assessment of adequacy of intakes of various population groups and for planning for intakes of populations or for groups with special needs. However, some uses for the different types of DRIs are described briefly in Chapter 9. A subsequent report is expected to focus on the uses of DRIs in various settings.

CRITERIA AND PROPOSED VALUES FOR
EARs, RDAs, AND AIs

Tables S-1 through S-5 present the criteria used for deriving the age-group specific EARs and AIs, as well as the values for EARs, AIs, and RDAs. For vitamin D, the same criterion was used for all the life stage groups; however, for calcium, phosphorus, and magnesium, different criteria were used for some of the life stage groups. For calcium for those ages one year and older, three lines of evidence were considered as described previously, yet due to a lack of experimental evidence for ages 1 through 3 and greater than 70 years, estimates of the AI were extrapolated from other age groups.

The DRIs presented in these tables do not differ by gender except for magnesium and fluoride (because of the gender difference in average body weight). For the other nutrients, differences by gender were not apparent. For calcium, vitamin D, and fluoride, AIs have been estimated. For calcium, phosphorus, vitamin D, and fluoride, the evidence indicated that the AIs or EARs for pregnant and lactating women were no different from those for adolescents and adults of the same age. For magnesium, there was a slight increase in the EARs during pregnancy, but not during lactation.

It is important to recognize that the major focus in the development of EARs and AIs has been the determination of the most appropriate indicator of adequacy, and then, from data available, the derivation of the EAR or AI. A key question is "adequate for what?" The value derived for the EAR, for example, would differ depending on the outcome criterion of nutrient adequacy that was judged to be the most relevant based on the scientific data available. Each EAR and AI is described in terms of the criterion(a) or outcome chosen.

CRITERIA AND PROPOSED VALUES FOR ULs

The model for deriving ULs is described in detail in Chapter 3 of the report. This is a risk assessment model that consists of a systematic series of scientific considerations and judgments to be used in deriving a UL. The hallmark of the risk assessment model is the requirement to be explicit in all the evaluations and judgments that must be made to document conclusions. Primarily due to limitations of the database, ULs are set for very broad age groups.

ULs for calcium, phosphorus, magnesium, vitamin D, and fluoride are presented in Chapters 4 through 8 and summarized in Table S-6. These UL values have been set to protect the most sensitive individuals in the healthy general population (such as elderly individuals who tend to have a decreased glomerular filtration rate). They are likely to be too high for persons with certain illnesses (such as renal glomerular disease) or genetic abnormalities that affect the utilization or decrease the elimination of the nutrient.

RESEARCH RECOMMENDATIONS

Nutrient-specific recommendations for future research needs are provided in detail at the end of each nutrient chapter. The following major research areas are considered the highest priority in order to more accurately determine the DRIs for calcium, phosphorus, magnesium, vitamin D, and fluoride in future reports:

a)   Epidemiological research that evaluates the impact of habitual (lifetime) nutrient intake on functional outcomes related to specific diseases is urgently needed in order to optimize nutrient recommendations. Examples of such research include:

• dietary calcium, peak bone mass and fracture risk
• dietary calcium and prostate cancer
• dietary calcium and renal stones

• exposure to fluoride from all sources with prevention of dental caries and risk of fluorosis

• role of dietary magnesium in the development of hypertension, cardiovascular disease and diabetes.

b)   Research is needed to assess methods for determining individual risk of chronic disease outcomes. For example, the potential relationship between allelic variation in the vitamin D receptor (VDR), bone mineral density, and osteoporosis within and between population groups requires further elucidation in order to determine if VDR polymorphisms are a variable influencing life-long calcium intake needs.

c)   For children ages 1 through 18 years, research is needed to evaluate the dietary intakes of calcium, phosphorus, magnesium, and vitamin D required to optimize bone mineral accretion, especially in relation to changing age ranges for the onset of puberty and growth spurts.

d)   With respect to dietary intake needs for vitamin D, information is required by geographical and racial variables that reflect the mix of the Canadian and United States populations and the influence of sunscreens on intake requirements.

TABLE S-1 Criteria and Dietary Reference Intake Values for
Calcium by Life Stage Group

Life Stage Group[a]	Criterion[b]	AI (mg/day)[c]
0 through 6 months	Human milk content	210
7 through 12 months	Human milk + solid food	270
1 through 3 years	Extrapolation of desirable calcium retention from 4 through 8 years	500
4 through 8 years	Calcium accretion/Δ BMC/calcium balance	800
9 through 13 years	Desirable calcium retention/ factorial/Δ BMC	1,300
14 through 18 years	Desirable calcium retention/ factorial/Δ BMC	1,300
19 through 30 years	Desirable calcium retention/ factorial	1,000
31 through 50 years	Calcium balance	1,000
51 through 70 years	Desirable calcium retention/ factorial/Δ BMD	1,200
> 70 years	Extrapolation of desirable calcium retention from 51 through 70 year age group/Δ BMD/fracture rate	1,200
Pregnancy		
≤ 18 years	Bone mineral mass	1,300
19 through 50 years	Bone mineral mass	1,000
Lactation		
≤ 18 years	Bone mineral mass	1,300
19 through 50 years	Bone mineral mass	1,000

[a] All groups except Pregnancy and Lactation are males and females.

[b] Criteria upon which the AI was based vary between life stage groups depending on the data available in the literature that were judged to be appropriate. The value for the AI reflects an approximation of the calcium intake that is judged to maintain calcium nutriture based upon all of the information examined. See Table 4-5 for a detailed summary of the specific approaches and data considered for each life stage group. Δ BMC is the change in bone mineral content. Δ BMD is the change in bone mineral density.

[c] AI = Adequate Intake. The experimentally determined estimate of nutrient intake by a defined group of healthy people. AI is used if the scientific evidence is not available to derive an EAR. For healthy infants fed human milk, AI is an estimated mean intake. Some seemingly healthy individuals may require higher calcium intakes to minimize risk of osteopenia and some individuals may be at low risk on even lower intakes. The AI is believed to cover their needs, but lack of data or uncertainty in the data prevent being able to specify with confidence the percentage of individuals covered by this intake.

TABLE S-2 Criteria and Dietary Reference Intake Values for Phosphorus by Life Stage Group

Life Stage Group[a]	Criterion	EAR (mg/day)[b]	RDA (mg/day)[c]	AI (mg/day)[d]
0 through 6 months	Human milk content	—	—	100
7 through 12 months	Human milk + solid food	—	—	275
1 through 3 years	Factorial approach	380	460	—
4 through 8 years	Factorial approach	405	500	—
9 through 13 years	Factorial approach	1,055	1,250	—
14 through 18 years	Factorial approach	1,055	1,250	—
19 through 30 years	Serum P_i[e]	580	700	—
31 through 50 years	Serum P_i	580	700	—
51 through 70 years	Extrapolation of serum P_i from 19 through 50 years	580	700	—
> 70 years	Extrapolation of serum P_i from 19 through 50 years	580	700	—
Pregnancy				
≤ 18 years	Factorial approach	1,055	1,250	—
19 through 50 years	Serum P_i	580	700	—
Lactation				
≤ 18 years	Factorial approach	1,055	1,250	—
19 through 50 years	Serum P_i	580	700	—

[a] All groups except Pregnancy and Lactation are males and females.
[b] EAR = Estimated Average Requirement. The intake that meets the estimated nutrient needs of 50 percent of the individuals in a group.
[c] RDA = Recommended Dietary Allowance. The intake that meets the nutrient need of almost all (97 to 98 percent) of individuals in a group.
[d] AI = Adequate Intake. For healthy infants fed human milk, AI is the estimated mean intake.
[e] P_i = Serum inorganic phosphate concentration.

TABLE S-3 Criteria and Dietary Reference Intake Values for Magnesium by Life Stage Group

Life Stage Group	Criterion	EAR (mg/day)[a] Male	EAR (mg/day)[a] Female	RDA (mg/day)[b] Male	RDA (mg/day)[b] Female	AI (mg/day)[c] Male	AI (mg/day)[c] Female
0 through 6 months	Human milk content	—	—	—	—	30	30
7 through 12 months	Human milk + solid food	—	—	—	—	75	75
1 through 3 years	Extrapolation of balance from older children	65	65	80	80		
4 through 8 years	Extrapolation of balance from older children	110	110	130	130		
9 through 13 years	Balance studies	200	200	240	240		
14 through 18 years	Balance studies	340	300	410	360		
19 through 30 years	Balance studies	330	255	400	310		
31 through 50 years	Balance studies	350	265	420	320		
51 through 70 years	Balance studies	350	265	420	320		
> 70 years	Intracellular studies; decreases in absorption	350	265	420	320		
Pregnancy							
≤ 18 years	Gain in lean mass		335		400		
19 through 30 years	Gain in lean mass		290		350		
31 through 50 years	Gain in lean mass		300		360		
Lactation							
≤ 18 years	Balance studies		300		360		
19 through 30 years	Balance studies		255		310		
31 through 50 years	Balance studies		265		320		

[a] EAR = Estimated Average Requirement. The intake that meets the estimated nutrient needs of 50 percent of the individuals in a group.
[b] RDA = Recommended Dietary Allowance. The intake that meets the nutrient need of almost all (97–98 percent) individuals in a group.
[c] AI = Adequate Intake. For healthy infants fed human milk, AI is the estimated mean intake.

TABLE S-4 Criteria and Dietary Reference Intake Values for Vitamin D by Life Stage Group

Life Stage Group[a]	Criterion	AI (µg/day)[b,c,d]
0 through 6 months	Serum 25(OH)D	5
7 through 12 months	Serum 25(OH)D	5
1 through 3 years	Serum 25(OH)D	5
4 through 8 years	Serum 25(OH)D	5
9 through 13 years	Serum 25(OH)D	5
14 through 18 years	Serum 25(OH)D	5
19 through 30 years	Serum 25(OH)D	5
31 through 50 years	Serum 25(OH)D	5
51 through 70 years	Serum 25(OH)D	10
> 70 years	Serum 25(OH)D	15
Pregnancy		
≤ 18 years	Serum 25(OH)D	5
19 through 50 years	Serum 25(OH)D	5
Lactation		
≤ 18 years	Serum 25(OH)D	5
19 through 50 years	Serum 25(OH)D	5

[a]All groups except Pregnancy and Lactation are males and females.

[b]As cholecalciferol. 1 µg cholecalciferol = 40 IU vitamin D.

[c]AI = Adequate Intake. The experimentally determined estimate of nutrient intake by a defined group of healthy people. AI is used if the scientific evidence is not available to derive an EAR. For healthy infants fed human milk, AI is the estimated mean intake. Some seemingly healthy individuals may require higher vitamin D intakes to minimize risk of low serum 25(OH)D levels and some individuals may be at low risk on lower dietary intakes of vitamin D. The AI is believed to cover their needs, but lack of data or uncertainty in the data prevent being able to specify with confidence the percentage of individuals covered by this intake.

[d] In the absence of adequate exposure to sunlight.

TABLE S-5 Criteria and Dietary Reference Intake Values for Fluoride by Life Stage Group

Life Stage Group	Criterion	AI (mg/day)[a]	
		Male	Female
0 through 6 months	Human milk content	0.01	0.01
7 through 12 months	Caries prevention	0.5	0.5
1 through 3 years	Caries prevention	0.7	0.7
4 through 8 years	Caries prevention	1	1
9 through 13 years	Caries prevention	2	2
14 through 18 years	Caries prevention	3	3
19 through 30 years	Caries prevention	4	3
31 through 50 years	Caries prevention	4	3
51 through 70 years	Caries prevention	4	3
> 70 years	Caries prevention	4	3
Pregnancy			
≤ 18 years	Caries prevention	—	3
19 through 50 years	Caries prevention	—	3
Lactation			
≤ 18 years	Caries prevention	—	3
19 through 50 years	Caries prevention	—	3

[a] AI = Adequate Intake. For healthy infants fed human milk, AI is the mean intake. The observed estimate of nutrient intake that reduces the incidence of dental caries maximally in a group of healthy people. The AI is used if the scientific evidence is not available to derive an EAR. The AI is believed to cover their needs, but lack of data or uncertainty in the data prevent being able to specify with confidence the percentage of individuals covered by this intake.

TABLE S-6 Tolerable Upper Intake Levels (UL[a]), by Life Stage Group

Life Stage Group	Calcium (g/day)	Phosphorus (g/day)	Magnesium (mg/day)[b]	Vitamin D (μg/day)[c]	Fluoride (mg/day)
0 through 6 months	ND[d]	ND	ND	25	0.7
7 through 12 months	ND	ND	ND	25	0.9
1 through 3 years	2.5	3	65	50	1.3
4 through 8 years	2.5	3	110	50	2.2
9 through 18 years	2.5	4	350	50	10
19 through 70 years	2.5	4	350	50	10
> 70 years	2.5	3	350	50	10
Pregnancy					
≤ 18 years	2.5	3.5	350	50	10
19 through 50 years	2.5	3.5	350	50	10
Lactation					
≤ 18 years	2.5	4	350	50	10
19 through 50 years	2.5	4	350	50	10

[a] UL = the maximum level of daily nutrient intake that is likely to pose no risk of adverse effects to members of the healthy general population. Unless specified otherwise, the UL represents total intake from food, water, and supplements.

[b] The UL for magnesium represents intake from pharmacological agents only and does not include intake from food and water.

[c] As cholecalciferol. 1 μg cholecalciferol = 40 IU vitamin D.

[d] ND. Not determinable due to lack of data of adverse effects in this age group and concern with regard to lack of ability to handle excess amounts. Source of intake should be from food only in order to prevent high levels of intake.

1
Dietary Reference Intakes

INTRODUCTION

The term *Dietary Reference Intakes* (DRIs) is new to the field of nutrition. It refers to a set of at least four nutrient-based reference values that can be used for planning and assessing diets and for many other purposes. The DRIs replace the periodic revisions of the *Recommended Dietary Allowances*, which have been published since 1941 by the National Academy of Sciences. This is a comprehensive effort being undertaken by the Standing Committee on the Scientific Evaluation of Dietary Reference Intakes of the Food and Nutrition Board (FNB), Institute of Medicine, National Academy of Sciences, with the involvement of Health Canada. See Appendix A for a description of the overall process and its origins.

WHAT ARE DIETARY REFERENCE INTAKES?

The reference values, collectively called the *DRIs*, include the Estimated Average Requirement (EAR), the Recommended Dietary Allowance (RDA), the Adequate Intake (AI), and the Tolerable Upper Intake Level (UL).

A *requirement* is defined as the lowest continuing intake level of a nutrient that, for a specified indicator of adequacy, will maintain a defined level of nutriture in an individual. The chosen criterion on which nutritional adequacy for a nutrient is based may differ according to the life stage or gender of the individual. Hence, partic-

21

ular attention is given throughout this report to the choice and justification of the criterion used to establish requirement values.

This approach differs somewhat from that used recently by the joint World Health Organization, Food and Agriculture Organization, and International Atomic Energy Agency (WHO/FAO/IAEA) Expert Consultation on *Trace Elements in Human Nutrition and Health* (WHO, 1996). That publication uses the term *basal requirement* to indicate the level of intake needed to prevent pathologically relevant and clinically detectable signs of a dietary inadequacy. The term *normative requirement* indicates the level of intake sufficient to maintain a desirable body store or reserve. In developing DRIs, emphasis is placed instead on the reasons underlying the choice of the criterion of nutritional adequacy used to establish the requirement. They have not been designated as basal or normative.

Unless otherwise stated, all values given for EARs, RDAs, and AIs represent the quantity of the nutrient or food component to be supplied by foods from the diet that are similar to those consumed by a life stage or gender group in Canada and the United States. If the food source of the nutrient is very different (as in the diets of some ethnic groups), or if the source is supplements, adjustments may need to be made for differences in nutrient bioavailability. When this is an issue, it is discussed for the specific nutrient under the heading "Special Considerations."

As has been the practice in the past with recommendations regarding dietary allowances from the FNB (NRC, 1980, 1989a), the DRIs included in this report are intended to apply to the healthy general population. RDAs and AIs are dietary intake values that should minimize the risk of developing a condition that is associated with that nutrient in question and that has a negative functional outcome. They could not necessarily be expected to replete individuals who are already malnourished, nor would they be adequate for certain disease states marked by increased requirements. Qualified medical and nutrition personnel must tailor recommendations for individuals who are known to have diseases that greatly increase requirements, or who have increased sensitivity to developing adverse effects associated with higher intakes. Although at times these reference intakes may serve as the basis for such individual recommendations, qualified professional adaptation that is specific to each situation is necessary.

CATEGORIES OF DRIs

Each type of DRI refers to average daily nutrient intake over time. Some deviation around this average value over a number of days is expected.

Estimated Average[1] Requirement

The *Estimated Average Requirement* (EAR) is the daily intake value that is estimated to meet the requirement, as defined by the specified indicator of adequacy, in 50 percent of the individuals in a life stage or gender group (see Figure 1-1). At this level of intake, the other 50 percent of individuals in a specified group would not have their nutritional needs met. The EAR is used in setting the RDA (see below).

Recommended Dietary Allowance

The *Recommended Dietary Allowance* (RDA) is the average daily dietary intake level that is sufficient to meet the nutrient requirements of nearly all (97 to 98 percent) healthy individuals in a specific life stage and gender group (see Figure 1-1). The RDA is intended primarily for use as a goal for daily intake by individuals.

The EAR forms the basis for setting the RDA. If the variation in requirements is well defined and the requirement is normally distributed, the RDA is set at 2 standard deviations (SD) above the EAR:

$$RDA = EAR + 2\ SD_{EAR}.$$

If the SDs reported in studies are inconsistent, or if sufficient data on variation in requirements are not available for other reasons, a standard estimate of variance will be applied. This estimate assumes

---

[1] It is recognized that the definition of EAR implies a median as opposed to a mean or average. The median and average would be the same if the distribution of requirements followed a symmetrical distribution, and would diverge as a distribution became skewed. Three considerations prompted the choice of the term estimated average requirement: (1) data are rarely adequate to determine the distribution of requirements, (2) precedent has been set by other countries that have used the same term for reference values similarly derived (COMA, 1991), and (3) the impreciseness of the data evaluated makes the determination of a statistically reliable median extremely unlikely.

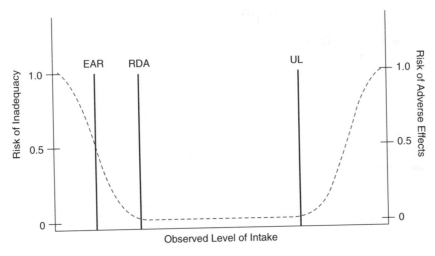

FIGURE 1-1 Dietary reference intakes. This figure shows that the Estimated Average Requirement (EAR) is the intake at which the risk of inadequacy is 0.5 (50%) to an individual. The Recommended Dietary Allowance (RDA) is the intake at which the risk of inadequacy is very small—only 0.02 to 0.03 (2 to 3%). The Adequate Intake (AI) does not bear a consistent relationship to the EAR or the RDA because it is set without being able to estimate the average requirement. It is assumed that the AI is at or above the RDA if one could be calculated. At intakes between the RDA and the Tolerable Upper Intake Level (UL), the risks of inadequacy and of excess are both close to 0. At intakes above the UL, the risk of adverse effect may increase.

a coefficient of variation (CV; SD divided by the mean × 100) of 10 percent, which is equal to 1 SD, such that

$$RDA = 1.2 \times EAR.$$

If the distribution of the nutrient requirements is known to be skewed for a population, other approaches will be used to find the ninety-seventh to ninety-eighth percentile.

The assumed CV of 10 percent is based on extensive data on the variation in basal metabolic rate (FAO/WHO/UNA, 1985; Garby and Lammert, 1984), which accounts for about two-thirds of the daily energy needs of many individuals residing in Canada and the United States (Elia, 1992), and on the similar CV of 12.5 percent estimated for protein requirements in adults (FAO/WHO/UNA, 1985). The assumption is made that the CV of requirements is similar for most nutrients if special outside factors do not apply. In all cases, the method used to derive the RDA from the EAR is stated.

Other Uses of the EAR

Together with an estimate of the variance of intake, the EAR may also be used in the assessment of the intake of groups or in planning for the intake of groups (Beaton, 1994) (see Chapter 9).

Adequate Intake

If sufficient scientific evidence is not available to calculate an EAR, a reference intake called an *Adequate Intake* (AI) is used instead of an RDA. The AI[2] is a value based on experimentally derived intake levels or approximations of observed mean nutrient intakes by a group (or groups) of healthy people. In the opinion of the DRI Committee, the AI for children and adults is expected to meet or exceed the amount needed to maintain a defined nutritional state or criterion of adequacy in essentially all members of a specific healthy population. Examples of defined nutritional states include normal growth, maintenance of normal circulating nutrient values, or other aspects of nutritional well-being or general health.

The AI is set when data are considered to be insufficient or inadequate to establish an EAR on which an RDA would be based. For example, for young infants for whom human milk is the recommended sole source of food for most nutrients for the first 4 to 6 months, the AI is based on the daily mean nutrient intake supplied by human milk for healthy, full-term infants who are exclusively breastfed. For adults, the AI may be based upon review of data from different approaches (e.g., dietary and experimental intakes of calcium) that each alone do not permit a reasonably confident estimate of an EAR.

The issuance of an AI is an indication that more research is needed to determine, with some degree of confidence, the mean and distribution of requirements for a specific nutrient. When this research is completed, it should be possible to replace AI estimates with EARs and RDAs.

---

[2] It should be emphasized that the AI is different from both the RDA as defined here and from the "lower limit of the population mean intake range for nutritional sufficiency" used in the WHO report *Trace Elements in Human Nutrition and Health* (1996), which are each derived from information about the EAR.

Comparison of the AI with the RDA

Similarities. Both the AI and RDA are to be used as a goal for individual intake. In general, the values are intended to cover the needs of nearly all persons in a life stage group. (For infants, the AI is the mean intake when consuming human milk by infants in the age group. Larger infants may have higher needs, which they meet by consuming more milk.) As with the RDAs, AIs for children and adolescents may be extrapolated from adult values if no other usable data are available.

Differences. There is much less certainty about the AI value than about the RDA value. Because AIs depend on a greater degree of judgment than is applied in estimating the EAR and subsequently an RDA, the AI may deviate significantly from the RDA, if it could have been determined, and may be numerically higher than the RDA, if it were known. For this reason, AIs must be used with greater care than is the case for RDAs. Also, the RDA is always calculated from the EAR, using a formula that takes into account the expected variation in the requirement for the nutrient (see previous section).

Tolerable Upper Intake Level

The *Tolerable Upper Intake Level* (UL) is the highest level of daily nutrient intake that is likely to pose no risks of adverse health effects in almost all individuals in the specified life stage group. As intake increases above the UL, the risk of adverse effects increases. It is based on an evaluation conducted using the methodology for risk assessment of nutrients described in Chapter 3 of this report. The need for setting ULs grew out of the increased fortification of foods with nutrients and the use of dietary supplements by more people and in larger doses.

The term *tolerable intake* was chosen to avoid implying a possible beneficial effect. Instead, the term connotes a level of intake that can, with high probability, be tolerated biologically. The UL is not intended to be a recommended level of intake, and there is no established benefit for healthy individuals if they consume a nutrient in amounts above the recommended intake (RDA or AI). As in the case of applying AIs, professionals should avoid very rigid use of ULs and first assess the characteristics of the individuals and/or group of concern; for example, source of nutrient, physiological state of the individual, length of sustained high intakes, etc.

For some nutrients there may be insufficient data on which to base a UL. This indicates a need for caution. It does not mean that high intakes pose no risk of adverse effects.

Determination of Adequacy

The major focus of the development of EARs and AIs has been the determination of the most appropriate indicator of adequacy, followed by the derivation, from available data, of the EAR or AI. A key question is "Adequate for what?" In many cases, a continuum of benefits can be ascribed to various levels of intake of the same nutrient. A specified marker or indicator may be deemed the most appropriate to determine risk of deficiency for a nutrient, while another indicator may be the best marker in determining risk of chronic degenerative disease for that nutrient.

Each EAR or AI is described in terms of the selected criterion or outcome. For example, the dietary intake recommended as the AI for vitamin D for older adults (> 70 years) is based on both a biochemical marker (circulating 25-hydroxyvitamin D) and a functional outcome marker (reduced fractures and bone loss). Using data from clinical studies, an intake of vitamin D associated with normal circulating 25-hydroxyvitamin D concentrations was derived. This intake was supported by clinical trials in which supplemental calcium and vitamin D were associated with a reduced risk of fracture over three years and a reduction in loss of bone mineral density at specific bone sites. Thus, two sets of data form the basis for the AI. Since the individual contributions of the added calcium and vitamin D to the attenuation of bone loss cannot be evaluated, an AI was established. Whether these higher intakes of vitamin D at younger ages will reduce risk of osteoporosis and fracture in later life remains to be determined.

USES OF DIETARY REFERENCE INTAKES

Imbedded in the framework of DRIs is the following approach. When requirements are estimated to decrease risk of disease, particularly chronic degenerative disease where associations may not be easily identified in short-term studies, there must be a preponderance of epidemiologic evidence that is supported by clinical trials and biologically plausible mechanisms before such associations are used to establish recommendations. Given that chronic degenerative diseases and developmental abnormalities may not be detectable for significant periods of time, it is quite possible that individuals who have increased risk due to diet may not be identifiable, and their long-term intake may be less than that which apparently decreases risk of the disease state.

If the strength of the data that associate risk of disease with the nutrient in question is sufficient to permit AIs to be based on such data, and national survey intake data indicate that the median intake is below the AI, then methods must be determined for individuals to increase consumption in order to decrease risk due to inadequate dietary intakes. Primary methods to accomplish this include educating consumers to change their food consumption behavior, increasing intake of fortified foodstuffs, providing dietary supplements, or a combination of these methods. It is not the function of this report, given the scope of work outlined, to analyze the potential impact of using these methods.

The benefits of food as the source of nutrients are well described in previous FNB reports (NRC, 1989a, 1989b). Obtaining RDAs and AIs from unfortified food continues to have the advantage of (1) providing intakes of other beneficial nutrients and food components, for which RDAs and AIs may not be determined, and (2) potentially enhancing intakes through interactions with other nutrients simultaneously. It is recognized, however, that the low energy intakes reported in recent national surveys and thought to result from decreased physical activity may mean that it would be unusual to see changes in food habits to the extent necessary to maintain intakes by all individuals at levels recommended in this report. Eating fortified food products represents one method by which to increase or maintain intakes without major changes in food habits. For some individuals at higher risk, nutrient supplements may be desirable in order to meet reference intakes.

It is not the function of this report, given the scope of the work (see Appendix A, Origin and Framework of the Development of Dietary Reference Intakes), to address applications of the DRIs, including assessment of the adequacy of intakes of various population groups and planning for intakes of populations or for groups with special needs. However, some uses for the different types of DRIs are described briefly in Chapter 9. A subsequent report will focus on uses of DRIs in various settings.

COMPARISON WITH OTHER COUNTRIES

Expert groups in many countries have developed reference values for nutrient intakes (Table 1-1). The number of life stage groups identified by these countries varies considerably. For example, the number of age categories identified within the first year of life rang-

TABLE 1-1 Reference Nutrient Values Used by Various Countries and Groups

Country/ Region	Year	Number of Life-Stage Groups[a]	Number of Infant Groups	Age at which Males and Females are First Treated Separately (years)	EAR RDI RDNI	AI RNI	PRI	RDA
Belgium	1994	4	2	11[b]		✓		
Canada	1990	17	2	7	✓			
European Community[c]	1993	9	1	11		✓		
Germany	1991	14	2	10	✓			
Netherlands	1992	14	2	10		✓		✓
Nordic countries	1989	13	2	11	✓			
Sweden	1989	13	2	11	✓			
United Kingdom	1991	14	4	11	✓	✓		
United States	1989	13	2	11				✓

NOTE: EAR, Estimated Average Requirement. United Kingdom: the required intake of a group of people for energy, protein, a vitamin, or a mineral. About half will usually need more than the EAR and half less.

RDI and RDNI, Recommended Daily Nutrient Intake: the average nutrient intake that meets the requirement needs of 50 percent of a group. The remaining 50 percent of the group will have requirements above the RDI.

RNI, Reference Nutrient Intake or AI, Adequate Intake. United Kingdom, Netherlands: an amount of the nutrient that is enough or more than enough to meet the needs of about 97 percent of people in a group. Canada: RNI = the recommended nutrient intakes of essential nutrients.

PRI, Population Reference Intake: the intake that is enough for virtually all healthy people within a group.

RDA, Recommended Dietary Allowance. United States: the intake that meets the nutrient needs of 97 to 98 percent of a group. Netherlands: the intake that meets the nutrient needs of practically all healthy people in a defined population/age category; applied to planning the food supply for the population group (similar to PRI).

[a] Males and females treated separately after age 7, 10, or 11.
[b] Except for energy.
[c] Adults >18 years all grouped together; age < 6 months not addressed.

SOURCES: Belgian National Council for Nutrition, 1994; COMA, 1991; European Community, 1993; German Society of Nutrition, 1991; Health Canada, 1990; National Food Administration, 1989; Netherlands Food and Nutrition Council, 1992; NRC 1989a; PNUN, 1989.

TABLE 1-2a Magnesium Nutrient Standards for Children Ages 1 to 3 Years and for Adult Females

	Magnesium Nutrient Standards	
Country/Region	Children 1–3 years (mg)	Adult Females (mg)
	Average Requirement or Equivalent	
Germany	80	300
Nordic countries	150	300
Sweden	150	300
United Kingdom	65	250
	Reference Nutrient Intake or Equivalent	
Belgium	80-85	330
Canada	40–50	200[a]
European Community	ND[b]	150–500
Netherlands	60–70[c]	250–300[c]
United Kingdom	85	270
United States	80	280

[a] Higher for women >51 years.
[b] ND = Not determined.
[c] Range given assuming a relationship with body weight.

SOURCES: Belgian National Council for Nutrition, 1994; COMA, 1991; European Community, 1993; German Society of Nutrition, 1991; Health Canada, 1990; National Food Administration, 1989; Netherlands Food and Nutrition Council, 1992; NRC 1989a; PNUN, 1989.

es from one to four. Although the United Kingdom (UK) (COMA, 1991) and The Netherlands (Netherlands Food and Nutrition Council, 1992) use two categories of reference values, and the UK includes an estimate of safe upper levels, the other countries listed in Table 1-1 provide only one each.

Two general types of reference values are used: (1) an estimate of the average requirement or (2) the intake that will meet the requirement of 97 to 98 percent (or virtually all) of the population. The reference values given differ by country. This is illustrated in Tables 1-2a and 1-2b, which give the magnesium and phosphorus values for children ages 1 to 3 years and for females (mainly of childbearing years). Average requirements specified by several countries exceed the values set by other countries for intakes that would meet the needs of virtually all the population within that age group. Criteria chosen for estimating average requirements vary from country to country, as do the judgments made where limited data are available.

TABLE 1-2b Phosphorus Nutrient Standards for Children
Ages 1 to 3 Years and for Adult Females

	Phosphorus Nutrient Standards	
Country/Region	Children 1–3 years (mg)	Adult Females (mg)
	Average Requirement or Equivalent	
Germany	ND[a]	ND
Nordic countries	800	800
Sweden	800	800
United Kingdom	214	406
	Reference Nutrient Intake or Equivalent	
Belgium	700	800
Canada	300–350	850
European Community	300	550
Netherlands	400–800[b]	700–1,400[b]

[a] ND = Not determined.

[b] Range depends on absorption expected.

SOURCES: Belgian National Council for Nutrition, 1994; COMA, 1991; European Community, 1993; German Society of Nutrition, 1991; Health Canada, 1990; National Food Administration, 1989; Netherlands Food and Nutrition Council, 1992; NRC 1989a; PNUN, 1989.

PARAMETERS FOR DIETARY REFERENCE INTAKES

Life Stage Categories

The life stage categories described below were chosen with all the nutrients to be reviewed in mind, rather than only those included in this report. Additional subdivisions within these groups may be added in later reports. For example, pregnancy may be subdivided into two or more periods to accommodate women's changing needs for certain nutrients. Differences will be indicated by gender when warranted by the data.

Infancy

Infancy covers the period from birth through 12 months of age and is divided into two 6-month intervals. The first 6-month interval was not subdivided further because intake is relatively constant during this time. That is, as infants grow, they ingest more food; however, on a body weight basis their intake remains the same.

During the second 6 months of life, growth velocity slows, and thus total daily nutrient needs on a body weight basis may be less than those during the first 6 months of life.

For a particular nutrient, average intake by full-term infants who are born to healthy, well-nourished mothers and exclusively fed human milk has been adopted as the primary basis for deriving the AI for most nutrients during the first 6 months of life. The value used is thus not an EAR; the extent to which intake of human milk may result in exceeding the actual requirements of the infant is not known, and ethics of experimentation preclude testing the levels known to be potentially inadequate. Therefore, the AI is not an estimated average requirement in which only half of the group would be expected to have their needs met.

Using the human milk-fed infant as a model is in keeping with the basis for estimating nutrient allowances of infants developed in the last RDA (NRC, 1989a) and RNI (Health Canada, 1990) reports. It also supports the recommendation that exclusive breastfeeding is the preferred method of feeding for normal full-term infants for the first 4 to 6 months of life. This recommendation has been made by the Canadian Paediatric Society (Health Canada, 1990), the American Academy of Pediatrics (1982) and in the FNB report *Nutrition During Lactation* (IOM, 1991).

In general, for this report, special consideration was not given to possible variations in physiological need during the first month after birth (when, for example, urinary phosphorus loss is lower due to immature glomerular filtration rate [Brodehl et al., 1982; Svenningsen and Lindquist, 1974]) or to the variations in intake of nutrients from human milk that result from differences in milk volume and nutrient concentration during early lactation.

Specific DRIs to meet the needs of formula-fed infants are not proposed in this report. The previously published RDAs and RNIs for infants have led to much misinterpretation of the adequacy of human milk because of a lack of understanding about their derivation for young infants. Although they were based on human milk composition and volume of intake, the previous RDA and RNI values allowed for lower bioavailability of nutrients from nonhuman milk. In order to assist in deriving appropriate intakes of infants fed foods other than human milk, considerations for applying the AIs to formulas are addressed under the "Special Considerations" sections in Chapters 4 through 8.

Ages 0 through 6 Months. To derive the AI value for infants ages 0 through 6 months, the mean intake of a nutrient was calculated based on the average concentration of the nutrient from 2 through

6 months of lactation using consensus values from several reported studies (Atkinson et al., 1995), and an average volume of milk intake of 780 ml/day as reported from studies of full-term infants by test weighing, a procedure in which the infant is weighed before and after each feeding (Butte et al., 1984; Chandra, 1984; Hofvander et al., 1982; Neville et al., 1988). Because there is variation in both of these measures, the computed value represents the mean. It is expected that infants will consume increased volumes of human milk as they grow.

Ages 7 through 12 Months. During the period of infants' growth acceleration and gradual weaning to a mixed diet of human milk and solid foods from ages 7 through 12 months, there is no evidence for markedly different nutrient needs within this period. The basis of the AI values derived for this age category was the sum of the specific nutrient provided by 600 ml/day of human milk, which is the average volume of milk reported from studies in this age category (Heinig et al., 1993), added to that provided by the usual intakes of complementary weaning foods consumed by infants in this age category (Specker et al., 1997). This approach is in keeping with the current recommendations of the Canadian Paediatric Society (Health Canada, 1990), the American Academy of Pediatrics (1982), and *Nutrition During Lactation* (IOM, 1991) for continued breastfeeding of infants through 9 to 12 months of age with appropriate introduction of solid foods.

One problem encountered in trying to derive intake data in infants was the lack of available data on total nutrient intake from a combination of human milk and solid foods in the second 6 months of life. Most intake survey data for the macrominerals do not identify the milk source, but the published values indicate that cow milk and cow milk formula were most likely consumed.

Toddlers: Ages 1 through 3 Years

The greater velocity of growth in height during ages 1 through 3 compared with ages 4 through 5 provides a biological basis for dividing this period of life. Because children in the United States and Canada from age 4 onwards begin to enter the public school system, ending this life stage prior to age 4 seemed appropriate. Data are sparse for indicators of nutrient adequacy on which to derive DRIs for these early years of life. In some cases, DRIs were derived from data extrapolated from studies of infants or of children aged 4 years or older.

Early Childhood: Ages 4 through 8 Years

Because major biological changes in velocity of growth and changing endocrine status occur during ages 4 through 8 or 9 years (the latter depending on onset of puberty in each gender), the category of 4 through 8 years is appropriate. For many nutrients, a reasonable amount of data are available on nutrient intake and various criteria for adequacy (such as nutrient balance measured in young children aged 5 through 7 years) that can be used as the basis for the EARs and AIs for this life stage group.

Puberty/Adolescence: Ages 9 through 13 Years and 14 through 18 Years

Recognizing that current data support younger ages for pubertal development, it was determined that the adolescent age group should begin at 9 years. The mean age of onset of breast development (Tanner Stage 2) for white females in the United States is 10.0 years (SD 1.8); this is a physical marker for the beginning of increased estrogen secretion (Herman-Giddens et al., 1997). In African American females, onset of breast development is earlier (mean 8.9 years (± 1.9). The reasons for the observed racial differences in the age at which girls enter puberty are unknown. The onset of the growth spurt in girls begins before the onset of breast development (Tanner, 1990). The age group of 9 through 13 years allows for this early growth spurt in females.

For males, the mean age of initiation of testicular development is 10.5 to 11 years, and their growth spurt begins 2 years later (Tanner, 1990). Thus, to begin the second age category at 14 years and to have different EARs and AIs for females and males for some nutrients at this age seemed biologically appropriate. All children continue to grow to some extent until as late as age 20; therefore, having these two age categories span the period 9 through 18 years of age seemed justified.

Young Adulthood and Middle Age: Ages 19 through 30 Years and 31 through 50 Years

The recognition of the possible value of higher nutrient intakes during early adulthood to achieving optimal genetic potential for peak bone mass was the reason for dividing adulthood into ages 19 through 30 years and 31 through 50 years. Moreover, mean energy expenditure decreases during this 30-year period, and needs for nutrients related to energy metabolism may also decrease. For some nutrients, the DRIs may be the same for the two age groups. However, for other nutrients, especially those related to energy metabolism, AIs or EARs (and RDAs) are likely to differ for these two age groups.

Adulthood and Older Adults: Ages 51 through 70 Years and > 70 Years

The age period of 51 through 70 years spans the active work years for most adults. After age 70, people of the same age increasingly display variability in physiological functioning and physical activity. A comparison of people over age 70 who are the same chronological age may demonstrate as much as a 15- to 20-year, age-related difference in level of reserve capacity and functioning. This is demonstrated by age-related declines in nutrient absorption and renal function. Because of the high variability in functional capacity of older adults, the EARs and AIs for this age group may reflect a greater variability in requirements for the older age categories. This may be most applicable to nutrients for which requirements are related to energy expenditure.

Pregnancy and Lactation

Recommendations for pregnancy and lactation may be subdivided because of the many physiological changes and changes in nutrient needs that occur during these life stages. In setting EARs and AIs for these life stages, however, consideration is given to adaptations to the increased nutrient demand—such as increased absorption and greater conservation of many nutrients. Moreover, there may be net losses of some nutrients that occur physiologically regardless of the nutrient intake. Thus, for some nutrients, there may not be a basis for EAR or AI values that are different during these life stages than they are for other women of comparable age.

Reference Weights and Heights

The reference weights and heights selected for adults and children are shown in Table 1-3. The values are based on anthropometric data collected during 1988–1994 as part of the Third National Health and Nutrition Examination Survey (NHANES III) in the United States.

The median heights for children aged 4 through 8, for adoles-

TABLE 1-3 DRI Reference Heights and Weights for Children and Adults[a]

Gender	Age	Median Body Mass Index, kg/m^2	Reference Height, cm (in)	Reference Weight,[b] kg (lb)
Male, female	2–6 months	—	64 (25)	7 (16)
	7–12 months	—	72 (28)	9 (20)
	1–3 years	—	91 (36)	13 (29)
	4–8 years	15.8	118 (46)	22 (48)
Male	9–13 years	18.5	147 (58)	40 (88)
	14–18 years	21.3	174 (68)	64 (142)
	19–30 years	24.4	176 (69)	76 (166)
Female	9–13 years	18.3	148 (58)	40 (88)
	14–18 years	21.3	163 (64)	57 (125)
	19–30 years	22.8	163 (64)	61 (133)

[a] Adapted from NHANES III, 1988-1994.
[b] Calculated from body mass index and height for ages 4 through 8 years and older.

cents aged 9 through 13 and 14 through 18, and for young adults aged 19 through 30 were identified, and the weights for those heights were based on Body Mass Index (BMI) for the same individuals within the group. Since there is no evidence that weight should change with aging if activity is maintained, the reference weights for 19- through 30-year-old young adults are applied to all adult age groups.

The most recent nationally representative data available for Canadians (from the 1970–1972 Nutrition Canada Survey [Demirjian, 1980]) were reviewed. In general, median heights of children from 1 year of age in the United States were greater by 3 to 8 cm (1 to 2 1/2 inches) compared to children of the same age in Canada measured two decades earlier (Demirjian, 1980). This could be partly explained by approximations necessary to compare the two data sets, but more possibly by a continuation of the secular trend of increased heights for age noted in the Nutrition Canada survey when it compared data from that survey to an earlier (1953) national Canadian survey (Pett and Ogilvie, 1956).

Similarly, median weights beyond age 1 year derived from the recent survey in the United States (NHANES III, 1988–1994) were also greater than those obtained from the older Canadian survey (Demirjian, 1980). Differences were greatest during adolescence, ranging from 10 to 17 percent higher. The differences probably reflect the secular trend of earlier onset of puberty (Herman-Giddens et al., 1997), rather than differences in populations. Calculations of BMI for young adults (for example, a median of 22.6 for Canadian women compared to 22.8 for American women) resulted in similar values, indicating that by adulthood there was greater concordance between the two surveys.

The reference weights chosen for this report were based on the most recent data set available from either country, recognizing that earlier surveys in Canada indicated shorter stature and lower weights during adolescence compared to those from surveys in the United States.

Reference weights are used primarily when setting the EAR, AI, or UL for children or when relating the nutrient needs of adults to body weight. For the 4- to 8-year-old age group, it can be assumed that a small 4-year-old child will require less than the EAR and that a large 8-year-old will require more than the EAR. However, the RDA should meet the needs of both.

SUMMARY

Dietary Reference Intakes is a generic term for a set of nutrient reference values that includes Estimated Average Requirement, Recommended Dietary Allowance, Adequate Intake, and Tolerable Upper Intake Level. These reference values are being developed for life stage and gender groups in a joint U.S.-Canadian activity. This report, which is the first in a series, covers the DRIs for calcium and four related nutrients: phosphorus, magnesium, vitamin D, and fluoride.

2

Calcium and Related Nutrients: Overview and Methods

OVERVIEW

This report focuses on five nutrients—calcium, phosphorus, magnesium, vitamin D, and fluoride, all of which play a key role in the development and maintenance of bone and other calcified tissues. Indeed, 99 percent of body calcium, 85 percent of body phosphorus, 50 to 60 percent of body magnesium, and 99 percent of body fluoride are found in bone or other calcified tissues. Vitamin D functions as the substrate for the synthesis of 1,25-dihydroxyvitamin D, which is the active hormone necessary for the regulation of calcium and phosphorus homeostasis.

Although the development and preservation of bone mass are key elements in the estimation of the needs for these five nutrients for the population of the United States and Canada, the evidence considered includes other biological roles for these nutrients and their possible relevance to human health and to decreasing risk of disease. For the most part, however, it is the functioning of these nutrients in bone and teeth that provided the most convincing criteria on which to base the new Dietary Reference Intakes (DRIs).

Other nutrients may be of biological significance to the development and maintenance of bone. These include the microminerals copper, zinc, manganese, and boron and the vitamins C and K. With the exception of boron, all these nutrients have been identified as required cofactors for enzymes that act in the synthesis or post-translational modification of constituents of bone matrix. Vitamin C is essential for collagen cross-linking, and vitamin K is essen-

38

tial for the gamma carboxylation of three bone matrix proteins (for example, osteocalcin, which facilitates calcium binding to hydroxyapatite). With the exception of boron, deficiencies of these nutrients in growing animals have been associated with bone lesions (Heaney, 1997). In humans, the primary biological function of these nutrients does not appear to be bone metabolism and maintenance of skeletal integrity. Bone fragility in humans related to deficiencies of these trace elements and vitamins has not been well described. Thus, these trace elements and vitamins will be covered in subsequent DRI reports that deal with their major functions.

The roles of boron in human health, in general, and in bone metabolism, in particular, are uncertain. Studies in animals suggest that boron contributes to the composition and strength characteristics of bone (Hunt and Nielsen, 1981). Boron may have an interactive role with vitamin D because it affects steroid hormone metabolism in humans (Nielsen, 1990; Nielsen et al., 1987). In studies in postmenopausal women, boron depletion was not consistently found to alter calcium and vitamin D homeostasis (Nielsen et al., 1987; Peace and Beattie, 1991). Epidemiological evidence of a relationship between dietary boron status and osteoporosis is not available. Thus, it was deemed premature to consider boron as a nutrient functionally related to bone health, and boron was not included in this report.

METHODOLOGICAL CONSIDERATIONS

The scientific data for developing the DRIs have come primarily from clinical, dose-response, balance, depletion-repletion, observational, and case-control studies. In general, only studies published in peer-reviewed journals have been utilized. However, studies published in other scientific journals or readily available reports were considered if they appeared to provide important information on health effects not documented elsewhere. In some cases they were used to estimate intakes. If applicable, original scientific studies were used for the critical determinants of endpoints for deriving the Estimated Average Requirement (EAR), Adequate Intake (AI), and Tolerable Upper Intake Level (UL) for each nutrient at each stage of the lifespan.

Based on a thorough review of the scientific literature, the possible criterion or outcomes of nutrient adequacy were identified for each nutrient and life stage or gender group. The choice of the indicator to utilize in determining the EAR or AI was based on scientific judgment. The strengths and weaknesses of each study considered in developing the EAR or AI were assessed. Chapters 4 through 8 describe the rationale for the inclusion or exclusion of evidence. Among the factors considered were the methods used to determine intake from food and supplements; methods used for measuring the indicator of adequacy; relationships among the indicator, dietary intake, and functional or physiologic outcome; any allowances for adaptation to changes in intake; and other aspects of the study design.

When applicable, the strength, consistency, and preponderance of the data and the degree of concordance among epidemiological, clinical, and laboratory evidence determined the strengths of the indicators that were used as the basis for EARs and AIs in each stage of the lifespan. As was adopted by the Surgeon General's *Report on Nutrition and Health* (DHHS, 1988) and the Food and Nutrition Board's *Diet and Health* (NRC, 1989b), the assessment of the strength of the data supporting a nutrient's role in decreasing risk of chronic debilitating disease or developmental abnormalities was based on the following criteria (Hill, 1971):

- strength of association, usually expressed as relative risk;
- dose-response relationship;
- temporally correct association, with exposure preceding the onset of disease;
- consistency of association;
- specificity of association; and
- biological plausibility.

The greatest weight was given to studies, if available, that were directly related to a determination of nutrient needs and that used an appropriate experimental design and outcome measure. Less weight was given to studies in which observed levels of nutrient intake were related to a specific criterion or criteria of nutriture. Neither average dietary intake data nor indicator of adequacy data alone provided a sufficient basis for deriving an EAR, although this approach, of necessity, was applied to the development of AIs for infants and for fluoride. If necessary, a factorial model could be used as a basis for estimating the physiological requirement, which could then be used to estimate the dietary requirement for a nutrient. This process was used to estimate the phosphorus requirements for some life stage groups.

In developing estimates of average requirements for minerals such as calcium, phosphorus, and magnesium, the available literature until the late 1980s consisted primarily of balance studies in which normal subjects with somewhat similar age, body size, and gender characteristics were tested while consuming different dietary intakes. A key concern in such studies was the significant body store represented by the skeletal tissues for these nutrients and the fact that the balance method could easily fail to detect, due to systematic bias or error, small changes in mineral status. In addition, balance studies tend to err toward a positive balance since intake is usually overestimated and excretion is underestimated. With the advent of readily available noninvasive and fairly inexpensive methods to detect changes in bone mineral content and bone mineral density, additional information relative to small changes became available to augment information from balance studies.

In general, in order to account for possible errors introduced through the use of available balance data, criteria and methods for compiling balance data that could be used to develop DRIs for calcium and magnesium included the following:

• Preferential use was made of studies on self-selected calcium intakes in order to avoid the bone remodeling transient as described in Chapter 4.

• For every situation, data from more than one reported investigation of calcium balance were considered.

• Only balance studies whose dietary periods were thought to be long enough to assure a reasonable degree of adaptation to the diet via urinary and fecal losses were used.

• In some instances (as for children ages 9 through 13 years), comparable data from individual investigations were combined to create a larger sample size in order to facilitate use of a statistical model which describes the relationship between calcium intake and retention over a range of intakes. Using the equation derived from this model (see Appendix E), a prediction of calcium intake required to attain a desirable calcium retention could be obtained.

• When investigators did not measure or estimate miscellaneous losses of calcium in balance studies, an adjustment for this was made in predicting the desirable calcium retention. When rate of expected growth or change in tissue mass was not accounted for in individual studies (particularly related to magnesium in children), adjustments for growth were made to the available balance data.

NUTRIENT INTAKE ESTIMATES

Methodological Considerations

When examining data on an individual's requirement for any nutrient, it is essential to consider the quality of the intake data. The most valid intake data are those collected from the metabolic study protocols in which all food is provided by the researchers, amounts consumed are accurately measured, and the nutrient composition of the food is determined by laboratory analyses. Such protocols can be used for balance studies with a small number of subjects, but they are seldom possible for larger studies. Thus, intake data are often self-reported (for example, 24-hour recalls of food intake, diet records, or food frequency questionnaires), which have inherent limitations. Potential sources of error in self-reported intake data include over- or under-reporting of portion sizes, omission of foods, and inaccuracies in tables of food composition. These and other sources of dietary intake errors have been discussed in several reviews (Kohlmeier et al., 1997; LSRO/FASEB, 1986; Thompson and Byers, 1994; Willett, 1990) and at two recent conferences on dietary assessment methods (Buzzard and Willett, 1994; Willett and Sampson, 1997). The general conclusion is that self-reported dietary data are subject to a number of inaccuracies and biases. Therefore, the values reported by nationwide surveys or studies that rely on self reporting may be somewhat inaccurate and possibly biased.

Because of day-to-day variation in dietary intakes, the distribution of 1-day (or 2-day) intakes for a group is wider than the distribution of usual intakes, even though the mean of the intakes may be the same. Statistical adjustments have been developed (NRC, 1986; Nusser et al., 1996) that require at least 2 days of dietary data from a representative subsample of the population of interest. These adjustments have been made to the U.S. population intake data from the 1994 U.S. Department of Agriculture (USDA) Continuing Survey of Food Intake of Individuals (CSFII) (Cleveland et al., 1996), which are used in this report to more accurately estimate intakes of specific life stage and gender groups. However, this method does not adjust for the underreporting of intake, which may be as much as 20 percent (Mertz et al., 1991).

Finally, food composition databases that are used to calculate nutrient intake from self-reported and observed intake data introduce errors due to random variability, genetic variation in content, and use of poor analytical methods. In general, when estimating nutrient intakes for groups, the effect of errors in the composition data is probably considerably smaller than the effect of errors in the self-reported intake data (NRC, 1986).

DIETARY INTAKES IN THE UNITED STATES AND CANADA

Sources of Dietary Intake Data

The major sources of intake data for the U.S. population are the national surveys conducted by the U.S. Department of Health and Human Services (USDHHS) and by the USDA. Partial results of two surveys from phase I (1988–1991) of the Third National Health and Nutrition Examination Survey (NHANES III), which was conducted from 1988 to 1994 by USDHHS (Alaimo et al., 1994), and the first two years of the 1994 to 1996 CSFII, which was conducted by USDA (Cleveland et al., 1996) have been released recently. NHANES III examined 30,000 subjects aged 2 months and older. A single 24-hour diet recall was collected for all subjects, and a second recall was collected for a 5 percent subsample. The 1994 to 1996 CSFII collected two nonconsecutive 24-hour recalls from approximately 16,000 subjects of all ages. Both surveys used a food composition database developed by USDA to calculate nutrient intakes (Perloff et al., 1990).

National survey data for Canada are not currently available, although data have been collected from two provinces and should be available shortly. The data regarding nutrient intakes for individuals in the United States may be applicable to Canada, but until comparable databases are available, the degree of similarity of intakes is unknown.

When comparisons are made in this report between intake and DRIs (AIs, EARs, RDAs, and ULs), only intakes from the recent CSFII survey that have been adjusted for day-to-day variation in intake are presented. In many cases, values available from the NHANES III survey are similar, which is noted. Values reported by CSFII are for intake from food only.

Table 2-1 gives the fifth, median, and ninety-fifth percentiles of intakes of calcium, phosphorus, and magnesium by age in the United States from the first phase of the CSFII survey, as adjusted by the method of Nusser et al. (1996). Because food composition data are not readily available for vitamin D, neither of the U.S. national surveys has attempted to estimate intakes for this nutrient. An analysis using NHANES II data (collected from 1976 to 1980) has estimated median 1-day vitamin D intakes by young women at 2.9 µg (114 IU)/day from food (maximum of 49 µg [1,960 IU]/day) (Mur-

TABLE 2-1 1994 CSFII Daily Intakes of Calcium, Phosphorus, and Magnesium by Life Stage and Gender

Life Stage[a]	Calcium (mg) (Percentiles)			Phosphorus (mg) (Percentiles)			Magnesium (mg) (Percentiles)		
	5th	50th	95th	5th	50th	95th	5th	50th	95th
All (5,576)	349	742	1,429	620	1,164	2,020	128	248	451
Males and Females									
0 to 6 months (69)	191	457	745	131	322	532	21	55	105
7 to 12 months (45)	351	703	1,177	302	612	1,086	61	109	171
1 through 3 years (702)	399	766	1,276	552	926	1,396	106	180	274
4 through 8 years (666)	455	808	1,325	677	1,059	1,596	128	205	315
Males, 9 + years (2,053)	431	865	1,620	874	1,445	2,282	177	310	516
9 through 13 years (180)	499	980	1,702	771	1,359	2,203	140	258	445
14 through 18 years (191)	554	1,094	2,039	956	1,582	2,534	166	298	522
19 through 30 years (328)	484	954	1,746	1,002	1,613	2,472	185	328	553
31 through 50 years (627)	429	857	1,588	907	1,484	2,312	194	329	529
51 through 70 years (490)	362	708	1,268	769	1,274	1,956	169	295	474
> 70 years (237)	368	702	1,185	721	1,176	1,712	160	275	429
Females, 9 + years (1,992)	316	625	1,109	620	1,001	1,510	134	222	342
9 through 13 years (200)	486	889	1,452	768	1,178	1,725	142	223	339
14 through 18 years (169)	348	713	1,293	632	1,097	1,727	123	217	352
19 through 30 years (302)	300	612	1,116	560	1,005	1,571	110	205	322
31 through 50 years (590)	297	606	1,082	593	990	1,516	133	229	363
51 through 70 years (510)	294	571	1,001	599	966	1,444	141	231	362
> 70 years (221)	277	517	860	521	859	1,282	118	206	314
Pregnancy (33)[b]	656	1,154	1,729	1,012	1,581	2,108	187	292	399
Lactation (16)[b]	794	1,050	1,324	1,211	1,483	1,822	244	315	396

NOTE: 1994 CSFII data from Cleveland et al. (1996) adjusted using the method developed by Nusser et al. (1996). Grouped data do not include pregnant or lactating women.

[a] Number of subjects measured given in parentheses.

[b] Estimates are less reliable than other life stage groups due to extremely small sample size.

phy and Calloway, 1986). A smaller study of older women estimated median food intakes of vitamin D at 2.3 μg (90 IU)/day, with a maximum of 12.5 μg (500 IU)/day (Krall et al., 1989). No estimates of the extent to which exposure to sunlight met part of the individual's requirements for vitamin D are available in these studies. Intakes of fluoride from foods are difficult to estimate due to wide variations in the fluoride content of local water supplies and inadvertent consumption of fluoride through dental products. As a result, none of the U.S. national surveys has attempted to estimate fluoride intake. Some data are available from relatively small samples of individuals, and these are provided in Chapter 8 which discusses fluoride.

Estimates of intakes for some of these nutrients can be made from per-capita food availability (disappearance data). For the United States, the most recent disappearance data (USDA, 1997) show 900 mg (22.5 mmol) of calcium per person, 1,420 mg (45.8 mmol) of phosphorus per person (which excludes the phosphorus used as a food additive in processed foods and beverages such as in soft drinks), and 320 mg (13.3 mmol) of magnesium per person. These daily average figures are lower than those shown in Table 2-1 for adults because intakes of all age groups are combined. In addition, they overestimate actual intakes of the population because spoilage, trimming, and plate waste are not subtracted from the per-capita estimates. However, the general magnitude of the intake estimates is confirmed by this alternative source of food consumption data.

Finally, drinking water may be an important source of some minerals other than fluoride. Although accounted for in most balance studies conducted in modern metabolic units, the contribution of calcium, magnesium, and phosphorus from water to the total estimated intake of subjects is frequently not included or estimated.

Sources of Supplement Intake Data

Although NHANES and CSFII ask subjects about the use of dietary supplements, neither collects quantified information on intakes from supplements. In 1986, the National Health Interview Survey (NHIS) queried 11,558 adults and 1,877 children on their intake of supplements during the previous 2 weeks (Moss et al., 1989). The composition of the supplement was obtained directly from the product label whenever possible. These data indicated that almost 25 percent of adults took a vitamin D supplement during the previous 2 weeks, 20 percent took a calcium supplement, and 15 percent took a magnesium supplement. Use of phosphorus

TABLE 2-2 Percentage Use of Supplements in the United States by Children and Adults: Calcium, Phosphorus, Magnesium, Vitamin D, and Fluoride

Nutrient	Percentage Who Reported Use in Previous 2 Weeks Median	Intake (mg/day) of Nutrient Supplements by Those Reporting Use in Previous 2 Weeks (Percentiles)		
		50th	95th	99th
Children				
Calcium (mg)	7.5	88	160	304
Phosphorus (mg)	6.2	48	128	200
Magnesium (mg)	7.9	23	70	117
Vitamin D (µg)	38.2	10	10	10
Fluoride	2 .5	ND[a]	ND	ND
Men				
Calcium (mg)	14.0	160	624	928
Phosphorus (mg)	9.2	120	264	448
Magnesium (mg)	13.5	102	200	350
Vitamin D (µg)	19.9	10	12	20
Fluoride	0	ND	ND	ND
Women				
Calcium (mg)	24.7	248	904	1,200
Phosphorus (mg)	11.2	128	264	448
Magnesium (mg)	17.1	100	240	400
Vitamin D (µg)	27.6	10	13	17
Fluoride	0.1	ND	ND	ND

[a] ND = not determined.

SOURCE: Moss et al. (1989).

supplements was less common (10 percent); virtually no adults used fluoride supplements. Children aged 2 to 6 years were less likely to take supplements of calcium, phosphorus, or magnesium (6 to 8 percent took these supplements) but they were more likely to take vitamin D (38 percent). The percentages of supplement use for adults and children, as well as the median, ninety-fifth, and ninety-ninth percentile of intake, are shown in Table 2-2 for calcium, phosphorus, magnesium, vitamin D, and fluoride.

The lack of accurate estimates of a population's intake from supplements plus food prevents accurate examination of the upper end of the nutrient intake distribution. This, in turn, limits the ability to identify intakes that approach or exceed the UL.

Use of Intake Data in This Report

Intake data from food, water, and, when available, supplements and some over-the-counter medications are used for several purposes in this report: to estimate the average requirement of a nutrient, to determine the lowest-observed-adverse-effect level (LOAEL) or the no-observed-adverse-effect level (NOAEL) of a nutrient, and to characterize the risk of exceeding the UL for a nutrient. They are also used in a few examples of applying DRIs to specific situations.

Food Sources of Calcium and Related Nutrients

Availability of nutrients from a range of foods provides useful information when setting nutrient requirements and ULs. Calcium in the United States and Canada is obtained primarily from dairy products (Cleveland et al., 1996; NIN, 1995). Household consumption data show that individuals in the United States consume the equivalent of 2 cups of milk per day (based on the calcium content of various dairy products), while Canadians consume approximately 1.6 cups per day (Cleveland et al., 1996; NIN, 1995).

Cross-Cultural Differences in Dietary Intake and Bioavailability

For this report, consideration of the dietary practices associated with intakes of calcium and related nutrients has been limited to observations within U.S. and Canadian populations. The recommendations for the DRIs may not be generalizable globally, especially where food intake and indigent dietary practices may result in very different bioavailability of mineral elements from sources not considered in traditional diets of Canadians and Americans. For example, both the consumption of bones from fish and meat foods and the practice of geophagia are more common in developing countries than in the United States or Canada. Population variations in the consumption of other diet components such as protein and sodium may significantly affect population calcium and magnesium needs and ULs.

With regard to the need for calcium and related nutrients for bone health, cross-cultural comparisons must also consider variability among populations in activity, weight-bearing practices, and sun exposure. Differences in hip axis length or other structural features may vary across cultures; hip axis length is directly associated with hip fracture risk (Cummings et al., 1993). Until more is learned about the prevalence of osteoporosis and hip fracture risk in other countries (Cooper et al., 1992), and about habitual intakes of calcium and related nutrients according to specific cultural dietary practices, the implementation of the published DRIs should be used with caution outside the United States and Canada.

USE OF ADEQUATE INTAKE RATHER THAN ESTIMATED AVERAGE REQUIREMENT

As defined in Chapter 1, the AI is used as a reference value when sufficient data are not available to estimate an average requirement. In this report, AIs rather than EARs and RDAs are developed for all nutrients for infants to age 1 year, and for calcium, vitamin D, and fluoride for all life stages. The method used to derive the AIs differs for infants and for each nutrient as follows.

Infants: Ages 0 through 6 Months

The AI is the intake by healthy breast-fed infants as obtained from average human milk nutrient composition and average milk volume. Since infants self-regulate milk intake from the breast, it is presumed that larger infants, who may require more milk than the average population intake, will achieve this by increasing milk intake volume.

Calcium

In this report, three major approaches were considered in deriving the AIs for calcium—calcium balance studies of subjects consuming variable amounts of calcium, a factorial model using calcium accretion based on bone mineral accretion data, and clinical trials which investigated the response of change in bone mineral content/density or fracture rate to varying calcium intakes. The prepublication version of this report estimated per cent maximal calcium retention derived from calcium balance data as one of the three major approaches considered to develop the recommended intakes for calcium. Subsequent comments received following the report's release in prepublication form indicated concerns with the statistical methodology used to obtain such estimates from the available balance data. In response to the technical issues raised, the DRI Committee determined for this final printed version that it would estimate *desirable* calcium retention in place of estimating the percent of maximal retention, using the same data and statistical methodology as was included in the prepublication version (see Appendix E).

Where sufficient data were available, values from balance studies for individual subjects within specific age groups were applied to a nonlinear mathematical model recently used by Jackman et al. (1997) which describes the relationship between varying calcium intakes and retention. The equation derived from this model was then solved to determine the calcium intake required to achieve retention of the desirable amount of calcium. The *desirable* retention varied by age group but for the most part reflected accretion of calcium in bone based on bone mineral accretion data available for some of the age groups.

Another major approach considered by the Committee to estimating intake needed to maintain calcium adequacy was the factorial method. This is based on combining estimates of losses of calcium via various routes by apparently healthy individuals and then assuming that these represent the degree to which calcium intake, as corrected by estimated absorption, will balance these losses. The weakness of using this approach alone is that the data come from different studies, in different subjects, and the variation in absorption, particularly depending on previous intake, may be significant. The third approach derives calcium requirements from the few available clinical trials in which addditional calcium was given and changes in bone mineral content or density or in fracture rate were measured over time.

Comparison of the intakes needed to achieve desirable calcium retention or maintain minimal calcium loss using each of these three methods gave reasonable confidence and concordance to the levels of intake recommended as AIs. Thus the recommended AI for each life stage group is an approximation of the calcium intake that would appear to be sufficient to maintain calcium nutriture for almost all the individuals in the specific group. It is also recognized that the ability to maximize calcium retention may not be limited by calcium intake alone since there are many other factors that affect calcium retention, such as growth velocity (in children), hormonal status, gender and ethnic backgrounds, other diet components, and genetic patterns. Evidence to support this is cited in the study by Jackman et al. (1997), which demonstrated that the further into puberty the teenage girls were, the lower their relative calcium retention was even though calcium intake remained the same. In addition, calcium retention would be expected to oscillate above and below a mean value at the calcium intake levels tested, which often were intended to approximate or exceed the subjects' usual intakes. Additional consideration of the approach used is included in Chapter 4.

The decision to set AIs rather than EARs and thus RDAs for calcium was based on the following concerns: (1) uncertainties in the methods inherent in and the precise nutritional significance of values obtained from the balance studies that form the basis of the desirable retention model, (2) the lack of concordance between observational and experimental data (mean calcium intakes in the United States and Canada are much lower than are the experimentally derived values required to achieve average desirable calcium retention), and (3) the lack of longitudinal data that could be used to verify the association of the experimentally derived calcium intakes for achieving a predetermining calcium retention with the rate and extent of long-term bone loss and its clinical sequelae, such as fracture. Taking all of these factors into consideration it was determined that an EAR for calcium could not be established at the present time. The recommended AI represents an approximation of the calcium intake that, in the opinion of the DRI Committee and its Panel on Calcium and Related Nutrients, would appear to be sufficient to maintain calcium nutriture while recognizing that lower intakes may be adequate for many; however, this evaluation will have to await additional studies on calcium balance over broad ranges of intakes and/or of long-term measures of calcium sufficiency.

Vitamin D

The AI is the intake value that appears to be needed to maintain, in a defined group of individuals with limited but uncertain sun exposure and stores, serum 25-hydroxyvitamin D concentration above a defined amount. The latter is that concentration below which vitamin D deficiency rickets or osteomalacia occurs. The intake value was rounded to the nearest 50 IU, and then doubled as a safety factor to cover the needs of all, regardless of their sun exposure.

Fluoride

The AI is the intake value that reduces the occurrence of dental caries maximally in a group of individuals without causing unwanted side effects. For fluoride, the data are strong on risk reduction, but the evidence on which to base an actual requirement is scant, thus driving the decision to adopt an AI as the reference value.

3

A Model for the
Development of Tolerable
Upper Intake Levels

BACKGROUND INFORMATION

The framework for developing Dietary Reference Intakes (DRIs) includes an evaluation of the Tolerable Upper Intake Level (UL) for nutrients. The UL in this context refers to an intake ordinarily in excess of the Recommended Dietary Allowance (RDA) or Adequate Intake (AI) and associated with negligible risk of adverse health effects; it does not include consideration of the level of intake with minimal risk of dietary deficiency. A model has been developed that is generally applicable to the problem of identifying upper levels of nutrient intake.

Like all chemical agents, nutrients can produce adverse health effects if intakes from any combination of food, water, nutrient supplements, and pharmacologic agents are excessive. It is also the case that some levels of nutrient intake above those associated with any documented benefit pose no likelihood or risk of adverse health effects in normal individuals. In actuality, it is not possible to identify a single "risk-free" intake level for a nutrient that can be applied with certainty to all members of a population. However, it is possible to develop intake levels that are unlikely to pose risks of adverse health effects to most members of the healthy population, including sensitive individuals, throughout the life stage, excepting in some cases discrete subpopulations (for example, those with genetic predispositions or certain disease states) that may be especially vulnerable to one or more adverse effects.

The term *Tolerable Upper Intake Level* is defined as the maximum

51

level of total chronic daily intake of a nutrient judged to be likely to pose no risk of adverse health effects to the most sensitive members of the healthy population. It is developed by applying the model described. The term *tolerable* is chosen because it connotes a level of intake that can, with high probability, be tolerated biologically by individuals, but it does not imply acceptability of that level in any other sense. Particularly, it should not be inferred that nutrient intakes greater than the RDA are recommended as being beneficial to an individual. The term *adverse effect* is defined as any significant alteration in the structure or function of the human organism (Klaassen et al., 1986) or any impairment of a physiologically important function, in accordance with the definition set by the joint World Health Organization, Food and Agriculture Organization of the United Nations, and International Atomic Energy Agency (WHO/FAO/IAEA) Expert Consultation in *Trace Elements in Human Nutrition and Health* (WHO, 1996).

A MODEL FOR DERIVATION OF TOLERABLE UPPER INTAKE LEVELS

The possibility that the methodology used to derive ULs might be reduced to a mathematical model that could be generically applied to all nutrients was considered. Such a model might have several potential advantages, including ease of application and assurance of consistent treatment of all nutrients. It was concluded, however, that the current state of scientific understanding of toxic phenomena in general, and nutrient toxicity in particular, is insufficient to support the development of such a model. (A fuller discussion of this problem is set forth in the section on "Risk Assessment and Food Safety".) Scientific information regarding various adverse effects and their relationships to intake levels varies greatly among nutrients, depending on the nature, comprehensiveness, and quality of available data and the uncertainties associated with the unavoidable problem of extrapolating from the circumstances under which data are developed (for example, in the laboratory or clinic) to other circumstances (for example, to the healthy population). Given the current state of knowledge, any attempt to capture in a mathematical model all the information and scientific judgments that must be made to reach conclusions regarding ULs would not be consistent with contemporary risk assessment practices.

An appropriate model for the derivation of ULs consists, then, not of a mathematical formula, but rather a set of scientific factors that always should be considered explicitly. The framework under which these factors are organized is called *risk assessment*. Risk assessment as first set forth by the National Research Council (NRC) in its 1983 report, and as affirmed by another NRC committee in 1994 (NRC, 1994), is a systematic means of evaluating the probability of occurrence of adverse health effects in humans from excess exposure to an environmental agent (in this case, a nutrient) (FAO/WHO, 1995; Health Canada, 1993). The hallmark of risk assessment is the requirement to be explicit in all of the evaluations and judgments that must be made to document conclusions.

RISK ASSESSMENT AND FOOD SAFETY

Basic Concepts

Risk assessment is a scientific undertaking having as its objective a characterization of the nature and likelihood of harm resulting from human exposure to agents in the environment. The characterization of risk typically contains both qualitative and quantitative information and includes a discussion of the significant scientific uncertainties in that information. In the present context, the agents of interest are nutrients, and the environmental media are food, water, and nonfood sources such as nutrient supplements and over-the-counter pharmaceutical preparations. Additional human exposure to some dietary agents, including nutrients, sometimes occurs through other media, such as air. For example, inhaling zinc oxide in an industrial setting is associated with metal fume fever (Hodgson et al., 1988). The applications of risk assessment to nutrients and other food components in general are the subject of this section, although the principles and methods discussed are more broadly applicable.

Performing a risk assessment results in a characterization, with due attention to scientific uncertainties, of the relationships between exposure(s) to an agent and the likelihood that adverse health effects will occur in members of exposed populations. Scientific uncertainties are an inherent part of the risk assessment process and are discussed below. Deciding whether the magnitude of exposure is "acceptable" or "tolerable" in specific circumstances is not a component of risk assessment; this activity falls within the domain of what is called *risk management*. Risk management decisions depend on the results of risk assessments but may involve additional considerations, such as the public health significance of the risk, the technical feasibility of achieving various degrees of risk control, and the economic and social costs of this control. Because there is no single, scientifically definable distinction between "safe" and "unsafe" exposures, risk management necessarily incorporates components of sound, practical decision making that are not addressed by the risk assessment process (NRC, 1983, 1994).

Although a risk assessment requires that information be organized in rather specific ways, its conduct does not require any specific scientific methodologies for evaluating that information. Rather, it asks risk assessors to evaluate scientific information using what are, in their judgments, appropriate methodologies and to make explicit the bases for their judgments. Risk assessment also requires explicit recognition of uncertainties in risk estimates and the acknowledgment, when appropriate, that alternative interpretations of the available data may be scientifically plausible (NRC, 1994; OTA, 1993).

Risk assessment is subject to two types of scientific uncertainties: (1) those related to data and (2) those associated with any inferences that are required when directly applicable data are not available (NRC, 1994). Data uncertainties arise in the evaluation of information obtained from the epidemiology and toxicology studies and investigations of nutrient intake levels that are the basis for risk assessments. The use of data from experimental animals to estimate responses in humans, and the selection of so-called uncertainty factors to estimate inter- and intraspecies variabilities in response to toxic substances are examples of the use of inferences in risk assessment. Uncertainties regarding the appropriate inferences to be made arise whenever attempts are made to estimate or predict adverse health effects in humans (in which there are often inadequate or nonexistent direct empirical data) based on extrapolations of data obtained under dissimilar conditions (for example, experimental animal studies). Data on nutrient toxicity are generally available from studies in human populations and, therefore, may not be subject to the same uncertainties (related to interspecies extrapolations) associated with the available data on nonessential chemicals. Options for dealing with uncertainties are discussed below and in detail in Appendix C.

Steps in the Risk Assessment Process

Although various terms are used to describe the specific organizing steps of the risk assessment process (for example, FAO/WHO, 1995), there appears to be widespread agreement among risk assessors on the content of those steps. The organization of risk assessment in this report is based on a model proposed by the NRC (1983,

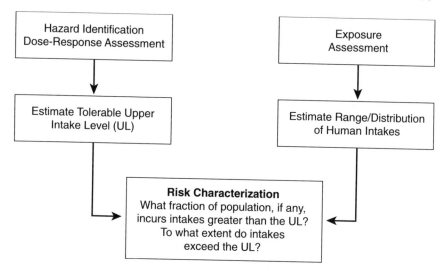

FIGURE 3-1 Risk assessment model for nutrient toxicity.

1994). The steps of risk assessment as applied to nutrients are as follows (see also Figure 3-1):

• Step 1. *Hazard identification* involves the collection, organization, and evaluation of all information pertaining to the toxic properties of a given nutrient. It concludes with a summary of the evidence concerning the capacity of the nutrient to cause one or more types of toxicity in humans.

• Step 2. *Dose-response assessment* determines the relationship between nutrient intake (dose) and adverse effect (in terms of incidence and severity). This step concludes with an estimate of the UL—the maximum level of total chronic daily nutrient intake judged unlikely to adversely affect the most sensitive individuals in a healthy population. ULs may be developed for various age groups within the population.

• Step 3. *Exposure assessment* evaluates the distribution of usual total daily nutrient intakes among members of a healthy population.

• Step 4. *Risk characterization* summarizes the conclusions from Steps 1 through 3 and evaluates the risk. Generally, the risk is expressed as the fraction of the exposed population, if any, having nutrient intakes (Step 3) in excess of the estimated UL (Steps 1 and 2). The characterization also discusses, where possible, the magnitude of any such excesses. Scientific uncertainties associated with both the UL and the intake estimates are described so that risk managers understand the degree of scientific confidence they can place in the risk assessment.

The risk assessment contains no discussion of recommendations for reducing risk; these are the focus of risk management.

Thresholds

A principal feature of the risk assessment process for noncarcinogens is the long-standing acceptance that no risk of adverse effects is expected unless a threshold dose (or intake) is exceeded. The adverse effects that may be caused by a nutrient almost certainly occur only when the threshold dose is exceeded. The critical issues concern the methods used to identify the approximate threshold of toxicity for a large and diverse human population. Because most nutrients are not considered to be carcinogenic in humans, the approach to carcinogenic risk assessment (EPA, 1996) will not be discussed here.

Thresholds vary among members of a healthy population (NRC, 1994). If, for any given adverse effect, the distribution of thresholds in the population could be quantitatively identified, then it would be possible to establish ULs by defining some point in the lower tail of the distribution of thresholds that would be protective for some specified fraction of the population. However, the current state of biomedical sciences is insufficiently developed to allow identification of the distribution of thresholds in all but a few, well-studied cases (for example, acute toxic effects or for chemicals such as lead, where the human database is very large). The method for identifying thresholds for a healthy population described here is designed to ensure that almost all members of the population will be protected, but it is not based on an analysis of the theoretical (but practically unattainable) distribution of thresholds. There is considerable confidence, however, that the threshold derived by application of the model, which becomes the UL for nutrients, lies very near the low end of the theoretical distribution, and is the end representing the most sensitive members of the population. Note that for some nutrients, there may be distinct subpopulations that are not included in the general distribution because of their unusual genetic predispositions to toxicity. Such distinct groups may not be protected by the UL.

The Joint FAO/WHO Expert Commission on Food Additives and various national regulatory bodies have identified certain factors that account for interspecies and intraspecies differences in response to the hazardous effects of substances and to account for other uncertainties (WHO, 1987). These factors are used to make inferences about the threshold dose of substances for members of a large and diverse human population from data on adverse effects obtained in epidemiological or experimental studies. These factors are applied consistently when data of specific types and quality are available. They are typically used to derive acceptable daily intakes for food additives and other substances for which data on adverse effects are considered sufficient to meet minimum standards of quality and completeness (FAO/WHO, 1982). These adopted or recognized factors have sometimes been coupled with other factors to compensate for deficiencies in the available data and other uncertainties regarding data.

The UL is generally based on a no-observed-adverse-effect level (NOAEL) that is identified for a specific circumstance in the hazard identification and dose-response assessment steps of the risk assessment. The NOAEL is the highest intake (or experimental dose) of a nutrient at which no adverse effects have been observed in the individuals studied. If there are no adequate data demonstrating a NOAEL, then a lowest-observed-adverse-effect level (LOAEL) may be used. A LOAEL is the lowest intake (or experimental dose) at which an adverse effect has been identified. The derivation of a UL from a NOAEL (or LOAEL) involves a series of choices about what factors should be used to deal with uncertainties. Uncertainty factors (UFs) are attempts both to deal with gaps in data (for example, lack of data on humans or lack of adequate data demonstrating a NOAEL) and with incomplete knowledge regarding the inferences required (for example, the expected variability in response within the human population). The problems of both data and inference uncertainties arise in all steps of the risk assessment. A discussion of options available for dealing with these uncertainties is presented below and in greater detail in Appendix C.

A UL is not, in itself, a description of human risk. It is derived by application of the hazard identification and dose-response evaluation steps (Steps 1 and 2) of the risk assessment model. To determine whether exposed populations are at risk requires an exposure assessment (Step 3, evaluation of their intakes of the nutrient) and a determination of the fractions of those populations, if any, whose intakes exceed the UL (for example, those whose intakes exceed the estimated threshold for toxicity). In the exposure assessment and risk characterization steps (Steps 3 and 4; described in the respective chapters for each nutrient), the ninety-fifth percentile intake level for exposed populations will be used as a basis in determining whether these populations are at risk. The remaining sections of this chapter deal with the derivation of ULs for nutrients (Steps 1 and 2).

APPLICATION OF THE RISK ASSESSMENT MODEL TO NUTRIENTS

This section provides guidance for applying the risk assessment framework (the "model") discussed above to the derivation of ULs for nutrients.

Special Problems Associated with Substances Required for Human Nutrition

Although the risk assessment model outlined above can be applied to nutrients to derive ULs, it must be recognized that nutrients possess some properties that distinguish them from the types of agents for which the risk assessment model was originally developed (NRC, 1983).

In the application of accepted standards for assessing risks of environmental chemicals to the risk assessment of nutrients, a fundamental difference between the two categories must be recognized: nutrients are essential for human well-being and often for life itself within a certain range of intakes, although they may share with other chemicals the production of adverse effects at excessive exposures. History has shown that the consumption of balanced diets is consistent with the development and survival of humankind over many millennia. This observation limits the need for some of the large uncertainty factors that have been found appropriate for risk assessment of nonessential chemicals. Moreover, data on nutrient toxicity are often available from studies in human populations and are therefore not usually subject to the degree of uncertainty associated with the types of data available on nonessential chemicals.

In addition, there is no evidence to suggest that nutrients consumed at the RDA or AI and as part of unfortified diets present a risk of adverse effects to the healthy population. Possible exceptions to this generalization relate to specific geochemical areas with excessive environmental exposures to certain trace elements (for example, selenium) and to rare case reports of adverse effects associated with highly eccentric consumption of specific foods. Data from such findings are not useful for setting ULs for the general U.S. population. It is clear, however, that the addition of high doses of nutrients to a diet, either through fortification or through nonfood sources such as nutrient supplements and over-the-counter pharmaceutical preparations, may at some level pose the risk of adverse health effects. The data available on such effects of specific nutrients pertain in some cases only to intakes from fortificants or nonfood sources; in other cases, they pertain to total intakes from all sources. Therefore, the derived ULs for some nutrients refer to total intakes and for others only to intakes from fortified foods or nonfood sources. Discussion of the UL for each nutrient clarifies which use of the term applies.

Differences in the effects of nutrients from fortified foods or nonfood sources and those that are endogenous constituents of foods may be due to factors such as the chemical form of the nutrient, the timing of the intake and amount consumed in a single bolus dose, the matrix supplied by the food, and the relation of the nutrient to the other constituents of the diet. Nutrient requirements and food intake are related to the metabolizing body mass, which is also a measure, although at times indirect, of the space in which the nutrients are distributed. This relation between food intake and space of distribution supports homeostasis, which maintains nutrient concentrations in that space within a range compatible with health. This is generally the case for individuals whose food intake corresponds to their energy needs and lean body mass. However, excessive intake of a single nutrient from nonfood sources can compromise this homeostatic mechanism. Such elevations alone may pose risks of adverse effects; imbalances among the concentrations of mineral elements (for example, calcium, iron, zinc, copper) can result in additional risks (Mertz et al., 1994). These reasons and those discussed previously support the need to include the form and pattern of consumption as an important component of the assessment of micronutrients.

Consideration of Variability in Sensitivity

The risk assessment model outlined in this chapter is consistent with classical risk assessment approaches in that it must consider variability in the sensitivity of individuals to adverse effects. A discussion of how variability is dealt with in the context of nutritional risk assessment is provided here.

Physiological changes and common conditions associated with growth and maturation that occur during an individual's lifespan may influence sensitivity to nutrient toxicity. For example, (1) sensitivity increases with declines in lean body mass and with declines in renal and liver function that occur with aging; (2) sensitivity changes in direct relation to intestinal absorption or intestinal synthesis of nutrients (for example, vitamin K, biotin); (3) in the unborn fetus and newborn infant, sensitivity increases due to active placental transfer, accumulation of certain nutrients in the amniotic fluid, rapid development of the brain, and with secretion of nutrients in human milk; and finally, (4) sensitivity increases with decreases in the rate of metabolism of nutrients. Therefore, to the extent possible, ULs are developed for each separate age or life stage group. Examples of life stage groups that may differ in terms of nutritional needs and toxicological sensitivity include infants and children, the elderly population, and women during pregnancy or lactation.

Even within relatively homogeneous life stage groups, there is a range of sensitivities to toxic effects. The model described below is directed at the derivation of ULs for members of the healthy population, divided into various life stage groups. It accounts for normally expected variability in sensitivity, but it excludes subpopulations with extreme and distinct vulnerabilities due to genetic predisposition or other considerations. Including data on subpopulations that have unusually high and distinct sensitivities to adverse effects would result in ULs that are significantly lower than are needed to protect most people. Subpopulations needing special protection are better served through the use of public health screening, health care providers, product labeling, or other individualized strategies. Such subpopulations may not be at "negligible risk" when their intakes reach the UL developed for the healthy population. The extent to which a subpopulation becomes significant enough to be assumed to be representative of a healthy population is an area of judgment and is discussed in the chapters for each nutrient.

Bioavailability

Bioavailability of a dietary nutrient can be defined as its accessibility to normal metabolic and physiological processes. Bioavailability determines a nutrient's beneficial effects at physiological levels of intake and affects the nature and severity of toxicity due to excessive intakes. Modulating components include: other dietary components; concentration and chemical form of the nutrient in food, water, nutrient supplements, and over-the-counter pharmaceutical preparations; the nutritional, physiological, and disease state of the individual; and excretory losses. Because of the considerable variability in nutrient bioavailability in humans, bioavailability data for specific nutrients must be considered and incorporated by the risk assessment process. Situations related to nutrient bioavailability, described in the following two sections, are relevant to establishing ULs.

Nutrient Interactions

It is well established that certain nutrients interact with each other to alter bioavailability. For example, dietary interactions can affect the chemical forms of elements at the site of absorption through ligand binding or changes in the valence state of an element (Mertz et al., 1994). Phytates, phosphates, and tannins are among the most powerful depressants of bioavailability, and organic acids, such as citric and ascorbic acid, are strong enhancers for some minerals and trace elements. Thus, dietary interactions strongly influence the bioavailability of elements by affecting their partition between the absorbed and the nonabsorbed portion of the diet. The large differences of bioavailability ensuing from these interactions support the need to specify the chemical form of the nutrient when setting ULs. Dietary interactions can also alter nutrient bioavailability through their effect on excretion. For example, dietary intake of protein, phosphorus, sodium, and chloride all affect urinary calcium excretion and hence calcium bioavailability (see Chapter 4). Interactions that significantly elevate or reduce bioavailability may represent adverse health effects.

Although it is critical to include knowledge of any such interactions in the risk assessment, it is difficult to evaluate the possibility of interactions without reference to a particular level of intake. This difficulty can be overcome if a UL for a nutrient or food component is first derived based on other measures of toxicity. Then an evaluation can be made of whether intake at the UL has the potential to affect the bioavailability of other nutrients.

Other Relevant Factors Affecting Bioavailability of Nutrients

In addition to nutrient interactions, other considerations have the potential to influence nutrient bioavailability, such as the nutritional status of an individual and the form of intake. These issues should be considered in the risk assessment. The absorption and utilization of most minerals, trace elements, and some vitamins are a function of the individual's nutritional status, particularly regarding the intake of other specific nutrients such as iron (Barger-Lux et al., 1995; Mertz et al., 1994).

With regard to the form of intake, minerals and trace elements often are less readily absorbed when they are part of a meal than when taken separately or when present in drinking water (NRC, 1989b). The opposite is true for fat-soluble vitamins whose absorption depends on fat in the diet. ULs must therefore be based on nutrients as part of the total diet, including the contribution from water. Nutrient supplements that are taken separately from food require special consideration, since they are likely to have different availabilities and therefore may present a greater risk of producing toxic effects.

STEPS IN THE DEVELOPMENT OF THE UL

Hazard Identification

The collection of scientific data for developing ULs is discussed in Chapter 2. Based on a thorough review of the scientific literature, the hazard identification step outlines the adverse health effects that have been demonstrated to be caused by the nutrient. As noted in the section above on nutrient interactions, interference with nutrient bioavailability is not considered an adverse effect at this stage; rather it is considered only after more conventional adverse responses are evaluated and a tentative UL is derived.

The primary types of data used as background for identifying nutrient hazards in humans are as follows:

- *Human studies.* Although data from controlled studies in humans are the basis for establishing nutritional requirements, the number of controlled human toxicity studies conducted in a clinical setting are, for ethical reasons, very limited and are useful for identifying only very mild and completely reversible adverse effects. Nevertheless, the available human data provide the most relevant kind of information for hazard identification and, when they are of sufficient quality and extent, are given greatest weight. Observational studies that focus on well-defined populations with clear exposures to diverse specific nutrient intake levels are useful for establishing a relationship between exposure and effect. Observational data in the form of case reports or anecdotal evidence are used for developing hypotheses that can lead to knowledge of causal associations.
- *Animal studies.* The majority of the available data used in regulatory risk assessments comes from controlled laboratory experiments in animals, usually mammalian species other than humans (for example, rodents). Such data are used in part because human data on nonessential chemicals are generally less available than human data on es-

sential substances. Because well-conducted animal studies can be controlled, establishing a causal relationship is not difficult.

Six key issues that are addressed in the data evaluation of human and animal studies are the following:

1. *Evidence of adverse effects in humans.* In the hazard identification step, all human, animal, and *in vitro* published evidence addressing the likelihood of a nutrient eliciting an adverse effect in humans is examined. Decisions regarding which observed effects are "adverse" are based on scientific judgments. Although toxicologists generally regard any demonstrable structural or functional alteration to represent an adverse effect, some alterations may be considered of little or self-limiting biological importance.

2. *Causality.* Is a causal relationship established by the published human data? Criteria for judging the causal significance of an exposure-effect association indicated by epidemiologic studies have been adopted by two reports, *Diet, Nutrition, and Cancer* (NRC, 1982) and *Diet and Health* (NRC, 1989b). These criteria include: demonstration of a temporal relationship, consistency, narrow confidence intervals for risk estimates, a biological gradient, specificity, biological plausibility, and coherence.

3. *Relevance of experimental data.* Consideration of the following issues can be useful in assessing the relevance of experimental data.

• *Animal data.* Animal data may be of limited utility in judging the toxicity of nutrients, because of highly variable interspecies differences in nutrient requirements. Nevertheless, all such data should be considered in the hazard identification step, and explicit reasons should be given whenever such data are judged not relevant to human risk.

• *Route of exposure.*[1] Data derived from studies involving ingestion exposure (rather than inhalation or dermal exposure) are most useful for the evaluation of nutrients. Data derived from studies involving inhalation or dermal routes of exposure may be considered relevant if the adverse effects are systemic and data are available to permit interroute extrapolation.

• *Duration of exposure.* Because the magnitude, duration, and fre-

---

[1]The terms *route of exposure* and *route of intake* refer to how a substance enters the body, for example, by ingestion, inhalation, or dermal absorption. These terms should not be confused with *form of intake,* which refers to the medium or vehicle used—for example, supplements, food, or drinking water.

quency of exposure can vary considerably in different situations, consideration needs to be given to the relevance of the exposure scenario (for example, chronic daily dietary exposure versus short-term bolus doses) to dietary intakes by human populations.

4. *Mechanisms of toxic action.* One active area of research in toxicology is the study of the molecular and cellular events underlying the production of toxicity. Knowledge of such mechanisms can assist in dealing with the problems of interspecies and high-to-low dose extrapolation. In the case of nutrients, it may also aid in understanding whether the mechanisms associated with toxicity are those associated with deficiency. In most cases, however, because knowledge of the biochemical sequence of events resulting from toxicity and deficiency is still incomplete, it is not yet possible to state with certainty whether or not these sequences share a common pathway. Iron, the most thoroughly studied trace element, may represent the only exception to this statement. Deficient to near-toxic exposures share the same pathway, which maintains controlled oxygen transport and catalysis. Toxicity sets in when the exposure exceeds the specific iron-complexing capacity of the organism, resulting in free iron species initiating peroxidation.

5. *Quality and completeness of the database.* The scientific quality and quantity of the database are evaluated. Human or animal data are reviewed for suggestions that the substances have the potential to produce additional adverse health effects. If suggestions are found, additional studies may be recommended.

6. *Identification of distinct and highly sensitive subpopulations.* Some highly sensitive subpopulations have responses (in terms of incidence, severity, or both) to the agent of interest that are clearly distinct from the responses expected for the healthy population. The risk assessment process recognizes that there may be individuals within any life stage group that are more biologically sensitive than others. The ULs derived for nutrients in this document are based on protecting the most sensitive members of a healthy population. For some substances, however, there may be distinct subgroups who have extreme sensitivities that do not fall within the range of sensitivities expected for the healthy population. Whenever data suggest the existence of such subgroups, the UL for the healthy population may not be protective for them. As indicated earlier, the extent to which a sensitive subpopulation will be included in the derivation of a UL for the healthy population is an area of judgment to be addressed on a case-by-case basis.

Dose-Response Assessment

The process for deriving the UL is described in this section and is summarized in Box 3-1. It includes selection of the critical data set, identification of a critical endpoint with its NOAEL (or LOAEL), and assessment of uncertainty.

Box 3-1
Development of Tolerable Upper Intake Levels (ULs)

HAZARD IDENTIFICATION

Components

- Evidence of adverse effects in humans
- Causality
- Relevance of experimental data
- Mechanisms of toxic action
- Quality and completeness of the database
- Identification of distinct and highly sensitive subpopulations

DOSE-RESPONSE ASSESSMENT

Components

- Data selection
- Identification of no-observed-adverse-effect level (NOAEL) (or lowest-observed-adverse-effect level [LOAEL]) and critical endpoint
- Uncertainty assessment
- Derivation of a UL
- Characterization of the estimate and special considerations

---

Data Selection

The data evaluation process results in the selection of the most appropriate or critical data set(s) for deriving the UL. Selecting the critical data set includes the following considerations:

- Human data are preferable to animal data.
- In the absence of appropriate human data, information from an animal species whose biological responses are most like those of humans is most valuable.
- If it is not possible to identify such a species or to select such

data, data from the most sensitive animal species, strain, or gender combination are given the greatest emphasis.

• The route of exposure that most resembles the route of expected human intake is preferable. This includes considering the digestive state, (for example, fed or fasted), of the subjects or experimental animals. Where this is not possible, the differences in route of exposure are noted as a source of uncertainty.

• The critical data set defines a dose-response relationship between intake and the extent of the toxic response known to be most relevant to humans. One additional issue examined during the evaluation of dose-response data concerns the bioavailability of the nutrient under review. For example, it is known that different metal salts can display different degrees of bioavailability. If the database involves studies of several different salts (for example, iron or chromium valence states), and the effect of the nutrient is systemic, then apparent differences in the degree and/or form of the toxic response among different salts may simply reflect differences in bioavailability. Data on bioavailability are considered and adjustments in expressions of dose-response are made to determine whether any apparent differences in response can be explained.

• The critical data set should document the route of exposure and the magnitude and duration of the intake. Furthermore, the critical data set should document the intake that does not produce adverse effects, the NOAEL, as well as the intake producing toxicity.

Identification of NOAEL (or LOAEL) and Critical Endpoint

The NOAEL can be identified from evaluation of the critical data set. If there are not adequate data demonstrating a NOAEL, then a LOAEL may be used. A nutrient can produce more than one toxic effect (or endpoint), even within the same species or in studies using the same or different exposure durations. The NOAELs (and LOAELs) for these effects will differ. The critical endpoint used in this report is the adverse biological effect exhibiting the lowest NOAEL (for example, the most sensitive indicator of a nutrient's toxicity). The derivation of a UL based on the most sensitive endpoint will ensure protection against all other adverse effects.

Uncertainty Assessment

As discussed previously and further elaborated in Appendix C, several judgments must be made regarding the uncertainties and thus uncertainty factor (UF) associated with extrapolating from the observed data to the healthy population. Applying UFs to a NOA-EL (or LOAEL) will result in a value for the derived UL that is less than the experimentally derived NOAEL, unless the UF is 1.0. The larger the uncertainty, the larger the UF and the smaller the UL, which represents a lower estimate of the threshold above which the risk of adverse effects may increase. This is consistent with the ultimate goal of the risk assessment: to provide an estimate of a level of intake that will protect the health of the healthy population (Mertz et al., 1994).

Although several reports describe the underlying basis for UFs (Dourson and Stara, 1983; Zielhuis and van der Kreek, 1979), the strength of the evidence supporting the use of a specific UF will vary. Because the imprecision of these UFs is a major limitation of risk assessment approaches, considerable leeway must be allowed for the application of scientific judgment in making the final determination. While the UFs selected for nonessential chemical agents are usually multiples of 10, the data on nutrient toxicity may not be subject to the same uncertainties as with nonessential chemical agents since data are generally available regarding intakes of human populations. The UFs for nutrients are typically less than 10 depending on the quality and nature of the data and the adverse effects involved. Also, smaller UFs may be used when the adverse effects are extremely mild and reversible.

In general, when determining a UF, the following potential sources of uncertainty are considered:

- *Interindividual variation in sensitivity.* Small UFs (in the range of 1 to 10) are used if it is judged that little population variability is expected for the adverse effect, and larger factors (greater than 10) are used if variability is expected to be great (NRC, 1994).
- *Experimental animal to human.* A UF is generally applied to the NOAEL to account for the uncertainty in extrapolating animal data to humans. Smaller or larger UFs (greater than 10) may be used if it is believed that the animal responses will over- or underpredict average human responses (NRC, 1994).
- *LOAEL to NOAEL.* If a NOAEL is not available, a UF may be applied to account for the uncertainty in deriving a UL from the LOAEL. The size of the UF involves scientific judgment based on the severity and incidence of the observed effect at the LOAEL and the steepness (slope) of the dose response.
- *Subchronic NOAEL to predict chronic NOAEL.* Scientific judgment is necessary to determine whether chronic exposure is likely to lead to adverse effects at lower intakes than those produc-

ing effects after subchronic exposures, when data are lacking on chronic exposures.

Selection of a UF for Calcium, Phosphorus, Magnesium, Vitamin D, and Fluoride

The selection of a UF of approximately 1.0 for fluoride and magnesium is primarily based on the very mild (and in the case of magnesium, reversible) nature of the adverse effects observed. A slightly larger UF (1.2) was selected for vitamin D intake in adults and other life stage groups except infants as the short duration of the study used (Narang et al., 1984) and the small sample size supports the selection of a slightly larger UF. For vitamin D in infants, a larger UF (1.8) was selected due to the insensitivity of the critical endpoint, the small sample sizes of the studies, and limited data about the sensitivity at the tails of the distribution. A UF of 2 was selected for calcium to account for the potential increased susceptibility to high calcium intake by individuals who form renal stones and the potential to increase the risk of mineral depletion in vulnerable populations due to calcium-mineral interactions. A UF of 2.5 was selected for phosphorus due to the lack of information on potential adverse effects in the range between normal phosphorus levels and levels associated with ectopic mineralization. The selection of a UF for phosphorus that is larger than those for the other nutrients evaluated is also due to the relative lack of human data describing adverse effects of excess phosphorus intake.

Derivation of a UL

The UL is derived by dividing the NOAEL (or LOAEL) by all the relevant UFs. The derivation of a UL involves the use of scientific judgment to select the appropriate NOAEL (or LOAEL) and UF. The framework or model outlined in this chapter for characterizing the potential risk (for example, scientific judgment used in deriving a UL from a NOAEL [or LOAEL]) is provided from a nutritional risk assessment perspective. This perspective is consistent with that of classical risk assessment in that it requires explicit consideration and discussion of all choices made, both regarding the data used and the uncertainties accounted for.

Characterization of the Estimate and Special Considerations

ULs are derived for various life stage groups utilizing relevant databases, NOAELs and LOAELs, and UFs. In cases where no data exist with regard to NOAELs or LOAELs for the group under consideration, extrapolations from data in other age groups and/or animal data are made on the basis of known differences in body size, physiology, metabolism, absorption, and excretion of the nutrient.

If the data review reveals the existence of subpopulations having distinct and exceptional sensitivities to a nutrient's toxicity, these subpopulations are considered under the heading "Special Considerations."

GLOSSARY

Bioavailability: The accessibility of a nutrient to participate in metabolic and/or physiological processes.

Dose-Response Assessment: The second step in a risk assessment in which the relationship between nutrient intake and adverse effect (in terms of incidence and/or severity of the effect) is determined.

Hazard Identification: The first step in a risk assessment, which is concerned with the collection, organization, and evaluation of all information pertaining to the toxic properties of a nutrient.

Lowest-Observed-Adverse-Effect Level (LOAEL): The lowest intake (or experimental dose) of a nutrient at which an adverse effect has been identified.

No-Observed-Adverse-Effect Level (NOAEL): The highest intake (or experimental dose) of a nutrient at which no adverse effects have been observed.

Risk: Within the context of nutrient toxicity, the probability or likelihood that some adverse effect will result from a specified excess intake of a nutrient.

Risk Assessment: An organized framework for evaluating scientific information, which has as its objective a characterization of the nature and likelihood of harm resulting from excess human exposure to an environmental agent (in this case, a dietary nutrient). It includes the development of both qualitative and quantitative expressions of risk. The process of risk assessment can be divided into four major steps: hazard identification, dose-response assessment, exposure assessment, and risk characterization.

Risk Characterization: The final step in a risk assessment, which summarizes the conclusions from Steps 1 through 3 of the risk assessment and evaluates the risk. This step also includes a characterization of the degree of scientific confidence that can be placed in the UL.

Risk Management: The process by which risk assessment results are integrated with other information to make decisions about the need for, method of, and extent of risk reduction. In addition to risk assessment results, risk management considers such issues as the public health significance of the risk, the technical feasibility of achieving various degrees of risk control, and the economic and social costs of this control.

Tolerable Upper Intake Level (UL): The maximum level of total chronic daily intake of a nutrient or food component that is unlikely to pose risks of adverse effects to the most sensitive members of the healthy population.

Uncertainty Factor (UF):   A number by which the NOAEL (or LOAEL) is divided to obtain the UL.   UFs are used in risk assessments to deal with gaps in data (for example, data uncertainties) and knowledge (for example, model uncertainties).   The size of the UF varies depending on the confidence in the data and the nature of the adverse effect.

4

Calcium

BACKGROUND INFORMATION

Overview

Calcium accounts for 1 to 2 percent of adult human body weight. Over 99 percent of total body calcium is found in teeth and bones. The remainder is present in blood, extracellular fluid, muscle, and other tissues, where it plays a role in mediating vascular contraction and vasodilation, muscle contraction, nerve transmission, and glandular secretion.

In bone, calcium exists primarily in the form of hydroxyapatite ($Ca_{10} (PO_4)_6 (OH)_2$), and bone mineral is almost 40 percent of the weight of bone. Bone is a dynamic tissue that is constantly undergoing osteoclastic bone resorption and osteoblastic bone formation. Bone formation exceeds resorption in growing children, is balanced with resorption in healthy adults, and lags behind resorption after menopause and with aging in men and women. Each year, a portion of the skeleton is remodeled (reabsorbed and replaced by new bone). The rate of cortical (or compact) bone remodeling can be as high as 50 percent per year in young children and is about 5 percent per year in adults (Parfitt, 1988). Trabecular (or cancellous) bone remodeling is about five-fold higher than cortical remodeling in adults. The skeleton has an obvious structural role and it also serves as a reservoir for calcium.

71

Physiology of Absorption, Metabolism, and Excretion

Calcium is absorbed by active transport and passive diffusion across the intestinal mucosa. Active transport of calcium into enterocytes and out on the serosal side is dependent on the action of 1,25-dihydroxyvitamin D (1,25(OH)$_2$D), the active form of vitamin D, and its intestinal receptors. This mechanism accounts for most of the absorption of calcium at low and moderate intake levels. Passive diffusion involves the movement of calcium between mucosal cells and is dependent on the luminal:serosal calcium concentration gradient. Passive diffusion becomes more important at high calcium intakes (Ireland and Fordtran, 1973).

It has long been recognized that fractional calcium absorption varies inversely with dietary calcium intake (Ireland and Fordtran, 1973; Malm, 1958; Spencer et al., 1969). For example, when calcium intake was acutely lowered from 2,000 to 300 mg (50 to 7.5 mmol)/day, healthy women increased their fractional whole body retention of ingested calcium, an index of calcium absorption, from 27 percent to about 37 percent (Dawson-Hughes et al., 1993). This adaptation required 1 to 2 weeks and was accompanied by a decline in serum calcium and a rise in serum parathyroid hormone (PTH) and 1,25(OH)$_2$D concentrations. In general, the adaptive rise in the fraction of calcium absorbed as intake is lowered is not sufficient to offset the loss in absorbed calcium that occurs with a decrease in calcium intake, however modest that decrease. This is clear from the demonstrations that absorbed calcium and calcium intake, throughout a wide intake range, are positively related (Gallagher et al., 1980; Heaney et al., 1975).

Fractional calcium absorption varies through the lifespan. It is highest (about 60 percent) in infancy (Abrams et al., 1997a; Fomon and Nelson, 1993) and rises again in early puberty. Abrams and Stuff (1994) found fractional absorption in Caucasian girls consuming a mean of about 925 mg (23.1 mmol)/day of calcium to average 28 percent in prepubertal children, 34 percent in early puberty (the age of the growth spurt), and 25 percent 2 years later. Fractional absorption remains at about this value (25 percent) in young adults, with the exception that it increases during the last two trimesters of pregnancy (Heaney et al., 1989). With aging, fractional absorption gradually declines. In postmenopausal women, fractional absorption declined by an average of 0.21 percent/year (Heaney et al., 1989). Bullamore and colleagues (1970) reported that men lose absorption efficiency with aging at about the same rate as women.

Renal calcium excretion is a function of the filtered load and the efficiency of reabsorption; the latter is regulated primarily by the PTH level. With aging, the urinary loss of calcium decreases (Davis et al., 1970), possibly because of an age-related decrease in intestinal calcium absorption efficiency and an associated reduction in filtered calcium load. Endogenous fecal calcium excretion does not change appreciably with aging (Heaney and Recker, 1994).

Racial differences in calcium metabolism have been noted in children and adults. In children and adolescents aged 9 to 18 years, Bell and colleagues (1993) found that African Americans had similar calcium absorption efficiency but lower urinary calcium excretion than Caucasians. Abrams and colleagues (1996a) found absorption efficiency to be similar in prepubertal African American and Caucasian girls or boys but greater in African American girls after menarche. In their study, urinary calcium excretion was lower in African American girls before menarche but similar in postmenarcheal African American and Caucasian girls. These metabolic differences may contribute to the widely observed higher bone mass in African American children (Bell et al., 1991; Gilsanz et al., 1991) and adults (Cohn et al., 1977; Liel et al., 1988; Luckey et al., 1989), and to lower fracture rates in African American adults in the United States (Farmer et al., 1984; Kellie and Brody, 1990). However, their implications for the calcium intake requirement are not clear, and observed differences do not warrant race-specific recommendations at this time.

Factors Affecting the Calcium Requirement

Bioavailability

When evaluating the food sources of calcium, the calcium content is generally of greater importance than bioavailability. Calcium absorption efficiency is fairly similar from most foods, including milk and milk products and grains (major food sources of calcium in North American diets). It should be noted that calcium may be poorly absorbed from foods rich in oxalic acid (spinach, sweet potatoes, rhubarb, and beans) or phytic acid (unleavened bread, raw beans, seeds, nuts and grains, and soy isolates). Soybeans contain large amounts of phytic acid, yet calcium absorption is relatively high from this food (Heaney et al., 1991). In comparison to calcium absorption from milk, calcium absorption from dried beans is about half and from spinach is about one tenth. Because diets used in metabolic studies and in the general population contain calcium from a variety of sources, and because the specific foods used in most of the published studies were not described, adjusting for varying bioavailability was not considered in setting the calcium intake requirements.

Bioavailability of calcium when measured from nonfood sources, or supplements, depends on the presence or absence of a meal and the size of the dose. Supplement solubility is not very important (Heaney et al., 1990a), but tablet disintegration (for example, breaking apart) is essential (Whiting and Pluhator, 1992). In studies that measured calcium absorption under similar test conditions, a 250 mg (6.2 mmol) elemental calcium load given with a standardized breakfast meal resulted in average fractional absorption rates of calcium from calcium citrate malate, calcium carbonate, and tricalcium phosphate of 35, 27, and 25 percent, respectively (Heaney et al., 1989, 1990a; Miller et al., 1988; Smith et al., 1987). Under the same conditions, absorption of calcium from milk was similar at 29 percent. Individuals with achlorhydria absorb calcium from calcium carbonate poorly unless the supplement is taken with a meal (Recker, 1985). The efficiency of absorption of calcium from supplements is greatest when calcium is taken in doses of 500 mg (12.5 mmol) or less (Heaney et al., 1975, 1988).

Physical Activity

The concept that weight-bearing physical activity or mechanical loading determines the strength, shape, and mass of bone is generally accepted (Frost, 1987). The mechanisms by which exercise influences bone mass and structure are currently under investigation (Frost, 1997). Although exercise and calcium intake both influence bone mass, it is unclear whether calcium intake influences the degree of benefit derived from exercise. Under the extreme condition of immobilization, rapid bone loss occurs despite consumption of 1,000 mg (25 mmol)/day of calcium (LeBlanc et al., 1995). In a 3-year calcium intervention study in children aged 6 to 14 years, both calcium and exercise influenced the rate of bone mineralization, but their effects appeared to be independent (Slemenda et al., 1994). Specker (1996) reviewed published prospective exercise studies in which calcium intake data were provided. Sixteen studies were identified, 15 conducted in women and 1 in men. High daily calcium intakes (over 1,000 mg [25 mmol]) enhanced the bone mineral density (BMD) benefits from exercise at the lumbar spine, but enhancement at the radius was less pronounced. Additional prospective studies are needed to test and compare individual and combined effects of calcium and exercise.

Currently, there is insufficient evidence to justify different calcium intake recommendations for people with different levels of physical activity.

Nutrient-Nutrient Interactions

Sodium. Sodium and calcium excretion are linked in the proximal renal tubule. High sodium chloride intake results in increased absorbed sodium, increased urinary sodium, and an increased obligatory loss of urinary calcium (Kurtz et al., 1987). Quantitatively, 500 mg of sodium as sodium chloride has been shown to draw about 10 mg (0.25 mmol) of calcium into the urine in postmenopausal women (Nordin and Polley, 1987). This linkage holds at moderate and high calcium intakes, but some dissociation occurs at low calcium intakes (Dawson-Hughes et al., 1996), probably because low calcium intakes induce higher PTH levels, and PTH promotes the reabsorption of filtered calcium in the distal renal tubule. In children and adolescents, urinary sodium is an important determinant of urinary calcium excretion (Matkovic et al., 1995; O'Brien et al., 1996). An association between salt intake (or sodium excretion) and skeletal development has not been demonstrated in children or adolescents, but one longitudinal study in postmenopausal women identified a correlation between high urinary sodium excretion and increased bone loss from the hip (Devine et al., 1995). Thus, although indirect evidence indicates that dietary sodium chloride has a negative effect on the skeleton, the effect of a change in sodium intake on bone loss and fracture rates has not been reported. Although there is some concern related to the effects of the high salt content of American diets (from processed foods, etc.), available evidence does not warrant different calcium intake requirements for individuals according to their salt consumption.

Protein. Protein increases urinary calcium excretion, but its effect on calcium retention is controversial. In balance studies involving use of formula diets in which the phosphorus content was stable, 1 g of dietary protein from both animal and vegetable sources increased urinary calcium excretion by about 1 to 1.5 mg (Linkswiler et al., 1981; Margen et al., 1974). Walker and Linkswiler (1972) found that urinary calcium increased by about 0.5 mg for each gram of dietary protein, as protein intake increased above 47 g/day. In a recent study, a high protein intake (2.71 ± 0.75 g/kg/day) had no measurable effect on urinary pyridinium cross-links of collagen, an index of bone resorption (Delmas, 1992), in young adults consuming 1,600 mg (40 mmol)/day of calcium, possibly because of the variability in this measure (Shapses et al., 1995). While dietary protein intake increases urinary calcium excretion, it should be recognized that inadequate protein intakes (34 g/day) have been associated with poor general health and poor recovery from osteoporotic hip fractures (Delmi et al., 1990). Similarly, serum albumin values have been shown to be inversely related to hip fracture risk (Huang et al., 1996). Available evidence does not warrant adjusting calcium intake recommendations based on dietary protein intake.

Other Food Components

Caffeine. Caffeine has a modest negative impact on calcium retention (Barger-Lux et al., 1990) and has been associated with increased hip fracture risk in women (Kiel et al., 1990). The association of caffeine consumption with accelerated bone loss has been limited to postmenopausal women with low calcium intakes (Harris and Dawson-Hughes, 1994). Specifically, associations with bone loss from the spine and total body were identified in women who consumed less than about 800 mg (20 mmol)/day of calcium and the amount of caffeine present in two or more cups of brewed coffee. Consistent with this is the observation that the negative effect of caffeine on BMD can be offset by the addition of dietary calcium (Barrett-Connor et al., 1994). Caffeine induces a short-term increase in renal calcium excretion (Massey and Wise, 1984) and may modestly decrease calcium absorption (Barger-Lux and Heaney, 1995); its effect on dermal calcium loss has not been evaluated. In summary, the skeletal effects of caffeine are modest at calcium intakes of 800 mg (20 mmol)/day and above. Available evidence does not warrant different calcium intake recommendations for people with different caffeine intakes.

Special Populations

Amenorrheic Women. Conditions that produce lower levels of circulating estrogen alter calcium homeostasis. Young women with amenorrhea resulting from anorexia nervosa have reduced net calcium absorption, higher urinary calcium excretion, and a lower rate of bone formation when compared with healthy eumenorrheic women (Abrams et al., 1993). Exercise-induced amenorrhea also results in reduced calcium retention and lower bone mass (Drinkwater et al., 1990; Marcus et al., 1985).

Menopausal Women. Decreased estrogen production at menopause is associated with accelerated bone loss, particularly from the lumbar spine, for about 5 years (Gallagher et al., 1987). During this period, women lose an average of about 3 percent of their skeletal mass per year. Lower levels of estrogen are accompanied by decreased calcium absorption efficiency (Gallagher et al., 1980; Heaney et al., 1989) and increased rates of bone turnover. These observations may be interpreted several ways. First, lowered estrogen levels primarily affect the skeleton, leading to increased bone resorption, an increase in circulating ionized calcium, a decrease in $1,25(OH)_2D$, and reduced stimulus for active intestinal transport of calcium (Gallagher et al., 1980). A second interpretation is that estrogen deficiency primarily reduces the efficiency of dietary calcium utilization and that this reduced efficiency produces a bone loss related to calcium substrate deficiency (Gallagher et al., 1980). A third interpretation is that estrogen has primary effects on both bone and the intestine. The impact on what the dietary calcium intake should be to meet requirements in the above scenarios differs. Increasing calcium intake would provide little skeletal benefit if the primary effect of estrogen withdrawal is at the skeleton. That is, increasing calcium intake would increase absorbed calcium but not the deposition of calcium in bone. The excess absorbed calcium would be excreted in the urine. In contrast, increasing calcium intake should correct the problem (for example, prevent bone loss) if estrogen deficiency primarily reduces calcium absorption efficiency.

Examination of the skeletal response to calcium supplementation in premenopausal and early postmenopausal women provides some insight. In a longitudinal calcium supplement trial in women aged 46 to 55 years, Elders et al. (1994) found that 2,000 mg (50 mmol)/day of supplemental calcium significantly reduced bone loss from the lumbar spine in premenopausal women but not in the early postmenopausal women. The effect of calcium supplementation on metacarpal cortical thickness was not significantly related to the menopausal status of the women in this study. In a different study of women with low usual calcium intakes, supplementation with 500 mg (12.5 mmol)/day of calcium had no significant impact on bone loss from the spine or other sites in early postmenopausal women, but it significantly reduced bone loss in women more than 5 years beyond menopause (Dawson-Hughes et al., 1990). From these and other studies (Aloia et al., 1994; Prince et al., 1991; Riis et al., 1987) (see Table 4-1), it is apparent that increasing calcium intake will not prevent the rapid trabecular bone loss that occurs in the first 5 years after menopause. Calcium responsiveness of cortical bone

TABLE 4-1 Randomized Controlled Calcium Intervention Trials in Postmenopausal Women

Site	N	Calcium Intake (mg/day) Diet	Supplement[a]	Relative Change in BMD or BMC in Calcium Group Compared with Placebo Year 1	Year 2 or More, Annualized	Statistically Significant Change in BMD or BMC in Calcium Group Compared with Placebo
Spine						
Early postmenopausal						
Aloia et al., 1994[b]	70	500	1,700	P[j]	S or N	no
Dawson-Hughes et al., 1990	67	<400	500	S[h] or N[i]	S	no
Elders et al., 1991[d]	248	1,150	1,000 and 2,000	P	S or N	yes
Riis et al., 1987	25	~1,000[c]	2,000	P	S or N	no
Late Menopausal						
Dawson-Hughes et al., 1990	169	<400	500 (CCM)	P	S or N	yes
			500 (CC)	P	S or N	no
		400–650	500 (CCM)	P	S or N	no
			500 (CC)	S or N	S or N	no
Prince et al., 1995	126	800	1,000	P	S or N	no
Reid et al., 1995	78	750	1,000	P	S or N	yes
Radius (Proximal)						
Early postmenopausal						
Aloia et al., 1994[b]	70	500	1,700	S or N	P	no
Dawson-Hughes et al., 1990	67	<400	500	P	P	no
Prince et al., 1991[e]	80	800	1,000	P	P	no
Riis et al., 1987	25	~1,000	2,000	P	P	yes
Late postmenopausal						
Dawson-Hughes et al., 1990	169	<400	500 (CCM)	P	P	yes
			500 (CC)	P	S or N	yes
		400–650	500 (CCM)	P	P	no
			500 (CC)	P	P	no
Recker et al., 1996:						
Prevalent vertebral fracture group	94	~450	1,200 (CC)	—	—	yes
Non-prevalent vertebral fracture group	99	~450	1,200 (CC)	—	—	no

TABLE 4-1 Continued

Site	N	Calcium Intake (mg/day) Diet	Supplement[a]	Relative Change in BMD or BMC in Calcium Group Compared with Placebo Year 1	Year 2 or More, Annualized	Statistically Significant Changes in BMD or BMC in Calcium Group Compared with Placebo
Femoral neck						
Early postmenopausal						
Aloia et al., 1994[b]	70	500	1,700	P	P	yes
Dawson-Hughes et al., 1990	67	<400	500	P	S	no
Late menopausal						
Chevalley et al., 1994	93	600	800	P[f]		no
Dawson-Hughes et al., 1990	169	<400	500 (CCM)	P	P	yes
			500 (CC)	P	P	no
		400–	500 (CCM)	P	S or N	no
		650	500 (CC)	P	S or N	no
Prince et al., 1995[g]	126	800	1,000	P	P	no
Reid et al., 1995	78	750	1,000	P	S or N	yes
Total Body						
Early postmenopausal						
Aloia et al., 1994[b]	70	500	1,700	P	P	yes
Late postmenopausal						
Reid et al., 1995	78	750	1,000	P	P	yes

[a] Calcium sources: Dawson-Hughes: citrate malate (CCM), carbonate (CC); Aloia, Ettinger, and Riis: CC; Prince: lactate-gluconate (1991, 1995), milk powder (1995); Elders and Reid: (lactate-gluconate + CC) or citrate; Chevalley: CC or osseino-mineral complex.
[b] All women treated with 400 IU (10 µg) vitamin D per day.
[c] Estimate based on national norm rather than on intake of study subjects.
[d] Randomized open trial.
[e] All women participated in exercise program.
[f] An 18-month study in 82 women and 11 men.
[g] Supplement tablets and milk powder significantly reduced bone loss at the trochanter.
[h] S = Similar change in BMD or BMC when compared with placebo.
[i] N = Negative, but not necessarily significant, change in BMC or BMD when compared with placebo.
[j] P = Positive, but not necessarily significant, change in BMC or BMD when compared with placebo.
SOURCE: Adapted, with permission, from Dawson-Hughes B. ©1996. Calcium. In: Marcus R, Feldman D, Kelsey J, eds. *Osteoporosis*. San Diego: Academic Press, Inc. Pp. 1103 and 1105.

appears to be less dependent on menopausal status. In summary, from available evidence, the calcium intake requirement for women does not appear to change acutely with menopause.

Lactose Intolerance. About 25 percent of adults in the United States have lactose intolerance and develop symptoms of diarrhea and bloating after ingestion of a large dose of lactose, such as the amount present in a quart of milk (about 46 g) (Coffin et al., 1994). Primary lactase deficiency begins in childhood and may become clinically apparent in adolescence. In adults, the prevalence of lactose intolerance, as estimated by a positive breath-hydrogen test, is highest in Asians (about 85 percent), intermediate in African Americans (about 50 percent), and lowest in Caucasians (about 10 percent) (Johnson et al., 1993a; Nose et al., 1979; Rao et al., 1994). Lactose-intolerant individuals often avoid milk products entirely although avoidance may not be necessary. Studies have revealed that many lactose-intolerant people can tolerate smaller doses of lactose, for example, the amount present in an 8 oz glass of milk (about 11 g) (Johnson et al., 1993b; Suarez et al., 1995). In addition, lactose-free dairy products are available. Although lactose-intolerant individuals absorb calcium normally from milk (Horowitz et al., 1987; Tremaine et al., 1986), they are at risk for calcium deficiency because of avoidance of milk and other calcium-rich milk products. Although lactose intolerance may influence intake, there is no evidence to suggest that it influences the calcium requirement.

Vegetarian Diets. Consumption of vegetarian diets may influence the calcium requirement because of their relatively high contents of oxalate and phytate, compounds that reduce calcium bioavailablity. In contrast to diets containing animal protein, however, vegetarian diets produce metabolizable anions (for example, acetate, bicarbonate) that lower urinary calcium excretion (Berkelhammer et al., 1988; Sebastian et al., 1994). On balance, lacto-ovovegetarians and omnivores appear to have fairly similar dietary calcium intakes (Marsh et al., 1980; Pedersen et al., 1991; Reed et al., 1994) and, on the same intakes, to have similar amounts of urinary calcium excretion (Lloyd et al., 1991; Tesar et al., 1992). BMD has been examined and compared in several cross-sectional studies of lacto-ovovegetarians and omnivores. Among premenopausal women, spinal BMD did not differ significantly in the two groups (Lloyd et al., 1991). Postmenopausal lacto-ovovegetarians are reported to have higher cortical bone mass than omnivores, as indicated by higher midradius density (Marsh et al., 1980; Tylavsky and Anderson,

1988). However, in a 5-year study, postmenopausal lacto-ovovege-tarians and omnivores with similar calcium intakes lost radius BMD at similar rates (Reed et al., 1994). Bone data on strict vegetarians (vegans) are not available, but there is evidence in this group to indicate lower intakes of calcium (among other nutrients) in pre-menopausal women (Janelle and Barr, 1995), and lower body weight in children (Sanders and Purves, 1981). In conclusion, available data do not support the need for a different calcium intake recom-mendation for vegetarians.

Intake of Calcium

The USDA 1994 Continuing Survey of Food Intakes by Individu-als (CSFII), showed that mean daily calcium intake, based on an adjusted 24-hour recall which allows for varying degrees of depar-ture from normality and recognizes the measurement error associ-ated with one-day dietary intakes (Nusser et al., 1996), was about 25 percent higher in males than in females aged 9 years and older in the United States (925 vs. 657 mg [23.1 vs. 16.4 mmol]) (Cleveland et al., 1996) (see Appendix D for data tables). The fifth percentiles of intake from the 1994 CSFII for males and females aged 9 and over were 431 and 316 mg (10.8 and 7.9 mmol)/day. The corre-sponding median intake was 865 and 625 mg (21.6 and 15.6 mmol)/day and the ninety-fifth percentile intakes were 1,620 and 1,109 mg (40.5 and 27.7 mmol)/day. In males, daily intake peaked in the age range of 14 through 18 years (at 1,094 mg [27.4 mmol]) whereas it was highest in females aged 9 through 13 years (at 889 mg [22.2 mmol]). After age 50, median daily calcium intake remained al-most constant for males aged 71 and above (708 to 702 mg [17.7 to 17.6 mmol]) and declined for women (571 to 517 mg [14.3 to 12.9 mmol]). Data from the first phase of the Third National Health and Nutrition Examination Survey (NHANES III) are similar (Alaimo et al., 1994). Unfortunately, national survey data from Canada are not currently available.

Food Sources of Calcium

According to data for 1994, 73 percent of calcium in the U.S. food supply is from milk products, 9 percent is from fruits and vegetables, 5 percent is from grain products, and the remaining 12 percent is from all other sources (CNPP, 1996). Grains are not particularly rich in calcium, but because they may be consumed in large quantities, they can account for a substantial proportion of dietary calcium. Among Mexican American adults, corn tortillas are the second most important food source of calcium, after milk (Looker et al., 1993), but calcium from tortillas may be poorly absorbed (Rosado et al., 1992). White bread is the second most important source among Puerto Rican adults (Looker et al., 1993). Milk products, the most calcium-dense foods in Western diets, contain about 300 mg (7.5 mmol) calcium per serving (for example, per 8 oz of milk or yogurt or 1.5 oz of cheddar cheese). Other calcium-rich foods include calcium-set tofu, Chinese cabbage, kale, calcium-fortified orange juice, and broccoli.

Calcium Intake from Supplements

Results from a National Health Interview Survey (NHIS) in 1986 show that almost 25 percent of women in the United States took supplements containing calcium (Moss et al., 1989). Usage by men (14 percent) and children 2 to 6 years of age (7.5 percent) was less. Women who used supplements also took higher doses (median of 248 mg [6.2 mmol]/day) than men who used supplements (160 mg [4 mmol]/day). Children who took supplements had a median supplemental intake of only 88 mg (2.2 mmol)/day. The ninety-fifth percentile of supplemental intake was 304 mg (7.6 mmol)/day for young children, 928 mg (23.2 mmol)/day for men, and 1,200 mg (30 mmol)/day for women.

Data from 11,643 adults who participated in the 1992 NHIS show that calcium intakes are higher for both men and women who take dietary supplements (of any kind) daily than those who seldom or never take them, but the differences are statistically significant only for women (Slesinski et al., 1996). However, those adults who specifically take calcium supplements do not have higher intakes of food calcium.

Effects of Inadequate Calcium Intake

Chronic calcium deficiency resulting from inadequate intake or poor intestinal absorption is one of several important causes of reduced bone mass and osteoporosis (DHHS, 1990; NIH, 1994; NRC, 1989b; Osteoporosis Society of Canada, 1993). A reduction in absorbed calcium causes the circulating ionized calcium concentration to decline, which triggers an increase in PTH synthesis and release. PTH acts on three target organs to restore the circulating calcium concentration to normal. At the kidney, PTH promotes the reabsorption of calcium in the distal tubule. PTH affects the intestine indirectly by stimulating the production of $1,25(OH)_2D$. PTH also induces bone resorption, thereby releasing calcium into the blood. Thus, although PTH maintains a normal circulating calcium concentration during calcium deprivation, it does so at the expense of skeletal mass.

Dietary Calcium and Osteoporosis

Osteoporosis is characterized by reduced bone mass, increased bone fragility, and increased risk of fracture (WHO, 1994). According to the World Health Organization (WHO), individuals with BMD more than 2.5 standard deviations (SD) below the mean for young adult women are *osteoporotic* (Kanis et al., 1994; WHO, 1994). By this definition, the prevalence of osteoporosis among postmenopausal women in the United States is 21 percent in Caucasian and Asian, 16 percent in Hispanic, and 10 percent in African American women (Looker et al., 1995). An additional 38 percent of American women aged 50 and older meet the WHO definition of *osteopenic* (for example, have BMD values 1.0 to 2.5 SD below the young adult reference mean) (Looker et al., 1995).

In the United States each year, approximately 1.5 million fractures are associated with osteoporosis, including 300,000 hip fractures, 700,000 vertebral fractures, 250,000 distal forearm fractures, and 250,000 fractures at other sites (Riggs and Melton, 1995). In Canada in 1993, approximately 76,000 fractures were associated with osteoporosis, including 21,000 hip fractures, 27,000 vertebral fractures, and 27,000 wrist fractures (Goeree et al., 1996). Incidence rates for most fractures rise exponentially with age (Cooper and Melton, 1992). For individuals at age 50, their risk of having a hip fracture at some point in the future is estimated at 17 percent for Caucasian women, 6 percent for African American women, 6 percent for Caucasian men, and 3 percent for African American men (Cummings et al., 1993; Melton et al., 1992). It has been estimated that a Caucasian woman's risk of a hip fracture is equivalent to her combined risk of developing breast, uterine, and ovarian cancer (Riggs and Melton, 1995). Health care costs associated with osteoporotic fractures in 1995 were estimated at $13.8 billion (Ray et al., 1997). Because of the expected increase in the number of individuals in the age range of highest risk, the incidence of hip fractures in the United States may triple by the year 2040 (Schneider and Guralnik, 1990).

ESTIMATING REQUIREMENTS FOR CALCIUM

Selection of Indicators for Estimating the Calcium Requirement

There is no biochemical assay that reflects calcium nutritional status. Blood calcium concentration, for example, is not a good indicator because it is tightly regulated. Only in extreme circumstances, such as severe malnutrition or hyperparathyroidism, is the serum ionized calcium concentration below or above the normal range. Search of the scientific literature reveals numerous potential indirect indicators of calcium adequacy, most of which are closely related to the skeletal calcium content.

Calcium Intake and Fracture Risk

Ideally, the optimal calcium intake for skeletal health would be defined as that which leads to the fewest osteoporotic fractures later in life. Attaining this information would require prospective determination of the influence of different increments in calcium intake on fracture rates in young and older subjects with a wide range of usual calcium intakes. Such studies are not available, would require that large numbers of subjects be studied for many years, and would be prohibitively expensive.

Several observational studies of calcium intake and fracture risk are available (Cumming et al., 1997; Cummings et al., 1995; Holbrook et al., 1988; Looker et al., 1993; Paganini-Hill et al., 1991; Wickham et al., 1989). Among these, no consistent association has been demonstrated between reported calcium intake over periods of up to 10 years and risk of fracture in peri- and postmenopausal women (Cumming et al., 1997). This is not surprising because osteoporosis results from complex interactions among genetic, dietary, and other environmental factors and has a long latency period. From a methodologic perspective, calcium intake may be underestimated by some survey methods and overestimated by others. More importantly, even if accurate estimates of calcium intake were available, intakes measured at one point in time do not reflect lifetime consumption. In addition, the influence of confounding factors such as frequency of falls and physical activity may vary over time. For these reasons observational studies cannot be used effectively to determine an Estimated Average Requirement (EAR) for calcium.

Another approach that has been attempted is to compare fracture rates across cultures that have different calcium intakes. This approach however, is severely limited by cross-cultural differences in bone structural features, genetic composition, diets (nutrients other than calcium), and other environmental factors that influence fracture rates. For example, a longer hip axis length (the distance from the greater trochanter to the inner pelvic brim [HAL]) is associated with an increased hip fracture incidence (Faulkner et al., 1993). Japanese women have shorter HALs than Caucasian Americans and this may partially account for why their hip fracture rates are lower (Nakamura et al., 1994). Genetic differences related to calcium homeostasis may also thwart efforts to estimate calcium requirements from cross-cultural studies. The prevalence of a vitamin D-receptor-gene genotype associated with reduced calcium absorption efficiency (Dawson-Hughes et al., 1995) is lower in Japanese women than in Caucasian American women (Yamagata et al., 1994). Finally, many environmental factors differ more between cultures than within cultures and these differences are not controlled for when independently conducted studies are compared. Thus the use of observational studies relating intakes to fracture risk as the primary determinant of requirements is not warranted at this time.

Bone Mass Measurements

Bone mineral content (BMC) is the amount of mineral at a particular skeletal site such as the femoral neck, lumbar spine, or total body. *Bone mineral density* (BMD) is BMC divided by the area of the scanned region. Recent studies have indicated that both measures are strong predictors of fracture risk (Black et al., 1992; Cummings et al., 1993; Melton et al., 1993a). In adults, a 1 standard deviation (SD) decrease (representing about a 15 percent decline) in femoral neck BMD is associated with a 2.5-fold increase in risk of hip fracture (Cummings et al., 1993). A 1 SD decrease in lumbar spine BMD increases vertebral fracture risk two fold (Cummings et al., 1993).

BMD and BMC are both measured by a variety of related techniques including dual-energy x-ray absorptiometry (DXA). The DXA method is precise, reasonably accurate, and, in the context of longitudinal calcium intervention trials that measure *change in BMC,* can provide data on the long-term impact of added calcium not only on the total skeleton but also on skeletal sites that are subject to osteoporotic fractures. In children, change in BMC is a useful indicator of calcium retention, but change in BMD is less suitable than BMC because BMD misses much of the change in skeletal size.

In adults, with their generally stable skeletal size, change in both BMD and BMC are useful outcome measures. The ability of DXA to measure specific skeletal regions such as the spine, hip, and forearm adds a potentially valuable refinement to the determination of the calcium requirement derived from balance studies (see "Calcium Retention" below). This technique has already revealed that the patterns and timing of acquisition of peak bone mass vary by skeletal site, and that bone loss from trabecular- and cortical-rich sites occurs at different rates in women at menopause (see Table 4-1). Available evidence from supplementation trials in postmenopausal women also suggests that the calcium intake needed for maximal bone preservation differs by skeletal site (see Table 4-1). This is addressed more specifically in the section on requirements for adults over age 50.

Calcium Intake and Bone Mass

Cross-sectional studies that relate dietary calcium intake to BMC or BMD are of modest value in establishing the calcium requirement. These studies are of limited value because calcium intake is not accurately measured, calcium intake at one point in time may not reflect lifetime calcium intake, and bone mass at a single point in time is the result of the lifelong influence of many confounding variables that are not measured.

In contrast, randomized, placebo-controlled calcium intervention studies that measure change in BMC or BMD provide valuable evidence for the calcium requirement. A major strength of such longitudinal studies is that the increment in calcium intake (the intervention) is known. In addition, their generally large sample sizes and subject randomization greatly reduce confounding of the results by other factors that influence bone mass. Limitations are that they require large sample sizes, are very expensive, and usually test only one or two doses of calcium per study. Assessment of dietary calcium intake (in contrast to the intervention) is subject to the usual inaccuracies.

An important consideration in the interpretation of longitudinal calcium intervention studies is the phenomenon of the *bone remodeling transient*, the one-time initial gain in bone mass that occurs in the first 3 to 12 months after increasing calcium intake (or administration of an antiresorptive drug) (Frost, 1973). Calcium supplementation trials of 1 to 2 years duration may overestimate the longer-term influence of calcium because of the effect of calcium (and all remodeling suppressers) in reducing the size of the remodeling space, the portion of total bone mass that is currently being remodeled. The remodeling rate in trabecular bone is four to five times greater than that in cortical bone. As a result, the remodeling transient is more apparent at the more highly trabecular spine than it is at the more cortical radius or the even more dominantly cortical total skeleton. Because of the bone remodeling transient, the long-term or cumulative effect of calcium can best be evaluated by examining the effect of added calcium in the second and later years of an intervention (Table 4-1).

Calcium Retention

In estimating the intake requirement for calcium, it is important to recognize that calcium is unique in several respects. First, 99 percent of body calcium is located in the skeleton which has an essential structural function. To maximize skeletal size and strength, one must have adequate calcium retention to provide the substrate (along with other minerals) for bone mineral expansion during growth and maintenance after peak bone mass has been achieved. To a great extent, the retention of calcium in bone is under strong homeostatic control, which is regulated by genetics, calciotropic hormones and weight bearing exercise. The target intake of dietary calcium to achieve the desirable and optimal calcium accretion in bone is difficult to estimate because of all of the other factors which play a role in bone mineral homeostasis.

In this report, classic metabolic studies of calcium balance were used to obtain data on the relationship between calcium intakes and retention from which a non-linear regression model was developed; and from this was derived an intake of calcium which would be adequate to attain a predetermined *desirable* calcium retention. This approach is a further refinement of an earlier approach suggested to determine the point at which additional calcium does not significantly increase calcium retention, called the *plateau intake* (Matkovic and Heaney, 1992; Spencer et al., 1984).

The predetermined desirable calcium retentions for adolescents and young adults were based on estimates of the calcium accretion in bone over either four years of adolescence or during the 3rd decade of life, to which were added estimates for sweat and other losses if not included in the experiment. For older adults, a value approximating zero balance was used for desirable retention assuming that no net positive accretion of bone at this age in replete individuals serves a functional advantage. Adults continue to lose bone despite high intakes of calcium for other reasons such as lack of estrogen, smoking, or sedentary lifestyle. Thus not all bone loss can be prevented by additional dietary calcium.

The balance studies used in this report were reviewed rigorously to meet specific criteria which included the following: subjects consumed a wide range of calcium intakes since variability in retention increases at higher intakes; the balance studies were initiated at least 7 days after starting the diet in order for subjects to approach a steady state as observed by Dawson-Hughes et al. (1988); and, where possible, the adult balance studies included were only for subjects who were consuming their usual calcium intakes unless otherwise indicated. By selecting studies conducted on such subjects, it obviates the concern about whether the *bone remodeling transient* might introduce bias in the calcium retentions observed. Such selection was not possible in studies in children where they have been randomized to one of two calcium intakes. However, in children the impact of the remodeling transient related to changing intake is overshadowed by their rapid and constantly changing rates of calcium accretion (for example, their modeling and remodeling rates are not in steady state even without an intake change).

The non-linear regression model describing the relationship between calcium intake and retention was solved to obtain a predicted calcium intake for a predetermined desirable calcium retention[1] which was specific for each age group. The basis of the value

---

[1] The Panel on Calcium and Related Nutrients proposed use of a recently described statistical model (Jackman et al., 1997) to estimate an intake necessary to support maximal calcium retention and from which to derive an EAR. In the original paper by Jackman et al. (1997), an estimate was made of the lowest level of calcium intake that was statistically indistinguishable from 100 percent maximal retention in some individuals. However, the Standing Committee on the Scientific Evaluation of Dietary Reference Intakes (DRI Committee) adopted a different interpretation of the data for the purpose of establishing an AI. The approach adopted is described in the prepublication version of this final report. The DRI Committee was subsequently advised that there were both statistical and biological concerns with the application of the percent maximal retention model (see Appendix E). After seeking input from the Panel on Calcium and Related Nutrients, the DRI Committee has chosen, for the final print of the report, to retain the statistical model described by Jackman et al. (1997), but to apply it to determine, from the same calcium balance data as was used in the prepublication report, an estimate of the calcium intake that is sufficient to achieve a defined, desirable level of calcium retention specific to the age groups considered. The mathematical modeling and basis of the equations were kindly provided for the report by Dr. George McCabe and Dr. Connie Weaver of Purdue University and are described in detail in Appendix E.

used for desirable calcium retention is delineated under each age-specific group. In general, for growing children and young adults, data on whole body bone mineral accretion using DXA technology were used to derive a value for calcium retention to support the reported bone accretion (assuming bone is 32.3 percent calcium). The major limitation of the data available is that bone mineral accretion during growth has not been studied over a wide range of calcium intakes.

Calcium Intake and Risk of Chronic Disease Other than Osteoporosis

Hypertension. Many studies have investigated a possible role of calcium in lowering the risk of hypertension. In a review of 22 randomized intervention trials, calcium supplementation was found to reduce systolic blood pressure modestly—by 1.68 mm Hg in hypertensive adults—and had no significant effect in normotensive adults (Allender et al., 1996). Diastolic blood pressure was not altered in either group. More recently, a diet with increased low-fat dairy products, fruits, and vegetables, and with reduced saturated and total fat, lowered blood pressure when fed to normotensive and hypertensive adults (Appel et al., 1997). In this study, the increase in dairy product consumption provided a mean dietary calcium increase from 443 to 1,265 mg (11.1 to 31.6 mmol)/day.

Little is known about the relationship of calcium intake and blood pressure in children. A recent randomized trial on 101 boys and girls with mean age 11 years (9.9 to 13.2 years) of African American, Caucasian, Asian, and Hispanic origin showed that calcium supplementation of 600 mg (15 mmol)/day could reduce blood pressure, although the effect was much larger in children who had lower baseline calcium intakes (150 to 347 mg [3.7 to 8.7 mmol]/1,000 kcal) (Gillman et al., 1995). No further reduction in blood pressure was observed in children already consuming over 1,000 mg (25 mmol)/day of calcium by supplementing them with 600 mg (15 mmol)/day.

The influence of dietary calcium on pregnancy-induced hypertension has been investigated extensively. A meta-analysis of 14 randomized controlled trials of calcium supplementation during pregnancy found that supplements of 1,500 to 2,000 mg (37.5 to 50 mmol)/day of calcium may result in a significant lowering of both diastolic and systolic blood pressure (Bucher et al., 1996). However, the randomized controlled trial of Calcium for Preeclampsia Prevention (CPEP) in 4,589 pregnant women found no effect of calcium supplementation on hypertension, blood pressure, or preeclampsia (Levine et al., 1997), perhaps because the intake of the control group was above a threshold value. In that study, women in the placebo group had a mean intake of 980 mg (24.5 mmol)/ day and women in the supplemental calcium group had a mean intake of 2,300 mg (57.5 mmol)/day.

Because the effect of dietary calcium on blood pressure may be modest and variable in the general population, and because the calcium intake needed to reduce blood pressure is very likely below the threshold necessary for desirable skeletal retention (McCarron et al., 1991), blood pressure will not be used as a primary indicator for estimating calcium requirements.

Colon Cancer. Colon cancer risk has been postulated as being influenced by dietary calcium intake, but the evidence is inconsistent. Bostick and colleagues (1993) reported a reduction in mucosal proliferation after calcium supplementation, whereas Kleibeuker and colleagues (1993) reported an increase. Greater mucosal proliferation has been observed in patients known to be at high risk of colon cancer as compared with those at low risk (Kanemitsu et al., 1985; Ponz de Leon et al., 1988; Roncucci et al., 1991). Data from observational and case-control studies are mixed (Garland et al., 1985; Meyer and White, 1993; Slattery et al., 1988), and prospective trials examining the effect of added calcium on colon cancer incidence are not available. Thus, colon cancer incidence is not a useful indicator for estimating calcium requirements at this time.

Limitations of the Evidence

In reviewing the scientific literature to provide the best estimate of calcium requirements for each stage of the lifespan, needed data were not always available. In most instances, calcium intake data could not be matched with the outcome criteria of both calcium retention and bone mass in the same subjects. For many of the age groups, available data did not adequately represent both genders and various ethnic groups. Although lower fracture rates have been reported in African American adults compared to those estimated in Caucasian adults (Farmer et al., 1984; Kellie and Brody, 1990) and in men compared to women (Cummings et al., 1993; Melton et al., 1992), the implications for calcium intake requirements are not clear at the present time. Because there is no sound basis for assigning different intake values according to gender or race/ethnic groups, findings have been extrapolated from one gender group to another and from a predominantly Caucasian population to other ethnic groups.

Summary

Desirable rates of calcium retention, determined from balance studies, factorial estimates of requirements, and limited data on BMD and BMC changes, will be used as the primary indicators of adequacy. These indicators will be used as reasonable surrogate markers to reflect changes in skeletal calcium content.

The decision to set AIs for calcium rather than EARs was based on the following concerns: (1) uncertainties in the methods inherent in and the precise nutritional significance of values obtained from the balance studies that form the basis of the desirable retention model; (2) the lack of concordance between observational and experimental data (mean calcium intakes in the United States and Canada are much lower than are the experimentally derived values predicted to be required to achieve a desirable level of calcium retention); and (3) the lack of longitudinal data that could be used to verify the association of the experimentally derived calcium intakes for achieving a predetermined level of calcium retention with the rate and extent of long-term bone loss and its clinical sequelae, such as fracture. Taking all of these factors into consideration, it was determined that an EAR for calcium could not be established at the present time. The recommended AI represents an approximation of the calcium intake that, in the judgment of the DRI Committee, would appear to be sufficient to maintain calcium nutriture while recognizing that lower intakes may be adequate for some, but this evaluation will have to await additional studies on calcium balance over broad ranges of intakes and/or of long-term measures of calcium sufficiency.

FINDINGS BY LIFE STAGE AND GENDER GROUP

Birth through 12 Months

Indicators Used to Set the AI

There are no functional criteria for calcium status that reflect response to dietary intake in infants. Thus recommended intakes of calcium are based on an *adequate intake* (AI) that reflects the derived mean intake of infants fed principally with human milk.

Human Milk. Human milk is recognized as the optimal source of nourishment for infants throughout at least the first year of life, and as a sole nutritional source for infants during the first 4 to 6 months of life (IOM, 1991). Further, there are no reports of full-term infants, who are exclusively and freely fed human milk and are vitamin D replete, who manifest any incidence of calcium deficiency. Therefore, consideration of the AI for calcium for infants is based on mean intake data from infants fed human milk as the principal fluid during the first year of life. This value was derived from studies where intake of human milk was measured by test weighing and where intake of food and formula by dietary records was determined for 3 days or more.

The concentration of calcium in human milk remains relatively constant, with a mean value of 264 mg (6.6 mmol)/liter throughout the first 6 months of nursing and with a small decrease during the second 6 months to about 210 mg (5.2 mmol)/liter (Atkinson et al., 1995). Variations in milk calcium content have been found between population groups. For example, in comparison with the above data from the United States, milk calcium concentrations were lower (by approximately 20 mg (0.5 mmol)/100 ml at 5 months of lactation) in mothers from the Gambia who usually have diets low in calcium (Prentice et al., 1995). Thus, for establishing values of milk calcium to use in setting the AIs, only studies on milk calcium from North America and the United Kingdom were considered to obtain a mean value.

Balance. Recently, calcium absorption using stable isotopes (Abrams et al., 1997a) was measured in 14 human milk-fed infants who were 5 through 7 months of age at the time of the study. Mean absorption was 61 ± 22 percent of intake when approximately 80 percent of the dietary calcium was from human milk. There was no significant relationship between calcium from solid foods and the fractional calcium absorption from human milk. This finding suggests that calcium from solid foods does not negatively affect the bioavailability of calcium from human milk. Using measured urinary calcium and estimates of endogenous excretion, net retention was calculated to be 68 ± 38 mg (1.7 ± 0.95 mmol)/day of calcium for those infants. At 61 percent calcium absorption from intake of the AI, this observed net retention (assuming small urinary and endogenous calcium losses) would easily be attained by infants fed the mixed diet of human milk and solid food.

Accretion. Total body calcium at birth in healthy, full-term infants is approximately 30 g (750 mmol) (Widdowson et al., 1951). Based on mineral accretion derived as a function of change in body weight, total body calcium increases to approximately 80 g (2,000 mmol) by 1 year of age (Leitch and Aitken, 1959). This change would lead to an average accretion rate of approximately 140 mg (3.5 mmol)/day during the first year of life. This greatly exceeds the accretion rate of approximately 30 to 35 mg (0.75 to 0.87 mmol)/day from 0 through 4 months of age and 50 to 55 mg (1.25 to 1.37 mmol)/day from 4 through 12 months of age derived from cadaveric sources (Fomon and Nelson, 1993; Koo and Tsang, 1997). A mean accretion rate of approximately 80 mg (2 mmol)/day during the first year of life was derived using metacarpal morphometry data (Garn, 1972; Weaver, 1994). Resolution of these different values for usual accretion rate is not currently possible.

Differences in calcium needs between infants fed human milk and those fed infant formula are discussed in the "Special Considerations" section.

0 through 6 Months

The AI for infants 0 through 6 months of age is based on the reported intake of milk (780 ml/day) determined by test weighing of full-term infants in three studies (Allen et al., 1991; Butte et al., 1984; Heinig et al., 1993) and by the reported average calcium concentration in human milk after 1 month of lactation of 264 mg (6.6 mmol)/liter (average of 10 studies from the United States and the United Kingdom as summarized in Atkinson et al. [1995]). Total calcium intake may be somewhat lower during the first month of life than in subsequent months because of a lower total volume of milk intake (Lonnerdal, 1997; Southgate et al., 1969; Widdowson, 1965). Using the mean value for intake of human milk of 780 ml/day and the average content of 264 mg (6.6 mmol)/liter of calcium, the AI for calcium is 210 mg (5.3 mmol)/day. The expected net retention of calcium from human milk assuming 61 percent absorption would be 128 mg (3.2 mmol)/day, which is in excess of the values predicted from calcium accretion based on cadaver and metacarpal analysis. This provides evidence that an AI of 210 mg (5.3 mmol)/day will result in retention of sufficient amounts of calcium to meet growth needs.

For infants in the first 4 months of life, balance studies suggest that 40 to 70 percent of the daily calcium intake is retained by the human milk-fed infant (Fomon and Nelson, 1993; Widdowson, 1965). In balance studies in human milk-fed infants, a mean calcium intake was 327 mg (8.2 mmol)/day, and the retention was 80 mg (2 mmol)/day (Fomon and Nelson, 1993). If infants consume the daily estimated AI, they would achieve a similar or greater calcium retention even if the efficiency of absorption was at the lower observed value of 40 percent. Thus, the AI should meet most infants' needs.

7 through 12 Months

During the 7- through 12-month age period, the intake of solid foods becomes more significant, and calcium intakes may increase substantially from these sources. Although limited data are available for typical calcium intakes from foods by human milk-fed older infants, mean calcium intakes from solid foods are 140 mg (3.5 mmol)/day for formula-fed infants (Abrams et al., 1997a; Specker et al., 1997). For the purpose of developing an AI for this age group, it is assumed that infants who are fed human milk have intakes of solid food similar to formula-fed infants of the same age (Specker et al., 1997). Based on data of Dewey et al. (1984), mean human milk intake during the second six months of life would be 600 ml/day. Thus, calcium intake from human milk with a calcium concentration of about 210 mg (5.3 mmol)/liter during this age span (Atkinson et al., 1995) would be approximately 130 mg (3.2 mmol)/day. Adding the intake from milk (130 mg [3.2 mmol]) and food (140 mg [3.5 mmol]), the total AI for calcium is 270 mg (6.8 mmol)/day.

In the presence of adequate supplies of vitamin D from the environment or supplemental sources, there is no evidence of calcium deficiency in the human milk-fed infant during the first year of life (Mimouni et al., 1993). How much the AI of 270 mg (6.8 mmol)/ day could be lowered and still meet the physiological needs for human milk-fed infants is unknown since mechanisms for adaptation to lower intakes of calcium are not well described for the infant population.

AI for Infants   **0 through 6 months   210 mg (5.3 mmol)/day**
                       7 through 12 months 270 mg (6.8 mmol)/day

Special Considerations

Infant Formulas. Intake of calcium from infant formulas may need to be greater than from human milk in order to achieve the same retention since absolute fractional absorption of calcium from cow milk or other formula may be lower than from human milk. Studies by Fomon and Nelson (1993) involving 40 human milk-fed, 252 cow milk formula-fed, and 135 soy protein formula-fed infants found absorption fractions of 58, 38, and 34 percent, respectively, for the three feeding types. However, the greater daily intake of calcium by the formula-fed infants (327 mg [8.2 mmol], 464 mg [11.6 mmol], and 652 mg [16.3 mmol] for human milk, cow milk, and soy milk infants, respectively) led to net calcium retention that was very similar among the three feeding types, with slightly higher values for the formula-fed infants. The bioavailability of minerals from protein hydrolysate formulas may be lower than from human milk, as indicated in studies in humans (Rigo et al., 1995) as well as in infant rhesus monkeys (Rudloff and Lonnerdal, 1990). However, since these studies were performed using a greater total intake of calcium from infant formulas compared with human milk, it is difficult to interpret the dietary bioavailability.

Numerous studies have compared whole body or regional bone mineral accretion in infants fed human milk, cow milk formula, or soy formula (Chan et al., 1987; Greer et al., 1982b; Hillman et al., 1988; Mimouni et al., 1993; Pittard et al., 1990; Specker et al., 1997; Steichen and Tsang, 1987). Results have varied, but there appears to be a greater bone mineral accretion in cow milk formula-fed infants compared with those fed human milk or soy formula. In spite of this trend, there is no evidence that this difference is beneficial or clinically significant.

No published studies indicate that increasing bone accretion using high calcium-containing formulas or cow milk during infancy leads to greater bone mineralization in later childhood or adolescence. In contrast, Bishop et al. (1996) suggested that premature infants fed human milk in early neonatal life, as opposed to cow milk formula with greater mineral content, may have greater BMC at 5 years of age. This finding is supported by a study in dogs suggesting that in forming stable bone, low calcium intakes early in life might be preferred to greater intakes (Gershoff et al., 1958). These findings need to be replicated to determine whether this effect is relevant to full-term infants. The possibility that "programming" of infants such that lower intakes and retention of calcium is beneficial to long-term mineralization is therefore possible but unproven. Further research is needed to define the risks and possible benefits of high calcium intakes during infancy.

Assuming an efficiency of calcium absorption of 38 percent from cow milk-based formula (Fomon and Nelson, 1993) with a calcium content approximately 50 percent higher than that from human milk, then a net calcium retention will be achieved that is at least comparable to that of the human milk-fed infant. Based on an average intake from human milk of 210 mg (5.3 mmol)/day, intakes of 315 mg (7.9 mmol)/day from formula should be adequate for infants 0 through 6 months of age. For infants ages 7 through 12 months, based on an average intake from human milk of 130 mg (3.2 mmol)/day, 195 mg (4.8 mmol)/day should be obtained from formula. When added to the average intake of calcium (by formula-fed infants) from solid food of 140 mg (3.5 mmol)/day, an intake of 335 mg (8.3 mmol)/day is adequate for infants ages 7 through 12 months who are fed formula and solid foods.

It is difficult to accurately estimate the calcium intake needed for infants fed the various special formulas, including soy protein-based and protein hydrolysate formulas. However, based on the data of Rigo et al. (1995) and Fomon and Nelson (1993), an additional 20 percent above the 315 mg (7.9 mmol) calculated above should be sufficient to compensate for decreased bioavailabilty from those sources. This added amount is likely to result in a net calcium retention comparable to that of infants fed formula with higher calcium concentrations.

Hypocalcemia. Hypocalcemia is a relatively common neonatal problem (Salle et al., 1990). However, this condition requires special evaluation, which is beyond the scope of an evaluation of the AI for calcium for a healthy population of infants.

Ages 1 through 3 and 4 through 8 Years

Indicators Used to Set the AI

Balance Studies. Much of the available data from balance studies of young children, which were principally conducted prior to 1960, have been compiled and reviewed (Matkovic, 1991; Matkovic and Heaney, 1992). In 2- to 8-year-old children, mean calcium intakes (± SD) of 821 ± 63 mg (20.5 ± 1.5 mmol)/day led to calcium retentions of 174 ± 81 mg (4.3 ± 2.0 mmol)/day (about 21 percent of intake).

A recent study used stable isotopes to estimate calcium retention from milk in girls 5 to 12 years of age (Abrams and Stuff, 1994). Calcium intake based on 3-day dietary records was 907 ± 188 mg (22.7 ± 4.7 mmol)/day, urinary calcium excretion was 78 ± 48 mg (2.0 ± 1.2 mmol)/day, and mean absorption fraction was 28 ± 8 percent. Using estimated values for endogenous fecal calcium excretion of 1.4 ± 0.4 mg/kg/day (Abrams et al., 1991), their calculated calcium retention was 130 mg (3.3 mmol)/day, a value somewhat lower than the 174 mg (4.3 mmol)/day obtained in the meta-analyses cited above (Matkovic, 1991; Matkovic and Heaney, 1992).

Although calcium balance with varying levels of intake is possibly a more useful method, few investigators have estimated it in children. Calcium retention averaged 76 mg (1.9 mmol)/day in five girls aged 3 to 5 years when the girls had an intake of 370 mg (9.3 mmol)/day for 8 weeks and increased to an average of 122 mg (3.0 mmol)/day when the girls consumed 615 mg (15.4 mmol)/day for the next 5 weeks (Outhouse et al., 1939). Calcium intakes of about 200 to 280 mg (5 to 7 mmol)/day in children from India resulted in absorption rates of approximately 50 percent of the calcium while maintaining a small positive balance of 50 to 60 mg (1.3 to 1.5 mmol)/day (Begum and Pereira, 1969).

Calcium Accretion. The few studies of usual calcium accretion rates in small children give generally comparable results to that derived from balance studies. Calcium accretion rate was estimated from body weight values during childhood and adolescence (Leitch and Aitken, 1959). Although the method was not independently validated, there is a very close correlation between BMC and body weight in small children (Ellis et al., 1996). Calcium accretion on the order of 60 to 100 mg (1.5 to 2.5 mmol)/day by boys and girls aged 2 to 5 years and 100 to 160 mg (2.5 to 4.0 mmol)/day by boys and girls aged 6 to 8 years was calculated.

Bone Mineral Content. Recently, total body BMC by DXA was used to calculate average mineral increments in a population of approximately 100 children aged 3 to 10 years (Ellis et al., 1997). The rate of accretion in Caucasian ($n = 46$) and Hispanic ($n = 23$) children increased from approximately 150 mg (3.8 mmol)/day of calcium at age 5 to approximately 200 mg (5 mmol)/day at age 8. Values for African Americans ($n = 36$) were approximately 20 to 30 mg (0.5 to 0.8 mmol)/day greater at each age.

Intervention trials in which children were randomized to different calcium intakes have resulted in short-term changes in BMC. In one of the few intervention trials conducted in young children, 22 prepubertal identical twin pairs averaging 7 years of age were randomized to receive either calcium supplements or placebo (Johnston et al., 1992). Those receiving supplements had an increase in their mean intake from approximately 900 to 1,600 mg (22.5 to 40 mmol)/day which resulted in a significant increase in BMD in the radius and lumbar spine after 36 months of treatment compared to the control twins. However, the increase in BMD was not sustained in a long-term follow-up study when those receiving supplements returned to their normal diets (Slemenda et al., 1997).

In another intervention study, 162 Chinese children who were 7 years of age with low daily calcium intakes (average 280 mg [7 mmol]) were randomly assigned to receive 300 mg (7.5 mmol)/day of a calcium supplement or placebo (Lee et al., 1994). After 18 months, the supplemented group had a significantly greater gain in BMC at the midshaft radius. In a follow-up study for another 18 months, the benefits of calcium supplementation disappeared after the supplements were withdrawn (Lee et al., 1996). In a similar study, greater increases in lumbar spine BMC were seen in 7-year-old children from Hong Kong with average calcium intakes of 570 mg (14.3 mmol)/day who were randomized to receive 300 mg (7.5 mmol)/day supplement compared with those who received a placebo (Lee et al., 1995).

Taken together, the above studies suggest that further evidence is needed regarding the length of time and level of supplementation necessary before a precise requirement value can be based on supplementation data in prepubertal children. There are no long-term studies in which the effects of supplemental calcium given to children prior to age 9 have been evaluated during adulthood.

AI Summary: Ages 1 through 3 and 4 through 8 Years

For females aged 1 through 8 years, calcium accretion in the range of 60 to 200 mg (1.5 to 5 mmol)/day has been predicted from both indirect estimates based on body weight (Leitch and Aitken, 1959) and direct estimates of bone mineral content using DXA (Ellis et al., 1997). The precise calcium intake needed to achieve such calcium accretion cannot be obtained from available data. From balance studies in the older age group, a calcium intake of 800 to 900 mg (20 to 22.5 mmol)/day would result in mean calcium retention up to 174 mg/day. Thus, for the 4- through 8-year-old age group, the AI for calcium is 800 mg (20 mmol)/day. As there are no balance studies available in boys, the data for girls has to be applied to both sexes.

The primary balance data described above for 4- through 8 year olds do not include adequate data applicable to younger children in the second and third years of life. Therefore, AIs for this period must be estimated from data for other age groups. Net accretion appears to be approximately 100 mg (2.5 mmol)/day during this life stage (Leitch and Aitken, 1959). Therefore, using an estimate of 20 percent net calcium retention in children based on the data from 4 through 8 year olds (Matkovic, 1991; Matkovic and Heaney, 1992), it is reasonable to set the AI for calcium at 500 mg (12.5 mmol)/day intake to achieve the 100 mg (2.5 mmol)/day retention. For this age group, there is a substantial need for further investigation using both balance techniques and bone densitometry to more precisely estimate calcium needs.

AI for Children   **1 through 3 years**   **500 mg (12.5 mmol)/day**
                                   4 through 8 years   **800 mg (20.0 mmol)/day**

Utilizing the 1994 CSFII data, adjusted for day-to-day variation (Nusser et al., 1996), the median calcium intake is 766 (19.2 mmol)/day for children aged 1 through 3 years (see Appendix D). Their AI of 500 mg (12.5 mmol)/day will fall between the tenth percentile (468 mg [11.7 mmol]/day) and the twenty-fifth percentile of calcium intake (599 mg [15 mmol]/day). For children aged 4 through 8 years, the median calcium intake is 808 mg (20.2 mmol)/day, which is very close to the AI of 800 mg (20 mmol)/day for this age group.

Special Considerations

Chronic Illness. Many chronic illnesses that affect children are associated with abnormalities of calcium metabolism and bone mineralization. Among the most significant of these are juvenile rheumatologic conditions (Reed et al., 1990), renal disease (Stapleton, 1994), liver failure (Bucuvalas et al., 1990), and endocrine disturbances, including insulin-dependent diabetes mellitus (Favus and Christakos, 1996). The value of adjustments in calcium intake for children with these conditions is beyond the scope of this report.

Ages 9 through 13 and 14 through 18 Years

Sexual Maturity

From 9 through 18 years of age, calcium retention increases to a peak and then declines. The peak calcium accretion rate typically occurs at mean age 13 years for girls and 14.5 years for boys (Martin et al., 1997). After menarche, calcium retention in girls declines rapidly (Weaver et al., 1995) as does bone formation and bone resorption (Abrams et al., 1996b; Wastney et al., 1996). Even though bone formation and resorption decrease exponentially after menarche, calcium intakes required to achieve desirable retention do not necessarily fall because calcium absorption efficiency decreases. This menarcheal change in absorption was not observed in African American girls (Abrams and Stuff, 1994). Measures of sexual maturity are better predictors of calcium retention than is chronological age during this developmental period.

In a cross-sectional evaluation in 136 males and 130 females aged 4 to 27 years, BMD of total body, lumbar spine, and femoral neck increased significantly with age until 17.5 years in males and 15.8 years in females (Lu et al., 1994). The later timing of peak BMD in boys may relate in part to the fact that BMD is more strongly correlated with weight than with age (Ponder et al., 1990; Teegarden et al., 1995).

Indicators Used to Set the AI

Calcium Retention. The desirable level of calcium retention for children in this age group was based upon new information on whole body bone mineral accretion for 228 children followed over 4 years between the ages of 9 and 19 years (Martin et al., 1997). The average peak velocity of bone mineral content which occurs between the ages 9.5 to 19.5 years was 320 g/year in boys and 240 g/year in girls. Using the assumption that bone mineral is 32.3 percent calcium, these values correspond to a daily calcium retention of 282 mg (7.1 mmol) in boys and 212 mg (5.3 mmol) in girls. One limitation of these data is that they do not provide information as to whether peak bone mineral accretion would be greater at higher calcium intakes than that consumed by the children studied; the mean intake for boys was 1,045 mg (26 mmol)/day at ages 10 to 12 years and 1,299 mg (32.5 mmol)/day at ages 13 to 15 years while for girls it was 903 mg (22.5 mmol)/day at 10 to 12 years and 954 mg (23.8 mmol)/day at ages 13 to 15 years (Martin et al., 1997). However, because the intakes of the children in the study were based on 24-hour recall data over 4 years, they are subject to under-reporting as previously observed (Livingstone et al., 1992), so actual intakes may have been higher.

In order to derive an estimate of calcium intake which would allow for the level of accretion of calcium in bone as derived above, a model for describing the relationship between calcium intake and retention was adopted. It had been applied to one set of calcium balance studies in girls (Jackman et al., 1997) (the method is described in detail in Appendix E).

The majority of the balance studies to which the model was applied are for girls aged 11 through 14 years, and all data are from Caucasians. For this report the nonlinear regression equation was derived by combining the optimally designed calcium balance studies of Jackman et al. (1997), Matkovic et al. (1990), and Greger et al. (1978) which represented 80 children aged 12 through 15 years. The measurements were made over the last 2 weeks of a 3-week balance study in girls consuming calcium intakes of 823 to 2,164 mg (20.6 to 54.1 mmol)/day. The retention of calcium was not corrected for sweat or skins losses of calcium in these studies.

The non-linear regression equation was solved to determine the calcium intake required to achieve a desirable retention of calcium of 282 mg (7.1 mmol)/day for boys and 212 mg (5.3 mmol)/day for girls based on peak whole body bone mineral accretion during adolescence (Figure E-1). The value used for sweat losses of 55 mg (1.4 mmol)/day (Peacock, 1991) was added to the desired retention value since these losses had not been accounted for in the calcium retention studies. The estimate of calcium intake that would result in a desirable level of retention was 1,070 mg (26.8 mmol)/day for females and 1,310 mg (32.8 mmol)/day for males. At this time there are insufficient data to subdivide the age range of 9 through 18 years for either bone mineral accretion or balance measures.

The approach used in this review results in a value which is midway between two other estimates of the calcium intake necessary to achieve a plateau balance. In applying a two-component split, linear regression model to balance studies published between 1922 and 1992, Matkovic and Heaney (1992) identified a plateau calcium intake of approximately 1,480 mg (37 mmol)/day during growth. Using the nonlinear regression model (Jackman et al., 1997) on the same data set of reported balances as was used by Matkovic and Heaney (1992) resulted in a lower plateau estimate of 820 mg (20.5 mmol)/day of calcium. It should be noted that included in this historical data set were balances which were measured in children who were not yet equilibrated to the study intake. For the analysis conducted for this report, data were included from published studies only if an adaptation period of at least 2 weeks had occurred before the balance period. Thus, the current recommendation is thought to be a more rigorous analysis of the data available.

Clinical Trials Measuring Bone Mineral Content. Several randomized trials have been conducted in children through adolescence which provide evidence that increasing dietary intakes of calcium of girls above their habitual intake of about 900 mg (22.5 mmol)/day is associated with positive effects on bone mineral accretion, especially during the pre-pubertal stage (Table 4-2). In the Lloyd et al. (1993) study, girls with a mean age of 11.9 years were supplemented (total daily intake of 1,370 ± 303 mg [34.2 ± 7.6 mmol]) and compared with a placebo group (total daily intake 935 ± 258 mg [23.4 ± 6.4 mmol]). After 18 months of supplementation, the girls had greater increases in lumbar spine BMD (18.7 versus 15.8 percent), lumbar spine BMC (39.4 versus 34.7 percent), and total body BMD (9.6 versus 8.3 percent). In the Chan et al. (1995) study, the girls (mean age 11 years) supplemented for 12 months (total daily intake 1,437 ± 366 mg [35.9 ± 9.2 mmol]) had significantly greater increases in lumbar spine BMD (22.8 ± 6.9 versus 12.9 ± 8.3 percent) and total body BMC (14.2 ± 7.0 versus 7.6 ± 6.0 percent) than control subjects (total daily intake 728 ± 321 mg [18.2 ± 8.0 mmol]). In a third study (Johnston et al., 1992), identical twins, aged 6 to 14 years, were given a supplement (total daily intake approximately 1,600 mg [40 mmol]) or a placebo (daily intake 900 mg [22.5 mmol]). When examined by pubertal status, the prepubertal twins (22 pairs) had a greater bone response to calcium supplementation than did the pubertal twins (23 pairs). The pubertal subjects in this study showed no significant effect of supplementation, unlike the pubertal girls in both the Lloyd et al. (1993) and Chan et al. (1995) studies.

Mounting evidence from randomized clinical trials suggests that the bone mass gained during childhood and adolescence through calcium or milk supplementation is not retained postintervention (Fehily et al., 1992; Lee et al., 1996; Slemenda et al., 1997). Upon cessation of the intervention, the component of calcium's effect due to reduction of the remodeling space disappears, as the space expands again. Further research is required to determine the long-term effects of higher calcium intakes during adolescence and the specific effect of calcium intake on bone modeling and achievement of genetically programmed peak bone mass.

Factorial Approach. For children ages 9 through 18 a more traditional factorial approach for estimating calcium requirements is to sum calcium needs for growth (accretion) plus calcium losses (urine, feces, and sweat) and adjust for absorption. Using this method, estimates for calcium requirements for adolescent girls and boys are 1,276 and 1,505 mg (31.9 and 37.6 mmol)/day, respectively (Table 4-3). Calcium accretion estimates, based on whole body bone mineral mass measurements by DXA, were obtained from a 4-year prospective study in 228 children aged 9.5 to 19.5 years (Mar-

TABLE 4-2 Differences in Mean Changes in Bone Mineral Content and Bone Mineral Density in Calcium Treated vs. Placebo Groups in Randomized, Controlled Trials in Adolescents

Source	No.	Age (y)	Sex	Length Study (mo)	Calcium Intake Controls (mg/day)	Calcium Intake Treatment (mg/day)	Site	Group Mean Differences BMC (g)	Change in BMD (%)
Chan et al., 1995	48	9–13	female	12	728	1,437	Total body	35.52	
Johnston et al., 1992	140	6–14	female and male	36	908	1,612	Midshaft radius		2.5
							Distal radius		3.3
							Lumbar spine		0.7
							Femoral neck		0.4
							Ward's triangle		1.2
							Greater trochanter		1.8
Lloyd et al., 1993	94	11.9 ± 0.5	female	18	960	1,314	Total body	13.32	

TABLE 4-3 Factorial Approach for Determining Calcium Requirements During Peak Calcium Accretion in White Adolescents

	Number of Observations	Females (mg/day)	Number of Observations	Males (mg/day)
Peak calcium accretion	507	212[a]	471	282[a]
Urinary losses	28	106[b]	14	127[c]
Endogenous fecal calcium	14	112[d]	3	108[e]
Sweat losses		55[f]		55[f]
Total		485		572
Absorption, percent	14	38[d]	14	38[d]
As adjusted for absorption		1,276		1,505

[a] Martin et al., 1997, using peak bone mineral content velocity.
[b] Weaver et al., 1995 and Greger et al., 1978.
[c] Matkovic, 1991.
[d] Wastney et al., 1996 for mean age 13 years on calcium intakes of 1,330 mg/day.
[e] Abrams et al., 1992.
[f] Taken from Peacock (1991) who adjusted the adult data of Charles et al. (1983) for body weight.

tin et al., 1997). The mean fractional absorption value of 38 percent was based on a study of girls, aged 13 ± 1 years, who consumed an average of 1,330 mg (33.3 mmol)/day of calcium (Wastney et al., 1996). It is unknown whether there are gender differences in absorption in this age range. The values for endogenous excretion and absorption in males in Table 4-3 are based on very few data points, and the values for sweat losses are extrapolated from adult data. Variability about these estimates is large. The values derived from the factorial approach are slightly higher than those obtained using the calcium retention model, but fall within the range of these values and those derived from the clinical trials described above. Because of the extrapolation of values from studies in girls to boys and from adults used in this approach, it was deemed inappropriate to use these values as a basis for an EAR.

Epidemiological Evidence. Several cross-sectional studies have identified a positive association between calcium consumption and bone density in children (Chan, 1991; Ruiz et al., 1995; Sentipal et al., 1991), whereas others have found no such association (Grimston et al., 1992; Katzman et al., 1991; Kröger et al., 1992, 1993). The studies showing the positive association tended to include a significant proportion of study subjects with low calcium intakes. A study of French children (Ruiz et al., 1995) found that 93 percent of the children with low vertebral BMD and 84 percent of those with low femoral neck BMD had dietary calcium intakes below 1,000 mg (25 mmol)/day; the investigators concluded that dietary calcium requirements for prepubertal and pubertal children were above 1,000 mg (25 mmol)/day.

Several retrospective studies suggest that higher calcium intakes in childhood are associated with greater bone mass in adulthood (Halioua and Anderson, 1989; Matkovic et al., 1994; Nieves et al., 1995; Sandler et al., 1985). As it appears now, and pending further research in this area, higher calcium intakes likely need to be maintained throughout growth in order to produce a higher peak bone mass.

AI Summary: Ages 9 through 13 and 14 through 18 Years

The three major lines of evidence for calcium needs in this age group—the factorial approach, calcium retention to meet peak bone mineral accretion, and clinical trials in which bone mineral content was measured in response to variable calcium intakes—provide estimates of calcium intake in the range of 1,100 to 1,600 mg (27.5 to 40 mmol)/day to attain a desirable level of calcium retention. Most of the data are based on balance studies and clinical intervention trials in girls. Thus, it is important to note that the value of peak bone mineral accretion for boys had to be used in the equation derived from balance studies in girls due to lack of data on boys. Given the extrapolation to boys for the balance data, the clinical trials being conducted primarily in girls, and the lack of data on bone mineral accretion at higher calcium intakes than that reported by Martin et al. (1997), it was inappropriate to establish a gender-specific AI for this age group. In considering collectively the evidence above, an AI of 1,300 mg (32.5 mmol)/day was judged as a reasonable goal for calcium intake for both boys and girls in this age group. Too few data exist in males to allow a gender difference to be established or to recommend different intakes within the age range.

AI for Boys	**9 through 13 years**	**1,300 mg (32.5 mmol)/day**
	14 through 18 years	**1,300 mg (32.5 mmol)/day**
AI for Girls	**9 through 13 years**	**1,300 mg (32.5 mmol)/day**
	14 through 18 years	**1,300 mg (32.5 mmol)/day**

Utilizing the 1994 CFSII data, adjusted for day-to-day variation

(Nusser et al., 1996), the median calcium intake for boys aged 9 through 13 is 980 mg (24.5 mmol)/day, the seventy-fifth percentile of intake is 1,245 mg (31.1 mmol)/day and the ninetieth percentile of intake is 1,520 mg (38 mmol)/day (see Appendix D). Thus, the AI for boys ages 9 through 13 years of 1,300 mg (32.5 mmol)/day is slightly above the seventy-fifth percentile of calcium intake. For girls in this age range, the median calcium intake is 889 mg (22.2 mmol)/day, and the ninetieth percentile of intake is 1,313 mg (32.8 mmol)/day. Thus, the AI for girls ages 9 through 13 years of 1,300 mg (32.5 mmol)/day, is slightly below the ninetieth percentile of calcium intake based on the 1994 CSFII data.

For boys aged 14 through 18 years, the median calcium intake is 1,094 mg (27.4 mmol)/day, and the seventy-fifth percentile is 1,422 mg (35.6 mmol)/day. Thus, for boys ages 14 through 18 years, the AI for calcium of 1,300 mg (32.5 mmol)/day would fall between the median and seventy-fifth percentiles of intake. For girls in this age range, the median calcium intake was 713 mg (17.8 mmol)/day, and the ninetieth percentile was 1,293 mg (32.3 mmol)/day. Thus, for girls ages 14 through 18 years, the AI for calcium of 1,300 mg (32.5 mmol)/day would be close to the ninety-fifth percentile of intake based on the 1994 CSFII data.

Ages 19 through 30 Years

Peak Bone Mass

During the age span of 19 through 30 years, peak bone mass is achieved. Growth of long bones has ceased, but consolidation of bone mass continues. The age at which peak mass is achieved appears to vary with the skeletal site. Using single measures of BMC by DXA on 247 females aged 11 to 32 years, 92 percent of the total body bone mass observed was present by age 17.9 years and 99 percent by age 26.2 years (Teegarden et al., 1995). In a cross-sectional study of 265 Caucasian females, only a 4 percent additional increase in total skeletal mass from age 18 to 50 years was reported (Matkovic et al., 1994). In a longitudinal study (with up to 5-year follow-up) of 156 women aged 18.5 to 26 years at entry and with a mean daily calcium intake from food and supplements of 786 mg (19.7 mmol), total body BMC increased by an average of 1.2 percent per year during the third decade of life, although within that age decade, the rate of gain slowed with age (Recker et al., 1992).

With regard to individual skeletal sites, no difference in subjects'

BMC at several sites was detected after the age of 18 except for the skull, which continued to gain mass (Matkovic et al., 1994). In a longitudinal study (Recker et al., 1992), lumbar BMC increased by a median gain of 5.9 percent, and the forearm increased by 4.8 percent during the third decade of life. In a smaller study of 45 females aged 9 to 21 years, BMC of the whole body, spine, and femoral neck plateaued at age 16 years (Katzman et al., 1991). Bone density of the hip decreased after age 17 years (Matkovic et al., 1994; Theintz et al., 1992). In summary, the age of peak bone mass appears to vary with skeletal site and sex. Nevertheless, taken all together, the data indicate that the skeleton continues to accrete mass for approximately 10 years after adult stature is achieved.

Indicators Used to Set the AI

Calcium Retention. A desirable level of calcium retention (the level of positive calcium balance) for the 19- to 30-year age group was set as the retention of calcium equivalent to the reported calcium accretion derived from studies of bone mineral accretion during the third decade (Peacock, 1991). The limitation of these data is that they were derived from metacarpal morphometry data (Garn, 1972). To date, there are no data on whole body bone mineral accretion using DXA technology nor for groups of subjects consuming variable amounts of dietary calcium. The accretion of calcium based on these data was 10 mg (0.25 mmol)/day for females and 50 mg (1.3 mmol)/day for males. This large discrepancy in calcium accretion between genders may reflect the older age at which males achieve peak bone mineral content velocity (Martin et al., 1997) or inaccuracies in the older bone densitometry methods.

The relationship between calcium intake and retention for this age group was computed from a compilation of balance studies in 163 young adults (26 males and 137 females), aged 18 to 30 years, from the literature between 1922 and 1992 as compiled by Matkovic and Heaney (1992). The non-linear regression approach of Jackman et al. (1997) was applied to these data (Appendix E) and the regression equation solved to determine the calcium intake at which a desirable daily calcium retention of 50 mg (1.3 mmol)/day for males and 10 mg (0.3 mmol)/day for females could be achieved. A value for sweat losses of 63 mg (1.6 mmol)/day (Charles et al., 1983) was added to the level of desired retention since these losses had not been corrected for in the calcium balance studies. The estimated calcium intake at which a desirable retention would be

TABLE 4-4 Factorial Approach for Determining Calcium
Requirements in Adults Aged 19 through 30 Years

	Females (mg/day)	Males (mg/day)
Peak calcium accretion	10^a	50^a
Urinary losses	203^b	162^e
Endogenous fecal calcium	132^b	156^f
Sweat losses	63^c	63^c
Total	408	431
Absorption, percent	30^d	30^d
As adjusted for absorption	1,360	1,437

a Taken from calculations by Peacock (1991) based on metacarpal morphometry
data of Garn (1972).
b Wastney et al. (1996).
c Charles et al. (1983).
d Heaney et al. (1988).
e Matkovic (1991).
f Heaney and Skillman (1964).

achieved was 1,026 mg (25.6 mmol)/day for females and 1,236 mg
(30.9 mmol)/day for males (Figure E-2).

Using the same database with data from men and women combined to determine the plateau intake using the two-component
split, linear-regression model of Matkovic and Heaney (1992), the
plateau retention of calcium was reached at an intake of 957 mg
(23.9 mmol)/day.

Factorial Approach. The factorial approach for estimating calcium
requirements for young adults is given in Table 4-4. This approach
gives higher daily estimates of requirements (1,360 mg [34 mmol]
for females and 1,437 mg [35.9 mmol] for males) than the desirable calcium retention approach (see above). The differences in
derived values for calcium intake may be a result of the correction
for endogenous fecal calcium applied in the factorial method which
is based on only one recent study (Wastney et al., 1996) and/or the
fact that a 30 percent absorption factor was applied. For the latter,
the absorption value is taken from a derivative report which included multiple study designs on 16 women and 6 men (Heaney et al.,
1988), and thus represents the average of all the subjects. Given
the variety of study designs, it isn't possible to apply the gender-
specific data.

AI Summary: Ages 19 through 30 Years

For this age group, estimates of average calcium requirements were hindered because of no reported randomized clinical trials testing multiple intakes of calcium, the lack of data on whole body bone mineral accretion, and the uncertainties in the values for endogenous fecal and sweat losses of calcium used in the factorial model. Thus, the estimate for the AI relies on using available calcium balance studies to determine intakes at which small gains in bone mineral content can be achieved. Because of the uncertainties related to the five-fold difference in estimated bone calcium accretion between genders during this time period, and the fact that the balance data are predominantly from women, the estimate of calcium intake from the calcium retention analysis for women was adopted for both genders. The estimate of an AI of 1,000 mg (25 mmol)/day was judged to be appropriate for this age group.

Based on desirable calcium retention data and with consideration of the estimates of calcium need from various methods, the AI requirement for both men and women ages 19 through 30 years is set at 1,000 mg (25 mmol)/day.

AI for Men   **19 through 30 years**   **1,000 mg (25 mmol)/day**
AI for Women **19 through 30 years**   **1,000 mg (25 mmol)/day**

Adjusting the 1994 CSFII data for day-to-day variation (Nusser et al., 1996), the median calcium intake for men aged 19 through 30 years is 954 mg (23.9 mmol)/day (see Appendix D), which is fairly close to the AI of 1,000 mg (25 mmol)/day for this age group. For women in this age range, the median calcium intake is 612 mg (15.3 mmol)/day, while the ninetieth percentile of intake is 985 mg (24.6 mmol)/day. Thus, an AI of 1,000 mg (25 mmol)/day is slightly above the ninetieth percentile of calcium intake based on the 1994 CSFII data.

Ages 31 through 50 Years

Indicators Used to Set the AI

Calcium Retention. For this age group, as for the others, balance studies were examined to identify the intake associated with a desirable calcium retention—the plateau intake, that at which there is no net loss of calcium. Two balance studies are available that examined estrogen-replete women on their usual calcium intakes (Heaney et al., 1978; Ohlson et al., 1952). Calcium balance was estimated in 25 women aged 30 to 39, with a mean calcium intake of 950 ± 300 mg (23.7 ± 7.5 mmol)/day and 34 women aged 40 to

49, with a mean intake of 840 ± 292 mg (21 ± 7.3 mmol)/day (Ohlson et al., 1952). In each age group, calcium intake and balance were positively correlated ($r = 0.43$ and $r = 0.44$). Only six women in the younger group and eight in the older group consumed more than 1,000 mg (25 mmol)/day. In the second study (Heaney et al., 1978) of 130 premenopausal women, aged 35 to 50 with a mean calcium intake of 661 ± 328 mg (16.5 ± 8.2 mmol)/day, calcium intake and balance were positively correlated ($r = 0.26$). This study included very few women with intakes over 1,000 mg (25 mmol)/day. From these data, it is apparent that the plateau intake is not below 1,000 mg (25 mmol)/day. However, the intake associated with a desirable retention so that no net loss will occur cannot be identified without additional balance studies in women with calcium intakes greater than 1,000 mg (25 mmol)/day. Available balance data from a large study in men (Spencer et al., 1984), with the wide age range of 34 to 71 years will be considered under the age group of 51 through 70 years.

Bone Mineral Density. The two available intervention trials in women in this age range (Baran et al., 1990; Elders et al., 1994) support a plateau intake at or above 1,000 mg (25 mmol)/day. In 37 premenopausal women aged 30 to 42 years randomly assigned to either their usual calcium intakes of 810 ± 367 mg (20.5 ± 9.2 mmol)/day or increased dairy product consumption to a total intake of 1,572 ± 920 mg (39.3 ± 24 mmol)/day, the group consuming extra dairy products had significantly reduced vertebral BMD loss over 3 years (Baran et al., 1990). Similarly, calcium supplementation of 1,000 and 2,000 mg (25 and 50 mmol)/day in premenopausal women aged 46 and older with a usual mean calcium intake of 1,100 mg (27.5 mmol)/day significantly reduced vertebral bone loss (Elders et al., 1994). In this study, the higher total intake (3,100 mg [77.5 mmol]/day) was no more effective than the 2,100 mg (52.5 mmol)/day intake.

Factorial Approach. If the needs for calcium accretion that are described for the young adults aged 19 through 30 years are removed from Table 4-4, the AIs based on a factorial approach would be 1,360 mg (34 mmol)/day and 1,270 mg (31.7 mmol)/day for females and males, respectively. Endogenous fecal calcium losses for 191 women aged 35 to 59 years averaged 102 ± 25 mg (2.6 ± 0.6 mmol)/day (Heaney and Recker, 1994), which if substituted in Table 4-4 would not appreciably reduce the net total calcium need. As indicated earlier, these values must be considered in light of the uncertainty of the values used for endogenous and sweat losses as well as efficiency of absorption.

AI Summary: Ages 31 through 50 Years

Based on available data from balance studies and BMD, the AI is placed at 1,000 mg (25 mmol)/day. Too few data for men are available to justify a separate AI for them.

AI for Men	**31 through 50 years**	**1,000 mg (25 mmol)/day**
AI for Women	**31 through 50 years**	**1,000 mg (25 mmol)/day**

Using the 1994 CSFII intake data, adjusted for day-to-day variation (Nusser et al., 1996), the median calcium intake for men, aged 31 through 50 years, is 857 mg (21.4 mmol)/day and their seventy-fifth percentile of intake is 1,112 mg (27.8 mmol)/day (see Appendix D). Their AI of 1,000 mg (25 mmol)/day falls between the median and seventy-fifth percentile of calcium intake. Median calcium intake for women in this age range is 606 mg (15.2 mmol)/day; their ninetieth percentile of intake is 961 mg (24 mmol)/day and their ninety-fifth percentile is 1,082 mg (27.1 mmol)/day. Thus, their AI of 1,000 mg (25 mmol)/day falls between the ninetieth and ninety-fifth percentile of calcium intake based on the 1994 CSFII data.

Ages 51 through 70 Years

Indicators Used to Set the AI for Men

Calcium Retention. Desirable retention of calcium in men aged 51 through 70 years is zero which assumes that no net positive accretion of bone at this age in replete individuals serves a functional advantage. The relationship between calcium intake and calcium retention was determined from 181 balance studies conducted in ambulatory males of mean age 54 years (range 34 to 71 years) (Spencer et al., 1984). The subjects could not be divided into different age categories based on the data reported. Six different calcium intake levels ranging from 234 to 2,320 mg (5.8 to 58 mmol)/day were studied. The distribution of intakes in the 181 balance studies were: 111 balance studies in subjects with daily calcium intakes below 1,200 mg (30 mmol), 22 at approximately 1,200 mg, and 48 at intakes above 1,200 mg. The nonlinear regression equation derived from these data (Appendix E) was solved for a desirable retention of zero balance plus 63 mg (1.6 mmol)/day of sweat loss (Charles et al., 1983) since the balance studies were not corrected for sweat losses. The estimated calcium intake at which this level of retention would be achieved is 995 mg (23.9 mmol)/day (Figure E-3). Thus, based on balance studies in men, a calcium intake to achieve the desired zero calcium retention is about 1,000 mg (25 mmol)/day.

Other investigators have contributed balance data in men. In long-term studies, Malm (1958) assessed balance in 39 men who had calcium intakes of 460 and 940 mg (11.5 and 23.5 mmol)/day. Balance was positively associated with calcium intake, but too few men were studied at high-enough calcium intakes to identify a plateau balance level. Although small sample sizes limit their usefulness in this context, older balance studies in males (Ackerman and Toro, 1953; Bogdonoff et al., 1953; Outhouse et al., 1941; Schwartz et al., 1964) indicate that a plateau retention of calcium would be achieved with a calcium intake of 1,000 to 1,200 mg (25 to 30 mmol)/day, which is similar to that derived using the desirable retention model based on the data of Spencer et al. (1984).

Bone Mineral Density. Only one randomized, controlled, calcium intervention study in men has been reported (Orwoll et al., 1990). In this 3-year study of 77 men aged 30 to 87 years (mean age 58 years) with a mean usual dietary calcium intake of 1,160 (29 mmol)/day, supplementation with an additional 1,000 mg (25 mmol)/day of calcium and 10 µg (400 IU) of vitamin D did not significantly reduce spinal or forearm bone loss. This finding, that increasing calcium intake above a mean intake of about 1,200 mg (30 mmol)/day did not reduce bone loss further, suggests that intakes less than or equal to 1,200 mg (30 mmol)/day are adequate to maximize maintenance of bone mass in this age group.

Indicators Used to Set the AI for Women

Calcium Retention. Women have been more widely studied regarding calcium retention because they are particularly prone to osteoporosis. Several balance studies are reported in postmenopausal women with mean calcium intakes under 1,000 mg (25 mmol)/day. In 61 women with varying degrees of osteoporosis and with calcium intakes ranging from 200 to 1,000 mg (5 to 25 mmol)/day, a positive linear correlation between calcium intake and balance was noted, and was similar in women with or without vertebral fractures

(Marshall et al., 1976). Calcium balance and usual calcium intake were positively correlated in 41 estrogen-deprived postmenopausal women with a mean usual calcium intake of 659 296 mg (16.5 ± 7.4 mmol)/day (Heaney and Recker, 1982; Heaney et al., 1977). In 76 women aged 50 to 85 years balance became more positive as calcium intake increased from 650 to 830 mg (16.2 to 20.7 mmol)/day (Ohlson et al., 1952). Only 10 women in that study had self-selected dietary calcium intakes over 1,000 mg (25 mmol)/day. Collectively, these studies consistently demonstrate that postmenopausal women with dietary calcium intakes under 1,000 mg (25 mmol)/day have less calcium loss when they increase their calcium intake.

Only two balance studies in postmenopausal women with average usual calcium intakes higher than 1,000 mg (25 mmol)/day were identified. Balance studies performed in 85 women with vertebral osteoporosis, aged 48 to 77 years, on a mean self-selected calcium intake of 1,116 mg (27.9 mmol)/day showed generally improved calcium balance in those subjects with higher calcium intakes (Hasling et al., 1990); very few subjects in this study had calcium intakes above 1,500 mg (37.5 mmol)/day. Calcium balance in 18 women and 7 men with osteoporosis (aged 26 to 70, mean 53 years) who consumed an average of 1,214 mg (30.3 mmol)/day of calcium was higher in those with higher calcium intakes (Selby, 1994). Notably, the men and women appeared to fit along the same regression line when intake was related to balance.

Several conclusions can be drawn from these balance studies. First, it is difficult to determine if the calcium intake needed for men over age 50 to minimize calcium loss is below 1,200 mg (30 mmol)/day as few studies have been done with intakes between 800 and 1,200 mg (20 and 30 mmol)/day. Second, available balance data indicate that the intake requirement of women over age 50 is at least 1,000 mg (25 mmol)/day and no evidence indicates that it differs substantially from that of similarly aged men. Finally, there are too few balance data at high calcium intakes to allow examination of subgroups, such as women in early menopause or subjects with and without fractures.

Bone Mineral Density. Many randomized, controlled, calcium intervention trials have been conducted in postmenopausal women. Several investigators have studied women within the first 5 years of menopause (designated as early postmenopausal), the period of most rapid bone loss (Aloia et al., 1994; Dawson-Hughes et al., 1990; Elders et al., 1991; Prince et al., 1995; Riis et al., 1987). Others have studied older or late postmenopausal women (Chevalley et al., 1994;

Dawson-Hughes et al., 1990; Reid et al., 1995). The main results of these studies are shown in Table 4-1. These studies reveal that the effectiveness of calcium varies by skeletal site, by menopausal age, and with the usual calcium intakes of the study subjects. Apart from the initial bone remodeling transient in year 1, added calcium offers little benefit in BMD at the spine. In contrast, calcium generally has more impact on BMD at the more cortical-rich proximal radius, femoral neck, and total body. Late postmenopausal women tend to be more responsive to supplemental calcium than early postmenopausal women. In addition, late postmenopausal women with very low calcium intakes generally gain more from calcium supplementation than do women with higher usual calcium intakes (Dawson-Hughes et al., 1990, Elders et al., 1994).

The positive impact of supplemental calcium on BMD in women with low-to-moderate usual mean calcium intakes is generally consistent with the observation that increasing calcium intake improves calcium balance. Trials involving women with the highest usual calcium intakes are more useful in this context, and they demonstrate that increasing calcium intake above 750 mg (18.7 mmol) (Reid et al., 1995), 800 mg (20 mmol) (Prince et al., 1995), or 1,000 mg (25 mmol) (Riis et al., 1987) reduces loss of bone mineral from cortical-rich skeletal sites. Since 80 percent of the skeleton is comprised of cortical bone, one would expect changes in cortical bone to parallel balance changes. Trials in women with even higher usual calcium intakes are needed to test the balance study estimate of 1,200 mg (30 mmol)/day.

AI Summary: Ages 51 through 70 years

The AI for men and women ages 51 through 70 is set at 1,200 mg (30 mmol)/day based primarily on the clinical trial data in women which demonstrated a positive reduction of bone loss with calcium intakes over 1,000 mg (25 mmol)/day. In addition, balance studies in women (Hasling et al., 1990) and women and men (Selby, 1994), showed that calcium intakes up to 1,500 mg (37.5 mmol)/day (mean intakes of 1,116 mg [27.9 mmol]/day and 1,214 mg [30.4 mmol]/day, for the cited studies, respectively), were associated with higher calcium retention. Although a value of about 1,000 mg (25 mmol)/day was derived from the calcium retention model using balance studies in men, there were no data for calcium intakes between 800 and 1,200 mg (20 and 30 mmol)/day. For the reported balance studies in women, a plateau calcium retention value could not be derived. The AI of 1,200 mg (30 mmol)/day was chosen for this age group assuming that their needs would be somewhat higher that the 19- through 30-year age group since calcium absorption is known to fall with advancing age.

AI for Men   **51 through 70 years**   **1,200 mg (30 mmol)/day**
AI for Women   **51 through 70 years**   **1,200 mg (30 mmol)/day**

Utilizing the 1994 CSFII data, adjusted for day-to-day variation (Nusser et al., 1996), the median intake for men aged 51 through 70 years is 708 mg (17.7 mmol)/day (see Appendix D). Their AI of 1,200 mg (30 mmol)/day falls between the ninetieth percentile of intake, 1,122 mg (28.1 mmol)/day, and the ninety-fifth percentile of calcium intake, 1,268 mg (31.7 mmol)/day. For women in this age range, the median calcium intake is 571 mg (14.3 mmol)/day. Their AI markedly exceeds the ninetieth percentile of calcium intake, 891 mg (22.3 mmol)/day.

Special Considerations

Estrogen Loss and Osteoporosis. Although diminished estrogen at menopause causes accelerated bone loss, estrogen deficiency-related bone loss cannot be prevented by increasing calcium intake (see earlier section "Factors Affecting the Calcium Requirement"). Estrogen does to some extent influence calcium absorption, but available evidence is not sufficient to support different AIs for women in this age range depending on their menopausal status or their use of hormone replacement therapy.

Ages > 70 Years

Indicators Used to Set the AI

Calcium Retention. Few men over age 70 have participated in balance studies. In the studies in which they have been included, it is not possible to separate their data from those of the younger men studied. Among women, there are too few balance data at high calcium intakes to identify a plateau intake value. To the extent that the age-related decline in calcium absorption efficiency is not offset by increased renal conservation of calcium, the intake requirement for men and women would be expected to increase with advancing age.

Fracture Rates. Several intervention studies have revealed a linkage between calcium intake and the clinically important outcome, fractures. In a large randomized trial in over 3,000 elderly retirement home residents (mean age 84 years), daily supplementation with 1,200 mg (30 mmol) of calcium and 20 µg (800 IU) of vitamin D reduced hip fracture and other nonvertebral fracture rates (Chapuy et al., 1992). In a randomized trial in younger men and women (aged 65 and older, mean age 71 years) residing at home, supplementation with 500 mg (12.5 mmol) of elemental calcium and 8.8 µg (352 IU) of vitamin D significantly reduced nonvertebral fracture rates (Dawson-Hughes et al., 1997). Notably, the men and women in this study had estimated usual dietary calcium and vitamin D intakes of 750 mg (18.8 mmol) and 5.0 µg (200 IU), respectively. Two other studies have assessed the effect of calcium alone on fracture rates (Chevalley et al., 1994; Recker et al., 1996). Among women with low usual daily calcium intakes (mean 450 mg [11.3 mmol]), calcium supplementation (1,200 mg [30 mmol]/day) reduced the vertebral fracture rate in women with prior vertebral fractures, but it did not reduce the risk of first vertebral fractures (Recker et al., 1996). In contrast, a reduction in first vertebral fractures with calcium supplementation of 800 mg (20 mmol)/day has been noted (Chevalley et al., 1994). Although these studies point to a favorable effect of calcium, additional studies are needed to estimate the magnitude of the impact of calcium intake on fracture rates. Available data do not allow use of fracture outcomes to identify the AI for calcium.

Bone Mineral Density. The randomized longitudinal trials (summarized in Table 4-5) that examined the effect of supplemental calcium (with or without vitamin D) on fracture incidence also assessed changes in BMD (Chapuy et al., 1992; Chevalley et al., 1994; Dawson-Hughes et al., 1997) or BMC (Recker et al., 1996). In each of these studies, there was a significant positive effect of calcium at one or more skeletal sites including the proximal femur (Chapuy et al., 1992; Dawson-Hughes et al., 1997), femoral shaft (Chevalley et al., 1994), spine (Dawson-Hughes et al., 1997), forearm (in women with prevalent vertebral fractures [Recker et al., 1996]), and total body (Dawson-Hughes et al., 1997).

AI Summary: Ages > 70 Years

Because there are too few data in men and women at high calcium intakes to allow estimation of the plateau intake, the AI is the same as that for 51 through 70 year olds—1,200 mg (30 mmol)/day.

AI for Men   > 70 years   1,200 mg (30 mmol)/day
AI for Women   > 70 years   1,200 mg (30 mmol)/day

Utilizing the 1994 CSFII intake data, adjusted for day-to-day variation (Nusser et al., 1996), the median calcium intake for men aged > 70 years is 702 mg (17.6 mmol)/day, and the ninety-fifth percentile of intake is 1,185 mg (29.6 mmol)/day (see Appendix D). Thus, the ninety-fifth percentile of calcium intake is very close to the AI of 1,200 mg (30 mmol)/day. For women in this age range, the median calcium intake is 517 mg (12.9 mmol)/day and the ninety-ninth percentile of intake is 1,037 mg (25.9 mmol)/day. Thus, nearly all women ages > 70 years are consuming less calcium than the AI.

Summary of Approaches Used for Adolescents and Adults

Desirable rates of calcium retention, determined from balance studies, factorial estimates of requirements, and limited data on BMD and BMC changes, have been used as the primary indicators of adequacy (Table 4-5). These indicators were chosen as reasonable surrogate markers to reflect changes in skeletal calcium content. In general, the decision to set AIs for calcium rather than EARs was based on the uncertainties in the these methods as discussed earlier, and the disparity between the estimates derived from these approaches and the limited observational data on calcium intakes of groups within the U.S. and Canadian populations.

Pregnancy

During pregnancy, approximately 25 to 30 g (625 to 750 mmol) of calcium are transferred to the fetus, with the majority of this transfer occurring during the third trimester (IOM, 1990). The major physiological adaptation of the mother to meet this increased calcium requirement is increased efficiency in intestinal absorption of calcium.

Both total and "free" (calculated as the molar ratio of $1,25(OH)_2D$ and vitamin D binding protein) serum $1,25(OH)_2D$ concentrations increase during pregnancy (Bouillon et al., 1981; Cross et al., 1995a; Kumar et al., 1979; Pitkin et al., 1979; Seki et al., 1991; Wilson et al., 1990) and may be responsible for the increase in calcium absorption that has been observed (Cross et al., 1995a; Heaney and Skillman, 1971; Kent et al., 1991). Whether the increase in $1,25(OH)_2D$ concentrations is a result of placental production or increases in serum PTH that may occur late in pregnancy (Pitkin et al., 1979) is

TABLE 4-5 Summary of Estimates of Calcium Needs Using Three Different Approaches

Age (y)	Desirable Retention (mg Ca/d)[a]	FactorialMethod (mg Ca/d)[b]
1–3	M/F - 100	M/F - 500
4–8	M/F - 200	No data
9–13 & 14–18	M - 282 (+55)	M - 1,505
	F - 212 (+55)	F - 1,276
19–30	M - 50 (+63)	M - 1,437
	F - 10 (+63)	F - 1,393
31–50	M - 0 (+0)	M - 1,270
	F - 0 (+102)	F - 1,360
51–70	M - 0 (+63)	M - 1,380
	F - 0 (+0)	F - 1,383
> 70	No data	No data

[a] Additional amount added to account for sweat losses given in parentheses.

[b] The factorial estimate was based on accretion values derived from measures of bone mineral content and the assumption that bone contains 32.3% calcium by weight (see text for details).

[c] The calcium retention model was based on balance studies from which the absolute intake and retention of individual subjects was modeled using non-linear regression analysis (Jackman et al., 1997). The derived equations were then solved to obtain an

Calcium Retention Model (mg Ca/d)[c]	Clinical Trials[d]
No data	No data
Calcium intake of 800–900 gave retention of +174	Calcium intakes (mg/d) of 600 vs. 300 (Lee et al., 1995); 1,600 vs. 900 (Slemenda et al., 1997) resulted in greater increase in spinal BMC for higher intake groups.
M - 1,310 F - 1,070	Calcium intakes (mg/d) of: 1,314 vs. 960 (Lloyd et al., 1993) 1,437 vs. 728 (Chan et al., 1995) 1,612 vs. 908 (Johnston et al., 1992) resulted in a mean increase in BMC for all higher intake groups.
M - 1,236 F - 1,026 M/F - 840–950 based on calcium balance	No data
M - 995	Calcium intakes (mg/d) of 1,572 vs. 810 resulted in reduced vertebral bone loss in premenopausal women (Baran et al., 1990). Calcium intake (mg/d) of > 1,200 resulted in no difference in bone loss in males.
F - 1200[e] as predicted from balance studies	Calcium intake (mg/d) of > 750, 800 and 1,000 showed less bone loss than lower intakes in females (see Table 4-1).
No data;[e] 1,200 mg extrapolated from data in 51–70 year olds	Calcium intake (mg/d) of 1,200 vs. 750 resulted in reduced fracture rate and lower bone loss measured by BMD at various sites (Chapuy et al., 1992; Dawson-Hughes et al., 1997).

estimate of the intake at which a desirable calcium retention would be attained (see text for specific values used for each age group; see Appendix E for equations).

[d] The major outcome evaluated from the clinical trials reviewed was change in BMD at various bone sites or fracture rate in the > 70 year age group.

[e] These estimates were not derived from statistical analysis of calcium intake and retention data to determine desirable calcium intakes due to limitations in the range of calcium intakes that had been studied.

not clear. Significant increases in maternal calcium accretion, bone turnover, and intestinal absorption early in pregnancy, prior to the mineralization of the fetal skeleton, have been observed in kinetic and histomorphometric studies (Heaney and Skillman, 1971; Purdie et al., 1988).

Results from balance and calcium kinetic studies in 15 women conducted during pregnancy demonstrated increased calcium retention well in advance of when most of the mineralization of the fetal skeleton occurs (Heaney and Skillman, 1971). The mean calcium intakes ranged from 920 to 2,020 mg (23 to 50.5 mmol)/day throughout pregnancy. Calcium retention exceeded the demand for fetal growth. A possible explanation for the increased calcium retention in these balance studies is that the mothers were still accreting bone regardless of their pregnancy state; the ages of the mothers ranged from 15 to 28 years.

Urinary calcium excretion increases during pregnancy and is related to the elevated serum $1,25(OH)_2D$ and increased intestinal absorption of calcium (Gertner et al., 1986). This physiologic absorptive hypercalciuria has led some investigators to consider pregnancy a "period of calcium feast rather than famine" (Gertner et al., 1986). Whether dietary calcium modulates the $1,25(OH)_2D$ response to pregnancy is not clear.

Indicator Used to Set the AI

Bone Mineral Mass. Whether significant bone resorption occurs during pregnancy to serve as a mineral supply for fetal skeletal needs is not clear. In a prospective study of six women, lumbar spine BMD decreased between prepregnancy and postpartum measurements but increased to baseline values after weaning (Drinkwater and Chesnut, 1991). Another study reported no change in BMD during pregnancy in the radius (Cross et al., 1995a). However, the radius is more cortical than trabecular bone and may not be sensitive to subtle changes in bone mass.

Dietary calcium intake does not appear to influence changes in maternal bone mass during pregnancy. A study in undernourished pregnant mothers found that supplementation with 300 mg (7.5 mmol)/day or 600 mg (15 mmol)/day of calcium did not increase the metacarpal bone density of the mothers during pregnancy when compared with unsupplemented mothers. However, the bone density (determined from radiographs using an aluminum wedge calibration) of the neonates of supplemented mothers was significantly greater (mean of 77 percent greater averaged over four bone sites) than neonates of the unsupplemented mothers (Raman et al., 1978). Unfortunately, the baseline calcium intake of the unsupplemented mothers was not provided in this study, so the calcium intake associated with the less well-mineralized fetal bone cannot be determined.

A final piece of evidence that supports no increased need for dietary calcium during pregnancy is the lack of a relationship between the number of previous pregnancies and BMD (Alderman et al., 1986; Koetting and Wardlaw, 1988; Kreiger et al., 1982; Walker et al., 1972; Wasnich et al., 1983) or fracture risk (Johansson et al., 1993). Moreover, some studies support a positive correlation between the number of children born and either radial BMD or total body calcium (Aloia et al., 1983), as well as a reduction in hip fracture risk (Hoffman et al., 1993). It was not stated in these studies whether calcium intake modified the relationship between the number of pregnancies and BMD or fracture risk.

AI Summary for Pregnancy

Taken together, the available data on bone mineral mass during pregnancy and the lack of correlation between the number of pregnancies and BMD or fracture risk provide sufficient information to support the concept that the maternal skeleton is not used as a reserve for fetal calcium needs. Adaptive maternal responses to fetal calcium needs include an enhanced efficiency of absorption, which is modulated through changes in calciotropic hormones. Thus, provided that dietary calcium intake is sufficient for maximizing bone accretion rates in the nonpregnant state, the AI does not have to be increased during pregnancy.

AI for	**14 through 18 years**	**1,300 mg (32.5 mmol)/day**
Pregnancy	**19 through 30 years**	**1,000 mg (25 mmol)/day**
	31 through 50 years	**1,000 mg (25 mmol)/day**

Based on the 1994 CSFII intake data from 33 pregnant women, as adjusted for day-to-day variation (Nusser et al., 1996), the median intake of calcium for pregnant women is 1,154 mg (28.9 mmol)/day, twenty-fifth percentile of calcium intake is 939 mg (23.5 mmol)/day, and the seventy-fifth percentile of intake is 1,382 mg (34.6 mmol)/day (see Appendix D). Thus, the AI of 1,300 mg (32.5 mmol)/day for pregnant women 14 through 18 years of age is between the median and seventy-fifth percentile of calcium intake and the AI of 1,000 mg (25 mmol)/day for pregnant women 19 through 50 years of age is between the twenty-fifth percentile and median intake of calcium.

Special Considerations

Adolescent Pregnancies. The pregnant adolescent woman, theoretically, could have an increased need for calcium because of her need to support her own bone consolidation as well as that of the fetus. Sowers and coworkers (1985) found in a study of 86 women (20 to 35 years of age) that although the number of pregnancies was not associated with BMD of the distal radius, history of a teenage pregnancy (< 20 years of age) was associated with low BMD. Moreover, a lower incidence of preterm delivery and low birth weight was observed in 94 pregnant adolescents (< 17 years of age) randomized to receive 2,000 mg (50 mmol)/day supplemental calcium or a control (*n* = 95) (Villar and Repke, 1990). Both groups had a mean baseline calcium intake of 1,200 mg (30 mmol)/day. The results of these studies indicate that pregnant adolescents may benefit from a high calcium intake. However, research is needed to establish the plateau dietary intake at which these benefits may occur.

Lactation

The source of calcium utilized by a lactating woman for milk production (approximately 210 mg [5.3 mmol]/day [IOM, 1991]) could be from higher dietary intake, increased fractional intestinal absorption, reduced renal excretion, or stimulation of bone resorption. Based on studies utilizing biochemical indicators of calcium metabolism in lactating women (see Table 4-6), measures of serum $1,25(OH)_2D$ concentrations offer the most, albeit conflicting, information. If there is an increase in calcium need, one would assume this need could be met by increased serum $1,25(OH)_2D$ leading to enhanced calcium absorption. Although investigators have reported high serum $1,25(OH)_2D$ concentrations in lactating women (Kumar et al., 1979; Specker et al., 1987), the majority of studies have found no difference in serum concentrations between lactating and nonlactating women (Cross et al., 1995b; Hillman et al., 1981; Kalkwarf et al., 1996; Kent et al., 1990; Wilson et al., 1990). Serum $1,25(OH)_2D$ concentrations are increased during pregnancy (Wilson et al., 1990), and mean $1,25(OH)_2D$ concentrations in both lactating and nonlactating postpartum women tend to be high in the early postpartum period. These higher concentrations do not persist during lactation, but may increase again following the initiation of weaning (Kalkwarf et al., 1996; Specker et al., 1991a). Consistent with the lack of an increase in serum $1,25(OH)_2D$ concentrations in lactating women, calcium absorption also does not appear to be increased during lactation (Kalkwarf et al., 1996; Kent et al., 1991; Specker et al., 1994), even among women consuming a relatively low intake (750 mg [18.8 mmol]/day of calcium) (Kalkwarf et al., 1996). A randomized trial of calcium supplementation at approximately 1,000 mg (25 mmol)/day for 5 days in lactating women accustomed to low calcium intakes (approximately 300 mg [7.5 mmol]/day) found no difference between calcium supplementation groups in percent fractional intestinal absorption (Fairweather-Tait et al., 1995).

Biochemical markers and kinetic measurements indicate that bone resorption is increased during lactation (Affinito et al., 1996; Dobnig et al., 1995; Kent et al., 1990) and that this increase is independent of calcium intake (Cross et al., 1995b; Sowers et al., 1995a; Specker et al., 1994). Renal conservation of calcium also has been observed during lactation (Kent et al., 1990; Specker et al., 1994), and both the increased mobilization of calcium from bone and decreased urinary calcium excretion are sufficient to provide calcium for milk production.

These adaptive changes in calcium homeostasis are independent of the calcium intake of the mother and appear to be more dependent on return of ovarian function (Kalkwarf et al., 1996; Sowers et al., 1995b). As a woman regains ovarian function or weans her infant, the serum $1,25(OH)_2D$ concentration increases (Kalkwarf et al., 1996; Specker et al., 1991a), intestinal calcium absorption increases (Kalkwarf et al., 1996), renal retention of calcium persists (Kent et al., 1990), and biochemical markers of bone turnover begin to return to normal levels (Kent et al., 1990; Sowers et al., 1995b).

Indicators Used to Set the AI

Bone Mineral Mass and Fracture. The primary source of calcium secreted in human milk appears to be from increased maternal bone resorption that occurs during lactation (Affinito et al., 1996; Dobnig et al., 1995; Kent et al., 1990), and this increase in resorption is independent of calcium intake (Cross et al., 1995b; Sowers et al., 1995a; Specker et al., 1994).

Data from kinetic studies of lactating and nonlactating women consuming a wide range of calcium intakes indicate that the differ-

124

TABLE 4-6 Biochemical and Absorption Studies in Women During Lactation

Author and Year	Number Lactating	Number Controls	PP[a] Controls	Ca Intake (mg/day)	Effects of Lactation	Comment
Serum 1,25(OH)₂D Concentrations						
Greer et al., 1982c	14	0	No	1,005	Increased over 6 months lactation	4-8 weeks pp[a]
Hillman et al., 1981	28	20	Yes	Not stated	Similar during lactation	
Kalkwarf et al., 1996	24	24	Yes	1,308	Similar during lactation	4.6 months pp
	24	24	Yes	1,213	Higher during weaning	9.6 months pp
Kent et al., 1990	40	40	No	Not stated	Similar during lactation Similar at 2 months post-weaning	
Kumar et al., 1979	6	0	No	Not stated	Higher during lactation	
Markestad et al., 1983	8	17	No	Not stated	Similar during lactation	3.5 months pp
Specker et al., 1987	23	23	Yes	486 1,038	Higher during lactation especially on low Ca intake	
Specker et al., 1991a	26	32	Yes	1,400	Similar during lactation Higher during weaning	
Wilson et al., 1990	27	7	No	Not stated	Similar during lactation	18 weeks pp
Intestinal Calcium Absorption						
Fairweather-Tait et al., 1995	60	0	No	283 997	No effect of Ca intake	3 and 12 months pp
Kalkwarf et al., 1996	24	24	Yes	1,308	Similar during lactation	4.6 months pp
	24	24	Yes	1,213	Higher during weaning	9.6 months pp

Study				Calcium intake	Finding	Duration
Kent et al., 1991	31	26	No	Not stated	Similar during lactation	2 weeks pp
Specker et al., 1994	8	6	No	370	Similar during lactation	8.5 weeks pp
				1,870	No effect of Ca intake	
Renal Calcium Excretion						
Cross et al., 1995a	10	0	No	1,068	Urine lower during weaning	Followed 3 months pw
Kent et al., 1990	40	40	No	Not stated	Lower during lactation and weaning	3.8 months pp
Kent et al., 1991	31	26	No	Not stated	Lower during lactation and weaning	2 and 6 months pw[b]
Specker et al., 1994	8	6	No	370	Lower during lactation especially with low Ca intake	18 weeks pp
				1,870		
Bone Turnover						
Affinito et al., 1996	18	18	Yes	1,490	Higher during lactation / Similar during weaning	followed 12 months pp
Cross et al., 1995b	15	0	No	1,300	Higher during lactation	30 months pp
				2,400	Unaffected by Ca inake	
Dobnig et al., 1995	35	35	No	Not stated	Higher during lactation	6 months pp
Kent et al., 1990	40	40	No	Not stated	Higher during lactation / Similar 6 month after weaning	5.6 months pp
Sowers et al., 1995b	65	20	Yes	1,730	Higher during lactation / Similar during weaning	followed 18 months pp
Specker et al., 1994	8	6	No	370	Resorption higher during lactation	18 weeks pp
				1,870		

[a] pp = postpartum.
[b] pw = postweaning.

ence between bone resorption and formation represents a net flow of calcium from bone into the extracellular fluid calcium compartment of approximately 2.72 mg (0.07 mmol)/kg/day (Specker et al., 1994). Approximately 0.68 mg (0.02 mmol)/kg/day is conserved through reduced renal excretion. The net result is 3.4 mg (0.09 mmol)/kg/day of calcium entering the body pool through stimulation of bone resorption and reduced renal excretion, with an estimated loss in milk of 3.08 mg (0.08 mmol)/kg/day.

Results from longitudinal studies of changes in BMD with lactation indicate that the loss of bone is site specific (see Table 4-7). Results regarding changes in the distal radius are inconsistent (Affinito et al., 1996; Chan et al., 1982a; Hayslip et al., 1989; Kalkwarf and Specker, 1995; Prentice et al., 1990), whereas the majority of studies found decreases in the lumbar spine and femoral neck (Affinito et al., 1996; Cross et al., 1995b; Hayslip et al., 1989; Kalkwarf and Specker, 1995; Kent et al., 1990; Lopez et al., 1996; Sowers et al., 1993). The bone loss observed during lactation appears to be regained upon return of ovarian function (Affinito et al., 1996; Cross et al., 1995a; Kalkwarf and Specker, 1995; Kent et al., 1990; Sowers et al., 1993). These findings during weaning are consistent with changes in biochemical indicators of calcium homeostasis and intestinal absorption that are occurring at this time and with the majority of retrospective studies showing no net deleterious effect of prior lactation on bone mass (see discussion below).

Whether dietary calcium influences the changes in bone mass observed during lactation or affects milk calcium concentrations has been addressed in a few studies (summarized in Table 4-8). The results indicate that the loss of bone mass observed during lactation is not different between women on placebo or supplemental calcium intakes (1,000 mg [25 mmol]/day) (Cross et al., 1995b; Kalkwarf et al., 1997; Prentice et al., 1995) and that milk calcium is unaffected by maternal calcium intake (Kalkwarf et al., 1997; Prentice et al., 1995). The changes in bone mass that occur at this time are likely to be more related to the effects of lack of estrogen than to the increased demand of calcium for milk production. Therefore, it does not appear that dietary calcium intakes above that recommended for nonlactating women minimizes the bone loss observed during lactation, nor does it augment the bone gain during weaning.

Epidemiological studies provide additional support for the assumption that the observed lactation-induced bone loss is a normal physiological response and that after weaning this bone loss is replaced. Many studies have found no association between previous lactation history and BMD (Koetting and Wardlaw, 1988; Walker et al., 1972; Wasnich et al., 1983) or fracture risk and previous lactation history, although there are studies that report either a decreased (Lissner et al., 1991; Wardlaw and Pike, 1986) or increased (Aloia et al., 1983; Feldblum et al., 1992; Hreshchyshyn et al., 1988; Melton et al., 1993b) BMD with history of lactation (see Table 4-9). A longitudinal prospective study of over 9,000 women over the age of 65 found that the risk of hip fracture was not associated with the number of children who were breast-fed (Cummings et al., 1995). Although most studies have found no increase in fracture risk with a history of lactation, Kreiger and coworkers (1982) found that women who later in life had hip fractures lactated for fewer months than did control women without hip fracture.

AI Summary for Lactation

The loss of calcium from the maternal skeleton that occurs during lactation is not prevented by increased dietary calcium, and the calcium lost appears to be regained following weaning. There is no evidence that calcium intake in lactating women should be increased above that of nonlactating women. Thus, the AIs for calcium during lactation are the same AIs for the nonlactating woman of the same age.

AI for Lactation 14 through 18 years 1,300 mg (32.5 mmol)/day
19 through 30 years 1,000 mg (25 mmol)/day
31 through 50 years 1,000 mg (25 mmol)/day

Utilizing data as adjusted for day-to-day variation (Nusser et al., 1996) from the 16 lactating mothers in the 1994 CSFII sample, the twenty-fifth percentile of intake for calcium is 982 mg (24.6 mmol)/day (see Appendix D), which is close to the AI of 1,000 mg (25 mmol)/day for lactating women ages 19 through 50 years. The median intake is 1,050 mg (26.3 mmol)/day, the ninety-fifth percentile of intake is 1,324 mg (33.1 mmol)/day, which is slightly above the AI of 1,300 mg (32.5 mmol/day) for lactating women 14 through 18 years of age.

Special Considerations

Closely Spaced Pregnancies. Women aged 20 to 40 years, who breast-feed their infants for at least 6 months and become pregnant within 18 months of initiating lactation have BMDs similar to those of lactating women who do not have a subsequent pregnancy in 18

TABLE 4-7 Longitudinal Studies of Changes in BMD with Lactation

Author	Lact	Non Lact (pp)[a]	Non Wean (pp)	Wean Non Lact	Wean Lact >6 mo	Wean Lact 0–1 mo	Wean Lact 0–1 mo	N	Site	1 mo	3 mo	6 mo	12 mo	Calcium Intake (mg/d)	Percent Change
Affinito et al., 1996	✓							18	LS[c]		✓	✓		1,790	−7.5
		✓						18	LS		✓	✓		1,185	0
	✓							18	R					1,790	−5
								18	R					1,185	0
			✓					18	LS					1,144	3
			✓					18	LS			✓	✓	954	0
				✓				18	R			✓	✓	1,144	2.5
				✓				18	R					954	0
Chan et al., 1982a	✓							39	R[b]			✓		unk	none
Cross et al., 1995b	✓							7	LS	✓	✓			2,400	−6.3
	✓							8	LS	✓	✓			1,300	−4.3
								7	LS	✓	✓			2,400	3.0
								8	LS	✓	✓			1,300	1.7
Hayslip et al., 1989	✓						✓	12	LS			✓		1,786	−6.5
								7	LS			✓		1,253	0
	✓							12	R			✓		1,786	0
								7	R			✓		1,253	0

Group / Postpartum

Study											
Kalkwarf and Specker, 1995	✓						✓	65	LS	✓	892	-3.9
		✓						48	LS	✓	723	1.5
			✓					65	R	✓	892	-0.6
				✓				48	R	✓	723	-0.5
					✓	✓		40	LS	✓	763	5.5
					✓	✓		43	LS	✓	732	1.8
								40	R	✓	763	-0.9
								43	R	✓	732	0
Lopez et al., 1996	✓						✓	30	LS ✓	✓	1,479	-4.5[f]
	✓							26	LS ✓	✓	536	0
								30	LS	✓	1,479	-4.5
								26	LS	✓	536	0
					✓			30	LS	✓ pw[e]	1,479	0.5
								26	LS	✓ pw	536	0
				✓		✓		30	FN ✓		1,479	-4.0[f]
						✓		26	FN ✓		536	0
			✓					30	FN	✓ pw	1,479	-7.0
								26	FN	✓ pw	536	0
		✓						30	FN	✓ pw	1,479	1.0
								26	FN	✓ pw	536	0
Sowers et al., 1993	✓			✓			✓	64	LS	✓	1,596	4.3
							✓	20	LS	✓	939	1.4
							✓	64	FN[d]	✓	1,596	2.1
							✓	20	FN	✓	939	0.1

[a] pp = postpartum.
[b] R = radius.
[c] LS = lumbar spine.
[d] FN = femoral neck.
[e] pw = postweaning.
[f] Change relative to controls.

TABLE 4-8 Effect of Calcium Supplementation During Lactation on Changes in BMD

Author	Group Lactating	Non Lactating (pp)[a]	Wean	Non Wean (pp)	Calcium (mg/day)	Number	Site	Postpartum Weeks 3 mo	6 mo	Percent Change in BMD
Cross et al., 1995b	✓				1,300	7	LS	✓		-4.3
	✓				2,400	8	LS	✓		-6.3
			✓		1,300	7	LS	✓		1.7
			✓		2,400	8	LS	✓		3.0
	✓				1,300	7	Rad (ultra)[e]	✓		~1.5
	✓				2,400	8	Rad (ultra)	✓		5.7
			✓		1,300	7	Rad (ultra)	✓		~-5.7
			✓		2,400	8	Rad (ultra)	✓		~-5.7
			✓		1,300	7	TB	✓		0
			✓		2,400	8	TB	✓		0
Kalkwarf et al., 1997	✓				843	42	LS[b]		✓	-4.9
	✓				1,868	45	LS		✓	-4.2
		✓			656	40	LS		✓	0.4
		✓			1,739	41	LS		✓	2.2
			✓		776	38	LS		✓	4.4
			✓		1,684	38	LS		✓	5.9

679	42	LS	✓		1.6
1,744	40	LS	✓		2.5
843	42	Rad(1/3)[c]	✓		-0.1
1,868	45	Rad(1/3)	✓		-0.3
656	40	Rad(1/3)	✓		-0.6
1,739	41	Rad(1/3)	✓		0
776	38	Rad(1/3)	✓		-0.4
1,684	38	Rad(1/3)	✓		-0.8
679	42	Rad(1/3)	✓		-0.1
1,744	40	Rad(1/3)	✓		-0.2
843	42	TB[d]	✓		-3.4
1,868	45	TB	✓		-2.4
656	40	TB	✓		-1.2
1,739	41	TB	✓		-1.7
776	38	TB	✓		0.2
1,684	38	TB	✓		-0.2
679	42	TB	✓		-0.2
1,744	40	TB	✓		0.4

Prentice et al., 1995

283	30	Rad (mid)[f]	13	✓	-1.1
997	30	Rad (mid)	13	✓	-1.1
283	30	Rad (mid)	52	✓	0
997	30	Rad (mid)	52	✓	0

[a] pp = postpartum.
[b] LS = lumbar spine.
[c] Rad(1/3) = one-third radius.
[d] TB = total body.
[e] Rad (ultra) = ultradistal radius.
[f] Rad (mid) = midshaft radius.

TABLE 4-9 Retrospective or Cross-Sectional Studies Concerning Lactation-Induced Bone Loss

Author	Year	N	Site
Alderman et al.	1986	355	Fracture
		562	Controls
Aloia et al.	1983	80	Radius
Cummings et al.	1995	173	Fracture
		137	Controls
Feldblum et al.	1992	352	Lumbar spine
			Radius
Hoffman et al.	1993	174	Fracture
			Controls
Hreshchyshyn et al.	1988	151	Lumbar spine
Kent et al.	1990	80	Radius
Koetting and Wardlaw	1988	28	Hip, Radius
Kreiger et al.	1982	98	Fracture
		884	Controls
Lissner et al.	1991	126	Lumbar spine
Melton et al.	1993b	304	Hip, Radius, Lumbar spine
Walker et al.	1972	102	Metacarpal
Wardlaw and Pike	1986	21	Radius
Wasnich et al.	1983	608	Radius

months (Sowers et al., 1995b). These findings support those from a cross-sectional study that found similar BMD among women with small or large families (Walker et al., 1972). Therefore, it does not appear, from the data available at this time, that closely spaced pregnancies lead to a lower bone mass in these women than in women with pregnancies less closely spaced.

Feeding More Than One Infant. A study in women breast-feeding twins found significantly higher serum PTH and $1,25(OH)_2D$ concentrations compared to women nursing singletons. The authors suggest that these findings reflect an increased mineral need in the mothers (Greer et al., 1984). No studies have been reported in

Major Findings

Women who lactated more than 2 years had similar risk of fracture as women who never lactated.

Higher radius BMC with lactation (45 to 55 years of age and postmenopausal); no effect of total body Ca.

No increased risk of fracture with history of lactation (>65 years of age).

Higher BMD associated with history of lactation in perimenopausal women 40 to 54 years of age.

No association between hip fracture in women >45 years of age and lactation history.

Higher BMD in women 35 to 65 years of age who lactated compared to no lactation.

BMD at ultradistal radius 7% lower in 40 lactating women at 5.6 months pp compared to 40 controls. No difference at distal or midradius; BMD regained 4 to 6 months pw in 19 women studied.

No association between BMD at 26 to 37 years of age and lactation history. Ca intake not associated with bone measurements.

45 to 74 year olds with hip fractures compared to controls. Cases lactated for less months than nontrauma controls (N = 81) and trauma controls (N = 83).

Lower BMC associated with greater months of lactation.

BMD at any site not associated with lactation. Higher BMD of hip associated with long-term lactation (age-stratified random sample of all adult women in Rochester, MN).

No association between radiograph measurements at 30 to 44 years of age and size of families. Ca intake not associated with bone measurements.

Lower BMC in women 30 to 35 years of age in those who had long-term versus short-term lactation.

BMC in postmenopausal women (44 to 80 years of age) not associated with months of lactation.

which calcium supplementation of lactating mothers of more than one infant was evaluated.

Lactating Adolescents. A study in lactating adolescents found that 15 mothers consuming 900 mg (22.5 mmol)/day calcium had a significant decrease in BMC of the distal radius over the first 16 weeks postpartum. No change was observed in 21 mothers who were consuming 1,850 mg (46.3 mmol)/day of calcium (Chan et al., 1982b). Although the results of these studies are intriguing, several concerns about the findings have been expressed, including not finding bone loss in the adult women, a higher rate of bone loss than that seen in any pathological condition, and bone mass measurements greater than 4 SD above normal at baseline in two of the women (Cunningham and Mazess, 1983; Greer and Garn, 1982). Moreover, it is not clear whether the adolescents were randomized to receive intensive counseling and why there were uneven sample sizes in the two groups of lactating adolescents ($n = 15$ and 21). Due to the small sample sizes and the uncertainties regarding this study, it is not clear whether the calcium AI in lactating adolescents should be higher than the AI of 1,300 mg (32.5 mmol)/day in the nonlactating adolescent.

TOLERABLE UPPER INTAKE LEVELS

Hazard Identification

Calcium is among the most ubiquitous of elements found in the human system. As stated earlier, calcium plays a major role in the metabolism of virtually every cell in the body and interacts with a large number of other nutrients. As a result, disturbances of calcium metabolism give rise to a wide variety of adverse reactions. Disturbances of calcium metabolism, particularly those that are characterized by changes in extracellular ionized calcium concentration, can cause damage in the function and structure of many organs and systems.

Currently, the available data on the adverse effects of excess calcium intake in humans primarily concerns calcium intake from nutrient supplements. Of the many possible adverse effects of excessive calcium intake, the three most widely studied and biologically important are: kidney stone formation (nephrolithiasis), the syndrome of hypercalcemia and renal insufficiency with and without alkalosis (referred to historically as milk-alkali syndrome when associated with a constellation of peptic ulcer treatments), and the interaction of calcium with the absorption of other essential minerals. These are not the only adverse effects associated with excess calcium intake. However, the vast majority of reported effects are related to or result from one of these three conditions.

Nephrolithiasis

Twelve percent of the U.S. population will form a renal stone over their lifetime (Johnson et al., 1979), and it has generally been assumed that nephrolithiasis is, to a large extent, a nutritional disease. Research over the last 40 years has shown that there is a direct relationship between periods of affluence and increased nephrolithiasis (Robertson, 1985). A number of dietary factors seem to play a role in determining the incidence of this disease. In addition to being associated with increased calcium intakes, nephrolithiasis appears to be associated with higher intakes of oxalate, protein, and vegetable fiber (Massey et al., 1993). Goldfarb (1994) argued that dietary calcium plays a minor role in nephrolithiasis because only 6 percent of the overall calcium load appears in the urine of normal individuals. Also, the efficiency of calcium absorption is substantially lower when calcium supplements are consumed (Sakhaee et al., 1994).

The issue is made more complex by the association between high sodium intakes and hypercalciuria, since sodium and calcium compete for reabsorption at the same sites in the renal tubules (Goldfarb, 1994). Other minerals, such as phosphorus and magnesium, also are risk factors in stone formation (Pak, 1988). These findings suggest that excess calcium intake may play only a contributing role in the development of nephrolithiasis.

Two recent companion prospective epidemiologic studies in men (Curhan et al., 1993) and women (Curhan et al., 1997) with no history of kidney stones found that intakes of dietary calcium greater than 1,050 mg (26.3 mmol)/day in men and greater than 1,098 mg (27.5 mmol)/day in women were associated with a reduced risk of symptomatic kidney stones. This association for dietary calcium was attenuated when the intake of magnesium and phosphorus were included in the model for women (Curhan et al., 1997). This apparent protective effect of dietary calcium is attributed to the binding by calcium in the intestinal lumen of oxalate, which is a critical component of most kidney stones. In contrast, Curhan et al. (1997) found that after adjustment for age, intake of supplemental calcium was associated with an increased risk for kidney stones. After adjustment for potential confounders, the relative risk among women who took supplemental calcium, compared with women who did not, was 1.2. Calcium supplements may be taken without food, which limits opportunity for the beneficial effect of binding oxalate in the intestine. A similar effect of supplemental calcium was observed in men (Curhan et al., 1993) but failed to reach statistical significance. Neither study controlled for the time that calcium supplements were taken (for example, with or without meals); thus, it is possible that the observed significance of the results in women may be due to different uses of calcium supplements by men and women. Clearly, more carefully controlled studies are needed to determine the strength of the causal association between calcium intake vis-à-vis the intake of other nutrients and kidney stones in healthy individuals.

The association between calcium intake and urinary calcium excretion is weaker in children than in adults. However, as observed in adults, increased levels of dietary sodium are significantly associated with increased urinary calcium excretion in children (Matkovic et al., 1995; O'Brien et al., 1996).

Hypercalcemia and Renal Insufficiency (Milk-Alkali Syndrome)

The syndrome of hypercalcemia and, consequently, renal insufficiency with or without metabolic alkalosis is associated with severe clinical and metabolic derangements affecting virtually every organ system (Orwoll, 1982). Renal failure may be reversible but may also be progressive if the syndrome is unrelieved. Progressive renal failure may result in the deposition of calcium in soft tissues including the kidney (for example, nephrocalcinosis) with a potentially fatal outcome (Junor and Catto, 1976). This syndrome was first termed milk-alkali syndrome (MAS) in the context of the high milk and absorbable antacid intake which derived from the "Sippy diet" regimen for the treatment of peptic ulcer disease. MAS needs to be distinguished from primary hyperparathyroidism, in which primary abnormality of the parathyroid gland results in hypercalcemia, metabolic derangement, and impaired renal calcium resorption. As the treatment of peptic ulcers has changed (for example, systemically absorbed antacids and large quantities of milk are now rarely prescribed), the incidence of this syndrome has decreased (Whiting and Wood, 1997).

A review of the literature revealed 26 reported cases of MAS linked to high calcium intake from supplements and food since 1980 without other causes of underlying renal disease (Table 4-10). These reports described what appears to be the same syndrome at supplemental calcium intakes of 1.5 to 16.5 g (37.5 to 412.5 mmol)/day for 2 days to 30 years. Estimates of the occurrence of MAS in the North American population may be low since mild cases are often overlooked and the disorder may be confused with a number of other syndromes presenting with hypercalcemia.

No reported cases of MAS in children were found in the literature. This was not unexpected since children have very high rates of bone turnover and calcium utilization relative to adults (Abrams et al., 1992). A single case of severe constipation directly linked to daily calcium supplementation of 1,000 mg (25 mmol) or more has been reported in an 8-year-old boy, but this may represent an idiosyncratic reaction of calcium ions exerted locally in the intestine or colon (Frithz et al., 1991).

Calcium/Mineral Interactions

Calcium interacts with iron, zinc, magnesium, and phosphorus (Clarkson et al., 1967; Hallberg et al., 1992; Schiller et al., 1989; Spencer et al., 1965). Calcium-mineral interactions are more difficult to quantify than nephrolithiasis and MAS, since in many cases the interaction of calcium with several other nutrients results in changes in the absorption and utilization of each. Thus, it is virtually impossible to determine a dietary level at which calcium intake alone disturbs the absorption or metabolism of other minerals. Nevertheless, calcium clearly inhibits iron absorption in a dose-dependent and dose-saturable fashion (Hallberg et al., 1992). However, the available human data fail to show cases of iron deficiency or even reduced iron stores as a result of calcium intake (Snedeker et al., 1982; Sokoll and Dawson-Hughes, 1992). Similarly, except for a single report of negative zinc balance in the presence of calcium supplementation (Wood and Zheng, 1990), the effects of calcium on zinc absorption have not been shown to be associated with zinc depletion or undernutrition. Neither have interactions of high levels of calcium with magnesium or phosphorus shown evidence of depletion of the affected nutrient (Shils, 1994).

Thus, in the absence of clinically or functionally significant depletion of the affected nutrient, calcium interaction with other minerals represents a potential risk rather than an adverse effect, in the sense that nephrolithiasis or hypercalcemia are adverse effects. Still, the potential for increased risk of mineral depletion in vulnerable populations such as those on very low mineral intakes or the elderly needs to be incorporated into the uncertainty factor in deriving a UL for calcium. Furthermore, because of their potential to increase the risk of mineral depletion in vulnerable populations, calcium-mineral interactions should be the subject of additional studies.

Dose-Response Assessment

Adults: Ages 19 through 70 Years

Data Selection. Based on the discussion of adverse effects of excess calcium intake above, the most appropriate data available for identifying a critical endpoint and a no-observed-adverse-effect level (NOAEL) (or lowest-observed-adverse-effect level [LOAEL]) concern risk of MAS or nephrolithiasis. There are few well-controlled, chronic studies of calcium that show a dose-response relationship. While there are inadequate data on nephrolithiasis to establish a dose-response relationship and to identify a NOAEL (or LOAEL), there are adequate data on MAS that can be used.

Identification of a NOAEL (or LOAEL) and Critical Endpoint. Using MAS as the clinically defined critical endpoint, a LOAEL in the range of 4 to 5 grams (100 to 125 mmol)/day can be identified for adults (Table 4-10). A review of these reports revealed calcium intakes from supplements (and in some cases from dietary sources as well) in the range of 1.5 to 16.5 g (37.5 to 412.5 mmol)/day. A median intake of 4.8 g (120 mmol)/day resulted in documented cases. Since many of these reports included dietary calcium intake as well as intake from supplements, an intake in the range of 5 g (125 mmol)/day represents a LOAEL for total calcium intake (for example, from both supplements and food). A solid figure for a NOAEL is not available, but researchers have observed that daily calcium intakes of 1,500 to 2,400 mg (37.5 to 60 mmol) (including supplements), used to treat or prevent osteoporosis, did not result in hypercalcemic syndromes (Kochersberger et al., 1991; McCarron and Morris, 1985; Riggs et al., 1996; Saunders et al., 1988; Smith et al., 1989; Thys-Jacobs et al., 1989).

Consideration of hypercalciuria may have additional relevance to the derivation of a UL for adults. Hypercalciuria is observed in approximately 50 percent of patients with calcium oxalate/apatite nephrolithiasis and is an important risk factor for nephrolithiasis (Lemann et al., 1991; Whiting and Wood, 1997). Therefore, it is plausible that high calcium intakes associated with hypercalciuria could produce nephrolithiasis. Burtis et al. (1994) reported a significant positive association between both dietary calcium and sodium intake and hypercalciuria in 282 renal stone patients and derived a regression equation to predict the separate effects of dietary calcium and urinary sodium on urinary calcium excretion. Setting urinary sodium excretion at 150 mmol/day and defining hypercalciuria for men as greater than 300 mg (7.5 mmol) of calcium/day excreted (Burtis et al., 1994), the calcium intake that would be associated with hypercalciuria was 1,685 mg (42.1 mmol)/day. For women, for whom hypercalcemia was defined as greater than 250 mg (6.2 mmol)/day excreted, it would be 866 mg (21.6 mmol)/day. The results of these calculations from the Burtis et al. (1994) equation suggest that calcium intakes lower than AI levels derived earlier in this chapter for females could result in hypercalciuria in susceptible individuals.

TABLE 4-10 Case Reports of Milk Alkali Syndrome (single dose/day)[a]

Studies	Ca Intake (g/d)[b]	Duration	Mitigating Factors
Abreo et al., 1993	9.6[c]	>3 mo	None reported
	3.6[c]	>2 y	None reported
	10.8[d]	Not stated	None reported
Brandwein and Sigman, 1994	2.7[c]	2 y, 8 mo	None reported
Bullimore and Miloszewski, 1987	6.5[d]	23 y	Alkali in antacid
Campbell et al., 1994	5[d]	3 mo	None reported
Carroll et al., 1983	4.2[d]	30 y	None reported
	2[c]	5 y	None reported
	3.8[d]	2 mo	Vitamins A and E
	2.8[d]	10 y	NaHCO$_3$, 5 g/d
French et al., 1986	8[c]	2 y	None reported
	4.2[c]	>2 y	Thiazide
Gora et al., 1989	4[c]	2 y	Thiazide
Hart et al., 1982	10.6[d]	Not stated	NaHCO$_3$, 2 g/d
Kallmeyer and Funston, 1983	8[d]	10 y	Alkali in antacid
Kapsner et al., 1986	10[d]	10 mo	None reported
	6.8[d]	7 mo	None reported
	4.8[c]	2 d	10-y history of antacid use
Kleinman et al., 1991	16.5[d]	2 wk	10-y history of antacid use
Lin et al., 1996	1.5[c]	4 wk	None reported
Muldowney and Mazbar, 1996	1.7[c]	13 mo (52 wk)	None reported
Schuman and Jones, 1985	9.8[d]	20 y	None reported
	4.8[d]	6 wk	10-y history of antacid intake
Whiting and Wood, 1997	2.4[c]	>1 y	None reported
Whiting and Wood, 1997	2.3–4.6[c]	>1 y	None reported
Number of Subjects	26		
Mean	5.9	3 y, 8 mo	
Median	4.8	13 mo	
Range	1.5–>16.5	2 d–23 y	

[a] Case reports of patients with renal failure are not included in this table.
[b] Intake estimates provided by Whiting and Wood (1997).
[c] Calcium intake from supplements only.
[d] Calcium intake from supplements and diet.

Although Burtis et al. (1994) identified what could be defined as LOAELs for hypercalciuria, 1,685 mg (42.1 mmol)/day in men and 866 mg (21.6 mmol)/day in women, these values are not considered as appropriate for use as the LOAEL for healthy adults as they were based on patients with renal stones. However, they support for the need for conservative estimates of the Tolerable Upper Intake Level (UL).

Uncertainty Assessment. An uncertainty factor (UF) of 2 is recommended to take into account the potential for increased risk of high calcium intake based on the following: (1) 12 percent of the American population is estimated to have renal stones, (2) hypercalciuria has been shown to occur with intakes as low as 1,700 mg (42.5 mmol)/day in male and 870 mg (21.7 mmol)/day in female patients with renal stones (Burtis et al., 1994), and (3) concern for the potential increased risk of mineral depletion in vulnerable populations due to the interference of calcium on mineral bioavailability, especially iron and zinc.

TABLE 4-11 Case Reports of Milk Alkali Syndrome (multi- and increasing doses)

	Ca Intake (Dose 1) (g/d)	Duration (mo)	Ca Intake (Dose 2) (g/d)	Duration
Beall and Scofield, 1995	1[a]	13	2.4[a]	2 wk
	1	13	4.2	2 wk
	0.3[a]	6	1.8[a]	1 mo
Carroll et al., 1983	2.5	13	3	13 mo
Dorsch, 1986	Not reported	13	2.1[a]	6 mo
Hakim et al., 1979	1[a]	13	2.5[a]	3.5 wk
Malone and Horn, 1971	Not reported	13	3[a]	4.5 wk
Newmark and Nugent, 1993	Not reported	13	8.4[a]	<1 y ("recent")
Schuman and Jones, 1985	Not reported	13	4.6	6 wk
Number of Subjects	9		9	
Mean	1.2	12	3.6	16.7
Median	1	13	3	4.5
Range	0.3–2.5	6–13	1.8–8.4	2–53 wk

[a] Data do not include intake of calcium from dietary sources.

Derivation of the UL. A UL of 2.5 g (62.5 mmol)/day is calculated by dividing a LOAEL of 5 g (125 mmol)/day by the UF of 2. The data summarized in Table 4-11 show that calcium intakes of 0.3 to 2.5 g (7.5 to 62.5 mmol)/day have not been shown to cause MAS and provide supportive evidence for a UL of 2,500 mg (62.5 mmol)/day for adults. The estimated UL for calcium in adults is judged to be conservative. For individuals who are particularly susceptible to high calcium intakes, such as those with hypercalcemia and hyperabsorptive hypercalciuria, this level or below should be protective.

UL for Adults   19 through 70 years   2,500 mg (62.5 mmol)/day

Infants: Ages 0 through 12 Months

The safety of calcium intakes above the levels provided by infant formulas and weaning foods has recently been studied by Dalton et al. (1997). They did not find any effect on iron status from calcium intakes of approximately 1,700 mg (42.5 mmol)/day in infants, which was attained using calcium-fortified infant formula. However, further studies are needed before a UL specific to infants can be established.

UL for Infants   0 through 12 months   Not possible to establish
                                         for supplementary calcium

Toddlers, Children, and Adolescents: Ages 1 through 18 years

Although the safety of excess calcium intake in children ages 1 through 18 years has not been studied, a UL of 2,500 mg (62.5 mmol)/day is recommended for these life stage groups. Although calcium supplementation in children may appear to pose minimal risk of MAS or hyperabsorptive hypercalciuria, risk of depletion of other minerals associated with high calcium intakes may be greater. With high calcium intake, small children may be especially susceptible to deficiency of iron and zinc (Golden and Golden, 1981; Schlesinger et al., 1992; Simmer et al., 1988). However, no dose-response data exist regarding these interactions in children or the development of adaptation to chronic high calcium intakes. After age 9, rates of calcium absorption and bone formation begin to increase in preparation for pubertal development, but a conservative UL of 2,500 mg (62.5 mmol)/day (from diet and supplements) is recommended for children due to the lack of data.

UL for Children   1 through 18 years   2,500 mg (62.5 mmol)/day

Older Adults: Ages > 70 Years

Several physiologic differences in older adults need to be considered in setting the UL for people over age 70. Because this population is more likely to have achlorhydria (Recker, 1985), absorption of calcium, except when associated with meals, is likely to be somewhat impaired, which would protect these individuals from the adverse effects of high calcium intakes. Furthermore, there is a decline in calcium absorption associated with age that results from changes in function of the intestine (Ebeling et al., 1994). However, the elderly population is also more likely to have marginal zinc status, which theoretically would make them more susceptible to the negative interactions of calcium and zinc (Wood and Zheng, 1990). This matter deserves more study. These effects serve to increase the UF on the one hand and decrease it on the other, with the final result being to use the same UL for older adults as for younger adults.

UL for Older Adults   > 70 years   2,500 mg (62.5 mmol)/day

Pregnancy and Lactation

The available data were judged to be inadequate for deriving a UL for pregnant and lactating women that is different from the UL for the nonpregnant and nonlactating female.

UL for Pregnancy   14 through 50 years   2,500 mg (62.5 mmol)/day

UL for Lactation   14 through 50 years   2,500 mg (62.5 mmol)/day

Special Considerations

Not surprisingly, the ubiquitous nature of calcium results in a population of individuals with a wide range of sensitivities to its toxic effects. Subpopulations known to be particularly susceptible to the toxic effects of calcium include individuals with renal failure, those using thiazide diuretics (Whiting and Wood, 1997), and those with low intakes of minerals that interact with calcium (for example, iron, magnesium, zinc). For the majority of the general population, intakes of calcium from food substantially above the UL are probably safe.

Exposure Assessment

The highest median intake of calcium for any age group found in the 1994 CSFII data, adjusted for day-to-day variation (Nusser et al., 1996), was for boys 14 through 18 years of age with a median intake of 1,094 mg (27.4 mmol)/day and a ninety-fifth percentile intake of 2,039 mg (51 mmol)/day (see Appendix D). Calcium supplements were used by less than 8 percent of young children, 14 percent of men, and 25 percent of women in the United States (Moss et al., 1989). Daily dosages from supplements at the ninety-fifth percentile were relatively small for children (160 mg [4 mmol]), larger for men (624 mg [15.6 mmol]), and largest for women (904 mg [22.6 mmol]) according to Moss et al. (1989).

Risk Characterization

Although the ninety-fifth percentile of daily intake did not exceed the UL for any age group (2,101 mg [52.5 mmol] in males 14 through 18 years old) in the 1994 CSFII, persons with a very high caloric intake, especially if intakes of dairy products are also high, may exceed the UL of 2,500 mg (62.5 mmol)/day.

Even if the ninety-fifth percentile of intake from foods and the most recently available estimate of the ninety-fifth percentile of supplement use (Moss et al., 1989) are added together for teenage boys (1,920 + 928 mg/day) or for teenage girls (1,236 + 1,200 mg/day), total intakes are just at or slightly above the UL. Although users of dietary supplements (of any kind) tend to also have higher intakes of calcium from food than nonusers (Slesinski et al., 1996), it is unlikely that the same person would fall at the upper end of both ranges. Furthermore, the prevalence of usual intakes (from foods plus supplements) above the UL is well below 5 percent, even for age groups with relatively high intakes. Nevertheless, an informal survey of food products in supermarkets in the Washington, D.C. metropolitan area between 1994 and 1996 showed that the number of calcium-fortified products doubled in the 2-year period (Park Y., February, 1997, personal communication). Therefore, it is important to maintain surveillance of the calcium-fortified products in the marketplace and monitor their impact on calcium intake.

RESEARCH RECOMMENDATIONS

Balance studies can be used to determine the amount of calcium needed in the diet to support desirable calcium retention. Such studies need to be expanded in the following ways:

• To the extent possible, balance studies should be augmented with stable or radioactive tracers of calcium to estimate aspects of calcium homeostasis with changes in defined intakes (i.e., fractional absorption, bone calcium balance, and bone turnover rates);

• Adaptations to changes in the amount of dietary calcium should be followed within the same populations for short-term (2 months) to long-term (1 to 2 years) studies. Different experimental approaches will be needed to define the temporal response to changes in dietary calcium. Short-term studies may be conducted in a metabolic unit whereas the longer-term studies will need to be carried out in confined populations (i.e., convalescent home patients) fed prescribed diets; human study cohorts followed carefully for years with frequent, thorough estimates of dietary intakes; or metabolic studies of individuals fed their usual diets who typically consume a wide range of calcium intakes. All studies should include a comprehensive evaluation of biochemical measures of bone mineral content or metabolism. Bone mineral content and density should be evaluated in long-term studies. Good surrogate markers of osteopenia could be used in epidemiological studies.

• Assessment of the effect of ethnicity and osteoporosis phenotype on the relationship between dietary calcium, desirable calcium retention, bone metabolism, and bone mineral content.

• Evaluation of the independent impact of diet, lifestyle (especially physical activity), and hormonal changes on the utilization of dietary calcium for bone deposition and growth in children and adolescents. These studies need to be done in populations for which the usual calcium intakes range from low to above adequate.

• Epidemiological studies of the interrelationships between calcium intake and fracture risk, osteoporosis, prostate cancer, and hypertension must be pursued to determine if calcium intake is an independent determinant of any of these health outcomes. Control of other factors potentially associated as other risk factors for these health problems is essential (for example, fat intake in relation to cancer and cardiovascular disease; weight bearing activity; and dietary components such as salt, protein and caffeine in relation to osteoporosis). Such epidemiological studies need to be conducted in middle-aged as well as older adult men and women.

• More carefully controlled studies are needed to determine the strength of the causal association between calcium intake vis-à-vis the intake of other nutrients and kidney stones in healthy individuals.

• Because of their potential to increase the risk of mineral depletion in vulnerable populations, calcium-mineral interactions should be the subject of additional studies.

5

Phosphorus

BACKGROUND INFORMATION

Overview

Phosphorus is most commonly found in nature in its pentavalent form in combination with oxygen, as phosphate (PO_4^{3-}). Phosphorus (as phosphate) is an essential constituent of all known protoplasm and its content is quite uniform across most plant and animal tissues. Except for specialized cells with high ribonucleic acid content, and for nervous tissue with high myelin content, tissue phosphorus occurs at concentrations ranging approximately from 0.25 to 0.65 mmol (7.8 to 20.1 mg)/g protein. A practical consequence is that, as organisms consume other organisms lower in the food chain (whether animal or plant), they automatically obtain their phosphorus.

Phosphorus makes up about 0.5 percent of the newborn infant body (Fomon and Nelson, 1993), and from 0.65 to 1.1 percent of the adult body (Aloia et al., 1984; Diem, 1970). Eighty-five percent of adult body phosphorus is in bone. The remaining 15 percent is distributed through the soft tissues (Diem, 1970). Total phosphorus concentration in whole blood is 13 mmol/liter (40 mg/dl), most of which is in the phospholipids of red blood cells and plasma lipoproteins. Approximately 1 mmol/liter (3.1 mg/dl) is present as inorganic phosphate (P_i). This inorganic phosphate component, while a tiny fraction of body phosphorus (< 0.1 percent), is of critical importance. In adults this component makes up about 15 mmol (465 mg) and is located mainly in the blood and extracellular fluid.

146

It is into this inorganic phosphate compartment that phosphate is inserted upon absorption from the diet and resorption from bone and from this compartment that most urinary phosphorus and hydroxyapatite mineral phosphorus are derived. This compartment is also the primary source from which the cells of all tissues derive both structural and high-energy phosphate.

Structurally, phosphorus occurs as phospholipids, which are a major component of most biological membranes, and as nucleotides and nucleic acids. The functional roles include: (1) the buffering of acid or alkali excesses, hence helping to maintain normal pH; (2) the temporary storage and transfer of the energy derived from metabolic fuels; and (3) by phosphorylation, the activation of many catalytic proteins. Since phosphate is not irreversibly consumed in these processes and can be recycled indefinitely, the actual function of dietary phosphorus is first to support tissue growth (either during individual development or through pregnancy and lactation) and, second, to replace excretory and dermal losses. In both processes it is necessary to maintain a normal level of P_i in the extracellular fluid (ECF), which would otherwise be depleted of its phosphorus by growth and excretion.

Physiology of Absorption, Metabolism, and Excretion

Food phosphorus is a mixture of inorganic and organic forms. Intestinal phosphatases hydrolyze the organic forms contained in ingested protoplasm, and thus most phosphorus absorption occurs as inorganic phosphate. On a mixed diet, net absorption of total phosphorus in various reports ranges from 55 to 70 percent in adults (Lemann, 1996; Nordin, 1989; Stanbury, 1971) and from 65 to 90 percent in infants and children (Wilkinson, 1976; Ziegler and Fomon, 1983). There is no evidence that this absorption efficiency varies with dietary intake. In the data from both Stanbury (1971) and Lemann (1996), the intercept of the regression of adult fecal phosphorus on dietary phosphorus is not significantly different from zero, and the relationship is linear out to intakes of at least 3.1 g (100 mmol)/day. This means that there is no apparent adaptive mechanism that improves phosphorus absorption at low intakes. This is in sharp contrast to calcium, for which absorption efficiency increases as dietary intake decreases (Heaney et al., 1990b) and for which adaptive mechanisms exist that improve absorption still further at habitual low intakes (Heaney et al., 1989).

A portion of phosphorus absorption is by way of a saturable, active transport facilitated by 1,25-dihydroxyvitamin D $(1,25(OH)_2D)$ (Chen et al., 1974; Cramer, 1961). However, the fact that fractional phosphorus absorption is virtually constant across a broad range of intakes suggests that the bulk of phosphorus absorption occurs by passive, concentration-dependent processes. Also, even in the face of dangerous hyperphosphatemia, phosphorus continues to be absorbed from the diet at an efficiency only slightly lower than normal (Brickman et al., 1974).

Phosphorus absorption is reduced by ingestion of aluminum-containing antacids and by pharmacologic doses of calcium carbonate. There is, however, no significant interference with phosphorus absorption by calcium at intakes within the typical adult range.

Excretion of endogenous phosphorus is mainly through the kidneys. Inorganic serum phosphate is filtered at the glomerulus and reabsorbed in the proximal tubule. The transport capacity of the proximal tubule for phosphorus is limited; it cannot exceed a certain number of mmol per unit time. This limit is called the tubular maximum for phosphate (TmP). TmP varies inversely with parathyroid hormone (PTH) concentration; PTH thereby adjusts renal clearance of P_i. At filtered loads less than the TmP (for example, at low plasma P_i values), most or all of the filtered load is reabsorbed, and thus plasma phosphate levels can be at least partially maintained. By contrast, at filtered loads above the TmP, urinary phosphorus is a linear function of plasma phosphate (Bijvoet, 1969; Lemann, 1996; Nordin, 1989). In the healthy adult, urine phosphorus is essentially equal to absorbed diet phosphorus, less small amounts of phosphorus lost in shed cells of skin and intestinal mucosa.

This regulation of phosphorus excretion is apparent from early infancy. In infants, as in adults, the major site of regulation of phosphorus retention is at the kidney. In studies of infants receiving different calcium intakes (DeVizia et al., 1985; Moya et al., 1992; Williams et al., 1970; Ziegler and Fomon, 1983), phosphorus retention did not differ even with high amounts of dietary calcium (calcium:phosphorus [Ca:P] molar ratios of 0:6, 1:1, or 1.4:1). Any reduction in absorption of phosphorus due to high amounts of dietary calcium were compensated for by parallel reductions in renal phosphorus excretion (DeVizia et al., 1985; Fomon and Nelson, 1993; Moya et al., 1992). The least renal excretory work to maintain normal phosphorus homeostasis would be achieved with human milk as the major source of minerals during the first year of life.

Regulation of the Serum Inorganic Phosphate Concentration

P_i levels are only loosely regulated. Normal P_i levels decline with age from infancy to maturity (Table 5-1). The most likely reason for the

TABLE 5-1 Normative Values for Serum Inorganic
Phosphorus (mmol/liter) for Age

Age (y)	Mean	2.5 Percentile	97.5 Percentile
0–0.5	2.15	1.88	2.42
2	1.81	1.43	2.20
4	1.77	1.38	2.15
6	1.72	1.33	2.11
8	1.67	1.29	2.06
10	1.63	1.24	2.01
12	1.58	1.19	1.97
14	1.53	1.15	1.92
16	1.49	1.10	1.88
20	1.39	1.01	1.78
Adult	1.15	0.87	1.41

higher P_i in newborn infants than in older children and adults is the lower glomerular filtration rate (GFR) of infants. GFR is about 32 ml/min/1.73 m^2 at about 1 week of age, and rises to 87 at 4 to 6 months (Brodehl et al., 1982; Svenningsen and Lindquist, 1974). In the first months of life, plasma P_i concentration appears to be a reflection both of renal glomerular maturity and of the amount of dietary intake. Mean serum P_i appears to decline by about 0.3 mmol/liter (0.9 mg/dl) across the second half of the first year of life (Specker et al., 1986). Human milk-fed, compared with formula-fed, infants have a slightly lower plasma P_i (2.07 versus 2.25 mmol/liter or 6.4 versus 7.0 mg/dl) which is simply a function of differences in intake (Greer et al., 1982c; Specker et al., 1986); Caucasian compared with African American infants have a slightly higher plasma P_i irrespective of type of milk feeding (Specker et al., 1986).

The general relationship between absorbed phosphorus intake and plasma P_i in adults is set forth in Figure 5-1, derived by Nordin (1989) from the infusion studies of Bijvoet (1969). (In Bijovet's studies, a neutral phosphate solution was infused intravenously at a steadily increasing rate and produced a controlled hyperphosphatemia.) The achieved plasma P_i could thus be directly related to the quantity entering the circulation. Plasma P_i rises rapidly at low intakes, since the filtered load will be below the TmP, and little of the absorbed phosphorus will be lost in the urine (Figure 5-1). The steep, ascending portion of the curve thus represents a filling up of the extracellular fluid space with absorbed phosphate. At higher intakes, urinary excretion rises to match absorbed input and plasma levels change much more slowly.

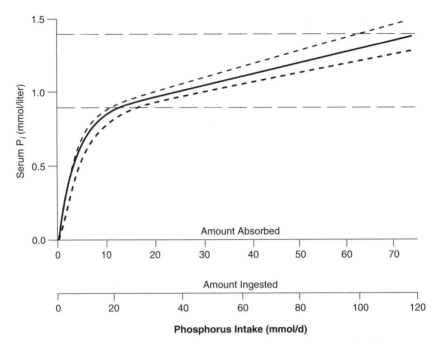

FIGURE 5-1 Relation of serum P_i to absorbed intake in adults with normal renal function. (See Nordin [1989] for further details.) The solid curve can be empirically approximated by the following equation: $P_i = 0.00765 \times AbsP + 0.8194 \times (1 - e^{(-0.2635 \times AbsP)})$, in which P_i = serum P_i (in mmol/liter), and AbsP = absorbed phosphorus intake (also in mmol). Solving this equation for the lower and upper limits of the normal range for P_i, as well as for its midpoint, yields the values presented in Table 5-1. The dashed horizontal lines represent approximate upper and lower limits of the normal range, while the dashed curves reflect the relationship between serum P_i and ingested intake for absorption efficiencies about 15 percent higher and lower than average. (© Robert P. Heaney, 1996. Reproduced with permission.)

The relationship shown in Figure 5-1 holds only in adult individuals with adequate renal function; that is, the slow rise of plasma P_i with rising phosphorus intake over most of the intake range applies only so long as excess absorbed phosphate can be spilled into the urine. However, in individuals with reduced renal function, phosphorus clearance remains essentially normal so long as GFR is at least 20 percent of mean adult normal values, largely because tubular reabsorption is reduced to match the reduction in filtered load. Below that level, excretion of absorbed phosphate requires higher and higher levels of plasma P_i to maintain a filtered load at least equal to the absorbed load. This is the reason for the hyperphosphatemia typically found in patients with end-stage renal disease.

Another process depleting the blood of P_i is mineralization of nucleated bone and cartilage matrix. The amorphous calcium phosphate formed in the first stages of mineralization exhibits a Ca:P molar ratio of about 1.33:1, or very close to the molar ratio of Ca:P in adult ECF. While outside of a mineralizing environment, ECF calcium and phosphorus concentrations are indefinitely stable at physiological pH and pCO_2, ECF is supersaturated in the presence of the hydroxyapatite crystal lattice. Hence, ECF supports calcium phosphate deposition only in the presence of a suitable crystal nucleus. As a consequence, in nonosseous tissues, ECF $[Ca^{2+}]$ and P_i concentrations will be essentially what can be measured in peripheral venous blood. However, at active bone-forming sites, ECF is depleted of both its calcium and its phosphate. Osteoblast function seems not to be appreciably affected by ECF $[Ca^{2+}]$, but like other tissues, the osteoblast needs a critical level of P_i in its bathing fluid for fully normal cellular functioning. Local P_i depletion both impairs osteoblast function and limits mineral deposition in previously deposited matrix. Finally, it should be noted that ECF P_i levels are indirectly supported by two mechanisms that amount to a weak, negative feedback type of control. One occurs via release of phosphate from bone, and the other via regulation of the renal 1-α hydroxylase. Still P_i concentration affects the responsiveness of the osteoclast to PTH: for any given PTH level, resorption is higher when P_i levels are low, and vice versa (Raisz and Niemann, 1969). High P_i values, by reducing bony responsiveness to PTH, lead to increased PTH secretion in order to maintain calcium homeostasis, and thereby to a lowering of ECF P_i. Similarly, high plasma P_i levels suppress renal synthesis of $1,25(OH)_2D$ (Portale et al., 1989), thereby slightly reducing net phosphorus absorption from the diet. Both mechanisms reduce phosphorus input into the ECF when P_i is high and augment it when P_i is low. However, in neither circumstance is the effect on plasma P_i more than modest. (See below for other special circumstances.)

Factors Affecting the Phosphorus Requirement

Bioavailability

Most food sources exhibit good phosphorus bioavailability. There is, however, one major exception. All plant seeds (beans, peas, cereals, nuts) contain a nonprotoplasmic, storage form of phosphate, phytic acid. The digestive systems of most mammals cannot hydrolyze phytic acid, and hence its phosphorus is not directly available. However, some foods contain phytase, as do some colonic bacteria. Thus, a variable amount of phytate phosphorus becomes available. However, in gnotobiotic animals, no phytate phosphorus is absorbed (Wise and Gilburt, 1982). In at least one study (Parfitt et al., 1964), up to 50 percent of phytate phosphorus was absorbed, representing the combined effect of food phytases and bacterial enzymes. Also, yeasts can hydrolyze phytate, and thus whole grain cereals incorporated into leavened bread products have higher phosphate bioavailability than cereal grains used, for example, in unleavened bread or breakfast cereals. Finally, unabsorbed calcium in the digestate complexes with phytic acid and interferes with bacterial hydrolysis of phytate (Sandberg et al., 1993; Wise and Gilburt, 1982). This may be a part of the explanation for calcium's interference with phosphorus absorption.

In infants, both the quantity of ingested phosphorus and the dietary bioavailability vary by type of milk fed. The efficiency of absorption is highest from human milk (85 to 90 percent) (Williams et al., 1970), intermediate from cow milk (72 percent) (Williams et al., 1970; Ziegler and Fomon, 1983), and lowest from soy formulas, which contain phytic acid (~59 percent) (Ziegler and Fomon, 1983). Because infant formulas contain substantially greater amounts of phosphorus than human milk, the absorbed phosphorus from cow milk and soy formulas is twice that attained by human milk-fed infants (Moya et al., 1992). The higher amounts of phosphorus (and also calcium and other mineral elements) in formulas that are based on cow milk or soy isolate protein effectively offset the lower mineral absorption of these formulas relative to human milk.

Relatively low intakes of phosphorus, as occur with human milk, may actually confer an advantage to the infant by virtue of the low residual phosphorus in the lower bowel. Low intestinal phosphorus concentrations lower the fecal pH (Manz, 1992), which in turn may reduce proliferation of potentially pathogenic microorganisms and provide an immune protective effect.

Nutrient-Nutrient Interactions

Calcium. In the past, considerable emphasis was placed on the Ca:P ratio of the diet (for example, Chinn, 1981), particularly in infant nutrition (for example, Fomon and Nelson, 1993). The concept has some utility under conditions of rapid growth (in which a large share of the ingested nutrients is converted into tissue mass), but it has no demonstrable relevance in adults. An optimal ratio ensures that, if intake of one nutrient is adequate for growth, the intake of the associated nutrient will also be adequate without a wasteful surplus of one or the other. However, the ratio by itself is of severely limited value, in that there is little merit to having the ratio "correct" if the absolute quantities of both nutrients are insufficient to support optimal growth.

Furthermore, the intake ratio, by itself, fails to take into account both differing bioavailabilities and physiological adaptive responses. For example, in term-born infants during the first year of life, a higher calcium content of soy-based formulas was found to reduce phosphorus absorption, but phosphorus retention was similar because of offsetting changes in renal phosphorus output (DeVizia et al., 1985). Substitution of lactose with sucrose and/or hydrolyzed corn syrup solids had no effect on the efficiency of phosphorus absorption from formulas based on cow milk (Moya et al., 1992) or soy protein (Ziegler and Fomon, 1983).

Estimates of optimal Ca:P intake ratios have frequently been based on the calcium and phosphorus needs of bone building. The molar ratio of Ca:P in synthetic hydroxyapatite is 1.67:1; in actual bone mineral, usually closer to 1.5:1; and in amorphous calcium-phosphate (the first mineral deposited at the mineralizing site), 1.3:1 (Nordin, 1976). However, during growth, soft tissue will be accreting phosphorus as well. On average, lean soft tissue growth accounts for about 1 mmol (31 mg) phosphorus for every 5 mmol (155 mg) added to bone (Diem, 1970). Since soft tissue accretion of calcium is negligible compared with skeletal calcium accretion, an absorbed Ca:P molar ratio sufficient to support the sum of bony and soft tissue growth would be ~1.3:1 (assuming equivalent degrees of renal conservation of both nutrients). The corresponding ingested intake ratio must consider the differing absorption efficiencies for dietary calcium and phosphorus. In infants, with net absorptions for calcium and phosphorus of approximately 60 and 80 percent respectively, the intake ratio matching tissue accretion would be ~2:1 (see also the section "Birth through 12 Months," below). This value is somewhat higher than the Ca:P molar ratio of human milk, which in most populations is in the range of 1.5:1 (Fomon and Nelson, 1993).

Human milk must be presumed to be optimal for the infant's nutritional needs. The disparity between its ratio of ~1.5:1 and the ingested ratio calculated above reflects both the uncertainties in the estimates on which the calculation is based and the limitations inherent in using such calculations.

If growth were the only consideration, the intake ratio would have to be substantially higher than 2:1 after infancy, because calcium absorption drops more sharply with age than does phosphorus absorption (Abrams et al., 1997b; Fomon and Nelson, 1993). However, as larger fractions of ingested food are used for energy (and a correspondingly smaller proportion for growth), the notion of a dietary Ca:P molar ratio has little meaning or value, particularly since, on a mixed diet, there is likely to be a relative surplus of phosphorus. Under such circumstances it would be inappropriate to conclude, simply on the basis of a departure from some theoretical Ca:P ratio, either that calcium intake should be elevated or, phosphorus intake reduced. In balance studies in human adults, Ca:P molar ratios ranging from 0.08:1 to 2.40:1 (a 30-fold range) had no effect on either calcium balance or calcium absorption (Heaney and Recker, 1982; Spencer et al., 1965, 1978a). Thus, for the reasons cited, there is little or no evidence for relating the two nutrients, one to the other, during most of human life.

Intake of Phosphorus

The USDA Continuing Survey of Food Intake of Individuals (CS-FII) in 1994, adjusted by the method of Nusser et al. (1996), indicated that the mean daily phosphorus intake from food in males aged 9 and over was 1,495 mg (48.2 mmol) (fifth percentile = 874 mg [28.2 mmol]; fiftieth percentile = 1,445 mg [46.6 mmol]; ninety-fifth percentile = 2,282 mg [73.6 mmol]) (see Appendix D for data tables). The mean daily intake in females aged 9 and over was 1,024 mg (33 mmol) (fifth percentile = 620 mg [20 mmol]; fiftieth percentile = 1,001 mg [32.3 mmol]; ninety-fifth percentile = 1,510 mg [48.7 mmol]). In both sexes, intakes decreased at ages 51 and over. The NHANES III data show similar median intake values (Alaimo et al., 1994). National survey data for Canada are not available.

Both extent of usage of phosphate salts as additives and the amount per serving have increased substantially over the past 20 years, and the nutrient databases may not reflect these changes (Calvo and Park, 1996). For that reason, phosphorus intake may be underestimated for certain individuals who rely heavily on processed foods. However, one comparison of calculated intakes with analyzed intake data from the U.S. Food and Drug Administration's Total Diet Study found slight overestimates of phosphorus intake (by an average of 61 mg [2 mmol]/day or 5 percent of the total intake) when intakes were calculated using USDA's nutrient database (Pennington and Wilson, 1990).

Because of the uncertainty about phosphorus values for processed foods in nutrient databases, trends in phosphorus intake may be difficult to ascertain. Daily intakes of women aged 19 to 50 years from USDA's national surveys averaged 965 mg (31.1 mmol) in 1977, 1,039 mg (33.5 mmol) in 1985, and 1,022 mg (33.0 mmol) in 1994 (Cleveland et al., 1996; USDA, 1985). Thus, it appears that intakes from foods increased about 8 percent between 1977 and 1985, but then decreased slightly between 1985 and 1994. Food supply data show a larger increase in phosphorus consumption: 12 percent from 1980 through 1994 (from 1,480 to 1,680 mg [47.7 to 54.2 mmol]/day per capita) (USDA, 1997). However, disappearance data may be unreliable for detecting trends because phosphate additives (such as those in cola beverages) are not included. Disappearance data on phosphorus-containing additives show that the use of these additives has increased by 17 percent over the last decade (Calvo, 1993). These figures also do not reflect actual consumption, because not all phosphates included in disappearance data are actually consumed, (for example, blends of sodium tripolyphosphate and sodium hexametaphosphate are used in brines for curing meat, but the brine is rinsed off and not consumed). Nevertheless, taken together, these data suggest a substantial increase in phosphorus consumption, in the range of 10 to 15 percent, over the past 20 years.

Food Sources of Phosphorus

Phosphates are found in foods as naturally occurring components of biological molecules and as food additives in the form of various phosphate salts. These salts are used in processed foods for nonnutrient functions, such as moisture retention, smoothness, and binding.

In infants, dietary intake of phosphorus spans a wide range, depending on whether the food is human milk, cow milk, adapted cow milk formula, or soy formula (see Table 5-2). Moreover, the phosphorus concentration of human milk declines with progressing lactation, especially between 4 and 25 weeks of lactation (Atkinson et al., 1995). By contrast, more of the variation in dietary intake of phosphorus in adults is due to differences in total food intake and less to differences in food composition. Phosphorus contents of adult diets average about 62 mg (2 mmol)/100 kcal in both sexes (Carroll et al., 1983), and phosphorus:energy ratios exhibit a coefficient of variation of only

TABLE 5-2 Average Phosphorus Content and
Calcium:Phosphorus Molar Ratio of Various Infant Feedings

Feeding Type	P (mmol/liter)	Ca:P Molar Ratio
Human milk[a]		
1 week	5.1 ± 0.9	1.3:1
4 weeks	4.8 ± 0.8	1.4:1
16 weeks	3.9 ± 0.5	1.5:1
Cows' milk formula	12	1.0:1
Soy formula[b]	15	1.2:1
Whole cows' milk	30	1.0:1

[a] Milk phosphorus at three different weeks of lactation (Atkinson et al., 1995).

[b] Phosphorus content of soy formula includes about 3 mmol/L, present as phytate phosphorus which is likely not to be bioavailable (DeVizia and Mansi, 1992).

about one-third that of total phosphorus intake. Nevertheless, individuals with high dairy product intakes will have diets with higher phosphorus density values, since the phosphorus density of cow milk is higher than that of most other foods in a typical diet. The same is true for diets high in colas and a few other soft drinks that use phosphoric acid as the acidulant. A 12-ounce serving of such beverages contains about 50 mg (< 2 mmol), which is only 5 percent of the typical intake of an adult woman. However, when consumed in a quantity of five or more servings per day, such beverages may contribute substantially to total phosphorus intake.

Intake from Supplements

Phosphorus supplements are not widely used in the United States. Based on a national survey in 1986, about 10 percent of U.S. adults and 6 percent of children aged 2 to 6 years took supplements containing phosphorus (Moss et al., 1989). Usage by men and women was similar, as was the dose taken by users: a median of about 120 mg (3.9 mmol)/day and a ninety-fifth percentile of 448 mg (14.5 mmol)/day. Young children who took supplements had a median supplemental intake of only 48 mg (1.5 mmol)/day and a ninety-fifth percentile of intake of 200 mg (6.5 mmol)/day.

Effects of Inadequate Phosphorus Intake

Hypophosphatemia and Phosphorus Depletion

Inadequate phosphorus intake is expressed as hypophosphatemia.

Only limited quantities of phosphate are stored within cells, and most tissues depend upon ECF P_i for their metabolic phosphate. When ECF P_i levels are low, cellular dysfunction follows. At a whole organism level, the effects of hypophosphatemia include anorexia, anemia, muscle weakness, bone pain, rickets and osteomalacia, general debility, increased susceptibility to infection, paresthesias, ataxia, confusion, and even death (Lotz et al., 1968). The muscle weakness, which involves especially proximal muscle groups when prolonged or severe, can lead to muscle fiber degeneration. The skeleton will exhibit either rickets in children or osteomalacia in adults. In both, the disorder consists of a failure to mineralize forming growth plate cartilage or bone matrix, together with impairment of chondroblast and osteoblast function (Lotz et al., 1968). These severe manifestations are usually confined to situations in which ECF P_i falls below ~0.3 mmol/liter (0.9 mg/dl).

Phosphorus is so ubiquitous in various foods that near total starvation is required to produce dietary phosphorus deficiency. However, movement of sugar into cells pulls P_i into the cells as well. Refeeding of energy-depleted individuals, either orally or parenterally, without adequate attention to supplying P_i, can precipitate extreme, even fatal, hypophosphatemia (Bushe, 1986; Dale et al., 1986; Knochel, 1977, 1985; Ritz, 1982; Silvis and Paragas, 1972; Stein et al., 1966; Travis et al., 1971; Young et al., 1985). Such outcomes can occur on recovery from alcoholic bouts, from diabetic ketoacidosis, and on refeeding with calorie-rich sources without paying attention to phosphorus needs. Also, aluminum-containing antacids, by binding diet phosphorus in the gut, can, when consumed in high doses, produce hypophosphatemia in their own right, as well as aggravate phosphate deficiency related to other problems (Lotz et al., 1968).

In full-term infants, severe hypophosphatemia from purely dietary causes is virtually unknown. It is likely to occur only in situations of poorly managed parenteral nutrition (in which intakes of phosphate are inadequate), with inappropriate administration of fluid and electrolyte therapy (which causes excessive renal phosphorus loss), or with rapid refeeding after prolonged dietary restriction (Koo and Tsang, 1997; Weinsier and Krumdieck, 1981). In the case of severely malnourished infants, especially with accompanying severe diarrhea, hypophosphatemia has been reported with an associated hypokalemia and hypotonia (Freiman et al., 1982).

ESTIMATING REQUIREMENTS FOR PHOSPHORUS

Selection of Indicators for Estimating the Phosphorus Requirement

In the past, indicators have not generally been used for the phosphorus requirement. Instead, phosphorus recommendations have been tied to calcium, usually on an equimass or equimolar basis. As noted above, that approach is unsatisfactory. The two indicators that will be considered here for the Estimated Average Requirement (EAR) are phosphorus balance and serum P_i.

Phosphorus Balance

Although phosphorus balance might seem to be a logical indicator of nutritional adequacy, it is not an adequate criterion, since an adult can be in zero balance at an intake inadequate to maintain serum P_i within the normal range. Even during growth, balance will be positive in direct proportion to soft tissue and bony accumulation, but so long as plasma P_i is high enough, the degree of positive balance will be limited either by the genetic programming or by availability of other nutrients. Furthermore, the balance data that would be needed to bracket the requirement during growth are not available. And during senescence, if there is loss of bone or soft tissue mass, phosphorus balance will be negative. However, so long as plasma P_i remains within normal limits, these balances will reflect other changes occurring in the body and will not be an indicator of the adequacy of dietary phosphorus.

Serum P_i

Because phosphorus intake directly affects serum P_i, and because both hypo- and hyperphosphatemia directly result in dysfunction or disease, the most logical indicator of nutritional adequacy of phosphorus intake is serum P_i. If serum P_i is above the lower limits of normal for age, phosphorus intake may be considered adequate to meet cellular and bone formation needs of healthy individuals. The relationship between P_i and phosphorus intake has, however, been clearly established only for adults (see "Regulation of the Serum Inorganic Phosphate Concentration"), and while the adverse effects of low serum P_i are well understood during growth, it is harder to define the critical values for phosphorus intake associated with the normal range of P_i values in infants and children. For that reason, estimates of requirements will be based on a factorial approach in infants, children, and adolescents and on serum P_i in adults.

There is a clear and absolute requirement for phosphorus during growth. At each growth stage, average net daily additions of bone and soft tissue mass can be approximated. Thus, the absorbed phosphorus intake needed to support such tissue accumulation can be readily estimated (see below for each relevant physiological state). In the mature adult, the requirement can be defined instead simply as the intake needed to maintain the plasma P_i within the normal range. As with all continuous clinical variables, there is a gray zone between the empirical normal range and values associated with evident deficiency disease. Thus, the lower end of the established normal range for serum P_i is 0.8 to 0.9 mmol/liter (2.5 to 2.8 mg/dl). Clear evidence of bony or soft tissue dysfunction are not common until serum P_i levels drop below 0.3 to 0.5 mmol/liter (0.9 to 1.6 mg/dl).

Although it is not likely that all levels of P_i within the normal range are equally salubrious for cell functioning, insufficient information exists to allow selection of any one value within the population normal range as superior to any other. The fact that growth and epiphyseal cartilage maturation in children are abnormal at even adult normal levels of P_i supports the assumption that subnormal P_i values are not adequate to sustain optimal tissue function. Therefore, in what follows, the requirement will be based on the intake associated with maintenance of serum P_i at the bottom end of the normal range. A limitation of this approach lies in the fact that available data on P_i apply mostly to the fasting state, whereas it is the integrated, 24-hour P_i that is most closely related to absorbed phosphorus intake and that constitutes the actual exposure that the tissues experience. Moreover, fasting serum P_i is only weakly correlated with current phosphorus intake (for example, Portale et al., 1987).

The approach is to define, as well as the available evidence will permit, the lower limit of normal for serum P_i in healthy individuals of various ages (Table 5-1). The exclusion of formula-fed babies from the infant data is essential since some formulas, and cow milk especially, have higher phosphorus levels than required, and hence they result in higher values for serum P_i. This fact precludes their use in establishing normative data for the requirement.

FINDINGS BY LIFE STAGE AND GENDER GROUP

Birth through 12 Months

There are no functional criteria for phosphorus status that reflect response to dietary intake in infants. Thus recommended intakes of phosphorus are based on Adequate Intakes (AIs) that reflect observed mean intakes of infants fed principally with human milk.

Indicators Used to Set the AI

Human Milk. Human milk is recognized as the optimal source of milk for infants throughout at least the first year of life and as a sole nutritional source for infants during the first 4 to 6 months of life (IOM, 1991). Furthermore, there are no reports of exclusively human milk-fed, vitamin D-replete, full-term infants manifesting any evidence of phosphorus deficiency. Therefore, consideration of the AI for phosphorus in infants is based on data from term-born healthy infants fed human milk as the principal fluid milk during the first year of life. The approach was to set the AI at the mean of usual intakes of phosphorus as derived from studies where intake of human milk was measured using test weighing, and intake of food was determined by dietary records for 3 days or more. The following limited data on infants were also reviewed and considered as supportive evidence for the derived AIs.

Serum P_i. Using the term-born infant fed human milk as the model, the target range for serum P_i (the most appropriate biochemical indicator of dietary phosphorus adequacy during early life), is 2.42 to 1.88 mmol/liter (7.5 to 5.8 mg/dl). This wide range is a function of the precipitous fall in serum P_i during the first 6 weeks of life (Greer et al., 1982b). The reasons for the well-documented decline in serum P_i in infants are: (1) an increase in GFR as the infant's kidneys mature postnatally (McCrory et al., 1950), (2) a decline in phosphorus concentration in breast milk with advancing lactation (Table 5-2), and (3) possibly an inappropriate PTH response to rising serum P_i during early neonatal life (DeVizia and Mansi, 1992). However, there is evidence that the parathyroid glands can respond in early life since high phosphorus feedings (Ca:P molar ratio 1:2.5) resulted in serum PTH, which was significantly higher than in breast-fed infants at 2, 7, and 14 days of age

(Janas et al., 1988). Similarly, in infants 4 to 6 months of age, the feeding of infant cereal in addition to standard infant formula, compared with formula alone, produced a significantly higher serum PTH in young infants. This result is often attributed to the dietary phosphorus load from the cereal (Bainbridge et al., 1996), but probably it is due to phytate complexation of food calcium with consequent reduction in calcium absorption.

Balance. Mean phosphorus intakes from human milk of 102 mg (3.3 mmol)/day in healthy infants (*n* = 33) supported a positive phosphorus balance; an efficiency of absorption of 85 percent provided a net retention of 59 mg (1.9 mmol)/day (Fomon and Nelson, 1993). In considering the possible functional indicators, positive rates of bone mineral accretion have been observed in human milk-fed infants over the first 6 months of life (Hillman et al., 1988; Mimouni et al., 1993; Specker et al., 1997). Although the absolute amount of bone mineral accrued over the first 6 months (measured both for the humerus alone and for the whole body) was less in infants fed human milk than in those fed modified formulas (Hillman et al., 1988; Specker et al., 1997), this difference does not have known long-term consequences. By 12 months of age whole body mineral content was similar among groups irrespective of feeding in the first 6 months (Specker et al., 1997). Perhaps the slower initial accretion of bone demonstrated in human milk-fed infants represents the physiological norm.

Accretion. Increments of body content of phosphorus over the first 6 months of life are estimated to range from 11 to 28 mg (0.35 to 0.9 mmol)/day (Fomon and Nelson, 1993); amounts that are easily obtained from human milk (Fomon and Nelson, 1993; Williams et al., 1970). Increments in whole body phosphorus between 6 and 12 months are calculated to be about 31 mg (1 mmol)/day. Assuming an efficiency of absorption of 52 percent (from high-calcium, soy-based formula) (DeVizia et al., 1985) or higher, intakes above 90 mg (2.9 mmol) are probably in excess of functional needs. Unfortunately no information exists on response of infants fed varying phosphorus intakes in the second 6 months of life.

Differences in phosphorus needs between infants fed human milk and those fed infant formula are considered in the "Special Considerations" section.

AI Summary: Ages 0 through 6 months

The estimate of the AI is based on two studies, Allen et al. (1991) and Butte et al. (1984), which reported mean intake of human milk of 780 ml/day based on test weighing of term-born infants, and a reported average phosphorus concentration in human milk after the first month of lactation of 124 mg/liter (4 mmol/liter) (Atkinson et al., 1995) (Table 5-2). Using the mean value for intake of human milk (780 ml/day), the AI would be 100 mg (3.2 mmol)/day for infants 0 through 6 months of age. Based on the available data on urinary and serum P_i, this phosphorus intake obtained from human milk over the first 6 months of life results in a circulating P_i concentration that does not require excessive renal excretion of phosphorus.

AI Summary: Ages 7 through 12 months

The basis of the AI for this age group is the average intake of phosphorus from human milk plus that obtained from infant foods. For infants over 6 months of age, there are no available data on dietary phosphorus intakes from the combination of human milk and solid foods. Thus, values for the phosphorus intake from solid food were derived from data on formula-fed infants, assuming that infants who are fed human milk have similar intakes of solid food during this time.

Based on the data from Dewey et al. (1984), mean milk intake by infants was 600 ml/day, and assuming a milk phosphorus concentration of 124 mg/liter (4 mmol/liter), the average phosphorus intake from human milk alone would be 75 mg (2.4 mmol)/day. To determine total phosphorus intake during the ages 7 through 12 months, an estimate of the contribution of solid foods must be made. Using the recent data of Specker et al. (1997), 40 infants fed standard formula and solid food had mean phosphorus intake from solid food of 151 mg (4.9 mmol) and 255 mg (8.2 mmol)/day at 9 and 12 months, respectively. This finding is comparable to the dietary phosphorus from solid foods estimated to be 155 to 186 mg (5 to 6 mmol)/day based on data from 24-hour dietary intakes from the 1976–1980 NHANES II for infants aged 7 to 12 months (Montalto and Benson, 1986).

Based on the literature cited above, the mean daily total phosphorus intake from human milk (75 mg [2.4 mmol]) and solid foods (200 mg [6.5 mmol]) is 275 mg (8.9 mmol) between the ages 7 and 12 months. The data are averaged for solid food intake based on the above observations of infants. Thus, the AI for infants ages 7 through 12 months is set at 275 mg (8.9 mmol)/day, which falls between the fifth and tenth percentiles for phosphorus intake of infants 7 to 11 months of age from the 1994 CSFII intake data. However, it must be emphasized that this database specifically excluded infants fed human milk, and thus the formula or cow milk in the infants' diets would elevate the population distribution and mean phosphorus intakes.

AI for Infants   **0 through 6 months**   **100 mg (3.2 mmol)/day**
                   7 through 12 months **275 mg (8.9 mmol)/day**

Special Considerations

Infant Formula. Much of the available data on phosphorus intake in infancy, particularly during the second 6 months of life, were collected prior to the 1980s when infants were often fed diluted evaporated milk formulas and/or undiluted cow milk, in addition to infant cereals and solid foods. These foods were introduced at an earlier age than is the general practice in the 1990s. If cow milk were fed instead of human milk, the phosphorus intake from milk and solid foods would be about 2.5-fold higher (Montalto and Benson, 1986). Although dietary phosphorus is generally well absorbed (72 percent from whole cow milk versus 85 percent from human milk [Fomon and Nelson, 1993]), there is evidence that dietary phosphorus intake above 310 mg (10 mmol) results in a linear increase in fecal excretion.

Several studies have reported significantly lower values for serum P_i in infants fed human milk versus modified cow milk-based formulas; this finding is logical since formulas provide about three times the amount of dietary phosphorus as human milk (Fomon and Nelson, 1993; Janas et al., 1988; Lealman et al., 1976; Specker et al., 1986). However, the mean serum P_i in the formula-fed infants fell within the range observed for human milk-fed infants within the first 6 months of life. Thus, the higher intakes from modified formulas are not likely to be of physiological significance. With maturation of the renal phosphate excretion mechanism sometime after 6 weeks of life (Brodehl et al., 1982), infants should be able to adapt to a wide range of phosphorus intakes. Mean phosphorus intake from a mixed diet of formula or cow milk and solid foods ranged between 490 and 800 mg (16 and 26 mmol)/day for infants 9 to 12 months of age (Specker et al., 1997). Since in this study there were no significant differences in weight, length, or bone mineral content between infant groups, the higher intakes conferred no benefit.

Ages 1 through 3 Years

Indicator Used to Set the EAR

Accretion. Since there are no data on serum P_i or phosphorus balance and limited information on bone mineral content for children aged 1 through 3 years, a surrogate indicator had to be adopted to set the EAR. An estimation of body accretion was used based on known tissue composition and growth rates. Rates of accretion of phosphorus in bone and soft tissue (for example, lean mass) during this period of growth were then corrected for predicted efficiency of absorption and urinary losses to derive an EAR using the factorial approach.

The phosphorus requirement for bone growth can be estimated from one of two methods: (1) the phosphorus content of bony tissue gained over this age range as derived from the body composition of Fomon et al. (1982), or (2) the known increments in whole body bone mineral content using the method of dual energy x-ray absorptiometry (DXA) (Ellis et al., 1997). For both approaches, a value of 19 percent by weight was used as the phosphorus content of bone. The phosphorus content of lean tissue is assumed to be 0.23 percent based on known composition of muscle (Pennington, 1994). The computations for tissue accretion are summarized in Table 5-3. The overall estimated mean value for both sexes combined is 54 mg (1.74 mmol) phosphorus accreted per day.

The value derived for phosphorus accretion in lean and osseous tissue is supported by estimates of phosphorus retention, 10 g (323 mmol)/kg body weight gained, derived from balance studies in children aged 4 to 12 years (Fomon et al., 1982), when corrected to the average weight gain for children aged 1 through 3 years. When males and females are averaged, a total of 2.36 kg of weight is gained over this period (Fomon et al., 1982); thus a total phosphorus increment of 23.6 g (768 mmol) is gained. A daily accretion of phosphorus is then predicted to be 62 mg (2.0 mmol), which is close to that calculated above for lean plus osseous tissue accretion.

The value derived for phosphorus accretion was then employed in a factorial model to obtain the EAR. It is known that phosphorus in urine increases with phosphorus intake, described by an equation derived by Lemann (1996) in adults. This approach was adopted here since no such relationship has been developed for children. Using the equation: $P_{urine} = 1.73 + 0.512 \times P_{intake}$ (in mmol/day), and an intake of 310 mg (10 mmol)/day, predicted urinary

TABLE 5-3 Accretion of Phosphorus (P) in Bone and Lean Tissue of Children Aged 1 to 3 Years Using Growth and Body Composition Data from Fomon et al. (1982)

Gender/ Age (y)	Change in Weight (g/y)	Change in Lean (FFBM-osseous) (g/y)	Lean-Tissue P[a] (g/y)	Osseous P (g/y)	Bone P[b] (g/y)	Total P Gain[c] (mg/d [mmol/ d])
Males						
1–2	2,440	1,539	3.54	94	17.8	58 (1.9)
2–3	2,085	2,001	4.60	84	16.0	56 (1.8)
Females						
1–2	2,730	2,397	5.51	75	14.2	54 (1.7)
2–3	2,190	1,950	4.48	67	12.7	47 (1.5)
Mean, both sexes						54 (1.7)

NOTE: Based on recent data (Ellis et al., 1997), the daily accretion of phosphorus in bone is calculated from cross-sectional measures of whole body bone mineral content in children. The values are almost identical to those calculated using Fomon et al. (1982) body composition data. Compared were the values listed vertically in the Bone P column above, the data from Ellis yield values of 16 g and 14 g for males, and 15 g and 12 g for females, at the respective ages. This comparability of values obtained by two very different methods gives credence to the method applied for this report in deriving the EARs.

[a] Assuming a phosphorus content of soft tissue of 0.23 percent.
[b] Assuming a phosphorus content of bone of 19 percent.
[c] Calculated from sum of accretion of P in lean and bone/year divided by 365 days.

excretion would be 213 mg (6.9 mmol)/day. At this intake of phosphorus, obligatory losses and predicted accretion values will be generously covered. Phosphorus intakes in excess of this amount would simply lead to increased urinary loss. When urinary excretion is added to the accrued phosphorus of 54 mg (1.74 mmol)/day (Table 5-3), there is a daily need for dietary phosphorus of 267 mg (8.6 mmol)/day.

A conservative estimate of efficiency of phosphorus absorption of 70 percent was used, as suggested for children aged 9 through 18 years, which is slightly higher than the 60 percent figure for adults (Lemann, 1996). No data are available that provide a value for percent efficiency of absorption from the typical mixed diet in early childhood. Using the equation: EAR = (accretion + urinary loss) divided by fractional absorption, an EAR of 380 mg (12.3 mmol)/day is derived by the factorial approach.

EAR Summary: Ages 1 through 3 Years

Based on the factorial estimate, an EAR of 380 mg (12.3 mmol)/day is set for children ages 1 through 3 years.

EAR for Children   1 through 3 years   380 mg (12.3 mmol)/day

Utilizing the 1994 CSFII intake data, adjusted for day-to-day variations (Nusser et al., 1996), the value derived for the EAR of 380 mg (12.3 mmol)/day represents a low dietary intake of phosphorus, as it falls below the first percentile (416 mg [13.4 mmol]/day) for phosphorus intake for children aged 1 through 3 years (see Appendix D). The EAR value will provide for the calculated physiological need for phosphorus accretion in lean and bone mass, accounting for the expected urinary phosphorus loss at that dietary intake. Because urinary excretion rises linearly with increasing dietary intake of phosphorus, it does not seem appropriate to set the EAR at an amount that exceeds the physiological needs for growth and maintenance.

Determination of the Recommended Dietary Allowance: Ages 1 through 3 Years

The variance in requirements cannot be determined from the available data. Thus, a coefficient of variation (CV) of 10 percent (1 standard deviation [SD]) is assumed, which results in an Recommended Dietary Allowance (RDA) of 460 mg (14.8 mmol)/day.

RDA for Children   1 through 3 years   460 mg (14.8 mmol)/day

Ages 4 through 8 Years

Indicator Used to Set the EAR

Accretion. The rationale for using a factorial approach based on the surrogate criteria of phosphorus accretion of bone and soft tissue is the same for children ages 4 through 8 years as for children ages 1 through 3 years. The surrogate indicator of tissue accretion was used since there are no data on phosphorus balance in this age group, with the exception of a study by Wang et al. (1930). These

TABLE 5-4 Accretion of Phosphorus (P) in Bone and Lean
Tissue of Children Aged 4 to 8 Years Using Growth and Body
Composition Data from Fomon et al. (1982)

Gender/ Age (y)	Change in Weight (g/y)	Change in Lean (FFBM-osseous) (g/y)	Lean-Tissue P[a] (g/y)	Osseous P (g/y)	Bone P[b] (g/y)	Total P Gain[c] (mg/d [mmol/ d])
Males						
4–6	2,000	1,841	4.2	89	16.9	58 (1.9)
6–8	2,305	1,957	4.5	99	18.8	64 (2.1)
Females						
4–6	1,780	1,500	3.45	54	10.3	38 (1.2)
6–8	2,660	1,647	3.79	57	10.8	40 (1.3)
Mean, both sexes						50 (1.6)

NOTE: Based on recent data (Ellis et al., 1997), the daily accretion of phosphorus in bone is calculated from cross-sectional measures of whole body bone mineral content in children. The values are almost identical to those calculated using Fomon et al. (1982) body composition data. Compared were the values listed vertically in the Bone P column above, the data from Ellis yield values of 16 g and 14 g for males, and 15 g and 12 g for females, at the respective ages. This comparability of values obtained by two very different methods gives credence to the method applied for this report in deriving the EARs.

[a] Assuming a phosphorus content of soft tissue of 0.23 percent.
[b] Assuming a phosphorus content of bone of 19 percent.
[c] Calculated from sum of accretion of P in lean and bone/year divided by 365 days.

data were thought to be inadmissible since the variations in intake were accomplished by adding a calcium and phosphorus salt, and the methods used to measure phosphorus were not those used currently and may have led to analytical differences that would have made the data not applicable today. No data are available on serum phosphorus or phosphorus balance at various phosphorus intakes in children aged 4 through 8 years.

To estimate tissue accretion of phosphorus, the compositions of lean and osseous tissue were calculated based on body weight of children growing from 4 through 8 years and known content of phosphorus in these tissues. (The computations are summarized in Table 5-4.) In calculating the accretion of phosphorus over this age interval, it is apparent that there are not great differences in phosphorus accumulation between ages 4 to 6 and 6 to 8 years. This provides support for combining the ages of 4 through 8 years in terms of phosphorus needs. The overall mean value for males of 62 mg (2.0 mmol)/day phosphorus accrued is in the same range as the value 68.2 mg (2.2 mmol)/day computed from the phosphorus composition of weight gain from Sheikh et al. as cited in the review by Lemann (1996). The slightly lower value of 40.8 mg (1.3 mmol)/day for females presumably reflects the differences in the amount of bone and lean tissue between the sexes at this age interval.

The value derived for phosphorus accretion of lean and osseous tissue is supported by estimates of phosphorus retention from balance studies in children aged 4 to 12 years; that is, phosphorus retention of 10 g (323 mmol)/kg body weight gained (Fomon et al., 1982), when applied to the average weight gain over this age interval. For males, ~2.15 kg are gained each year over this period (Fomon et al., 1982); thus a total increment of 21.6 g (697 mmol) of phosphorus is gained each year. Daily accretion of phosphorus is then predicted to be 60 mg (1.9 mmol). For females, daily phosphorus accretion calculated in this manner would be 62 mg (2.0 mmol). These estimates are similar to those calculated by summing phosphorus accretion in lean and bony compartments (Table 5-4).

For the factorial estimate of the EAR for children ages 4 through 8 years, as outlined previously for children ages 1 through 3 years, and an accretion value of 62 mg (2.0 mmol)/day, a value of 405 mg (13.1 mmol)/day was derived. The assumptions for efficiency of phosphorus absorption and urinary loss of phosphorus are identical to that used for the 1 through 3 years age group.

EAR Summary: Ages 4 through 8 Years

The estimated EAR for boys and girls ages 4 through 8 years is 405 mg (13.1 mmol)/day.

EAR for Children   4 through 8 years   405 mg (13.1 mmol)/day

Utilizing the 1994 CSFII intake data, adjusted for day-to-day variations (Nusser et al., 1996), this value derived for the EAR again represents a low dietary intake of phosphorus, as it falls below the first percentile of intake, 537 mg (17.3 mmol)/day, for phosphorus intakes of children aged 4 through 8 years (see Appendix D). Since excess phosphorus intake will be excreted, consuming intakes in excess of physiological needs by such a magnitude is not likely of any consequence.

Determination of the RDA: Ages 4 through 8 Years

The variance in requirements cannot be determined from the available data. Thus, a CV of 10 percent (1 SD) is assumed, resulting in an RDA of 500 mg (16.1 mmol)/day.

RDA for Children   4 through 8 years   500 mg (16.1 mmol)/day

Ages 9 through 13 and 14 through 18 Years

Indicators Used to Set the EAR

During the rapid growth period of adolescence, the most logical basis for estimating the phosphorus requirement would be from observation of the balance plateau, that is, the intake level above which no further phosphorus retention occurs, just as was done for the calcium requirement (see Chapter 4). Unfortunately, only a few phosphorus balance studies have been conducted in this age group, and insufficient data exist across a range of intakes to determine maximal retention. As an alternative, the same approach using tissue accretion used for the 1 through 3 and 4 through 8 years age groups was employed.

Accretion. Phosphorus intakes necessary to meet the needs for the addition of bone and soft tissue during this period of rapid growth can be calculated and adjusted for by urinary output and absorptive efficiency. The main limitation of this approach for this age category is that tissue accretion values are not available for adolescents beyond 14 years; thus, predicted needs for older adolescents may not be optimal to support any growth spurts beyond this age.

To estimate phosphorus requirement from tissue accretion, longitudinal data and a large database of cross-sectional data are available and represent very recent databases. Slemenda and colleagues (1994) conducted a 3-year longitudinal study in 90 white children aged 6 to 14 years at baseline. They showed increases in weight during this time of 10.9 ± 4.3 kg for the 44 prepubertal children, 19.6 ± 0.9 kg for the 38 peripubertal children, and 6.98 ± 4.54 kg for the 8 postpubertal children. The growth rate is higher and later in boys than in girls. Weight gain during this period amounts to approximately 50 percent of the ideal adult weight. However, there is enormous variability in the timing and extent of this growth acceleration.

To estimate tissue accretion of phosphorus, knowledge of both

TABLE 5-5 Accretion of Phosphorus (P) in Bone and Lean Tissue During Peak Adolescent Growth Spurt

Gender/ Age (y)	Change in Weight[a] (g/y)	Change in Lean[b] (FFBM- osseous) (g/y)	Lean- Tissue P[c] (g/y)	Osseous P[d] (g/y)	Bone P[e] (g/y)	Total P Gain[f] (mg/d [mmol/ d])
Males 13.3	5,000	3,970	9.1	320	60.8	192 (6.2)
Females 11.4	5,000	3,750	8.6	240	45.6	149 (4.8)
Mean, both sexes						171 (5.5)

[a] See Table 1-3.
[b] Body fat values from Deurenberg et al., 1990.
[c] Assuming a phosphorus content of soft tissue of 0.23 percent.
[d] Martin et al., 1997.
[e] Assuming a phosphorus content of bone of 19 percent.
[f] Calculated from sum of accretion of P in lean and bone/year divided by 365.

lean and osseous tissue gains is required. Gains in lean mass were determined by subtracting fat from total weight gain. Percentage body fat for pubertal boys aged 13.2 (standard error [SE] 1.3) was 14.2 (95 percent confidence interval [CI] 13.0 to 15.4), and 20.2 (95 percent CI 19.3 to 21.1) for pubertal girls aged 10.5 (SE 1.6) (Deurenberg et al., 1990). Osseous tissue gains were based on a study of 228 children in Canada where mean peak bone mineral content velocity was 320 g/year in boys at age 13.3 years and 240 g/ year in girls at age 11.4 years (Martin et al., 1997). The computations are summarized in Table 5-5. Assuming a phosphorus content of bone mineral of 19 percent and a phosphorus content of soft tissue of 0.23 percent (Pennington, 1994), daily phosphorus needs during peak growth would approximate 200 mg (6.5 mmol) for boys and 150 mg (4.8 mmol) for girls.

Similar to younger children, the value derived for phosphorus excretion was then employed in a factorial model to obtain the EAR. Urinary phosphate excretion rises linearly with phosphorus intake according to the equation derived by Lemann (1996) in adults. This approach was adopted here since no such relationship has been developed for adolescents. Using the equation: $P_{urine} = 1.73 + 0.512 \times P_{intake}$ (in mmol/day), and an intake of 1,000 mg

(32.3 mmol)/day, predicted urinary excretion would be 565 mg (18.2 mmol)/day. When urinary phosphorus is added to the mean accrued phosphorus for both boys and girls of 175 mg (5.6 mmol) (Table 5-5), there is a daily need for dietary phosphorus of 740 mg (23.9 mmol)/day. Absorption efficiency in the few balance studies performed in this age group (Greger et al., 1978; Lutwak et al., 1964) averaged 60 to 80 percent. This is consistent with the range of absorption efficiencies (60 to 65 percent) found in adults (Lemann, 1996). Using a midpoint value of absorption efficiency of 70 percent, ingested phosphorus to cover tissue accretion and urinary loss would need to be 1,055 mg (34 mmol)/day for both boys and girls. Although these phosphorus intakes cover tissue accumulation needs of the observed average adolescent, these intakes may not be optimal at the peak of the adolescent growth spurt.

The small amount of balance data available supports this estimate of phosphorus needs for children up to 14.5 years of age. Greger et al. (1978) studied 14 girls aged 12.5 to 14.5 years. Their balances averaged +82 ± 124 mg (+2.6 ± 4 mmol)/day on phosphorus intakes of 820 ± 10 mg (26.5 ± 0.3 mmol)/day. On phosphorus intakes of 925 mg (29.8 mmol)/day, 8 of 11 girls aged 12.5 to 14.2 years were in positive phosphorus balance with zinc intakes of 11.3 mg/day (Greger et al., 1979). In other studies, five adolescents aged 9 to 13 years and 18 adolescents aged 8 to 11 years were in positive phosphorus balance at intakes exceeding 1 g (32.3 mmol)/day (Lutwak et al., 1964; Sherman and Hawley, 1922). Of these 23 individuals, 4 boys and 13 girls aged 8 to 12 years were in positive phosphorus balance at daily phosphorus intakes above 34.5 mg (1.1 mmol)/kg body weight or 693 mg (22.4 mmol).

Serum P_i. An attempt was also made to estimate the EAR during adolescence by using the approach employed for adults, for example, using ECF P_i as the functional indicator, and estimating the intake needed to sustain ECF P_i at the lower limit of normal for the age concerned (see below for corresponding approach in adults). As Table 5-1 shows, the interpolated 2.5 percentile for P_i at age 9 is approximately 1.25 mmol/liter (3.9 mg/dl), falling to approximately 1.05 mmol/liter (3.3 mg/dl) by age 18. The curve in Figure 5-1 relates to adults and hence cannot be used directly. However, the lack of effective regulation of ECF P_i and the fact that it rises and falls with intake means that the rise in P_i for any given increment will be a function of the volume of the ECF into which the absorbed phosphorus is inserted, or in other words, a function of body size. Thus, a straightforward adjustment for body weight may permit a first approximation of the requirement for this age group. A number of assumptions related to serum P_i during adolescence and growth needs were necessary to complete this calculation, and the resulting value was not dissimilar from that determined using tissue accretion and the factorial method.

EAR Summary: Ages 9 through 13 and 14 through 18 Years

The EAR for children ages 9 through 13 years can be set based on the factorial approach at 1,055 mg (34 mmol)/day. Although accretion data are not available for ages 14 through 18 years, it seems reasonable to maintain this EAR value for the older adolescent since a similar value was obtained using the serum phosphorus curve extrapolated from adults. It should be noted, however, that this age range (9 through 18 years) brackets a period of intense growth, with growth rate, absorption efficiency, and normal values for ECF P_i changing during this time. Because of the similarity of these sex-specific estimates and the uncertainties involved, a single value of 1,055 mg (34 mmol)/day is selected for both males and females ages 9 through 18 years.

EAR for Boys	**9 through 13 years**	**1,055 mg (34 mmol)/day**
	14 through 18 years	**1,055 mg (34 mmol)/day**
EAR for Girls	**9 through 13 years**	**1,055 mg (34 mmol)/day**
	14 through 18 years	**1,055 mg (34 mmol)/day**

Utilizing the 1994 CSFII intake data, adjusted for day-to-day variations (Nusser et al., 1996), this EAR of 1,055 mg (34 mmol)/day is slightly below the twenty-fifth percentile (1,090 mg [35.2 mmol]) of phosphorus intake for boys, aged 9 through 13 years, and slightly above the twenty-fifth percentile of intake (1,005 mg [32.4 mmol]) for girls in this same age range (see Appendix D). For boys ages 14 through 18, the EAR of 1,055 mg (34 mmol)/day is close to the tenth percentile (1,072 mg [34.6 mmol]) of phosphorus intake. The EAR of 1,054 mg (34 mmol)/day for girls ages 14 through 18 is slightly below the fiftieth percentile (1,097 mg [35.4 mmol]) of phosphorus intake.

Determination of the RDA: Ages 9 through 13 and 14 through 18 Years

The variance in requirements cannot be determined from the available data. Thus, a CV of 10 percent (1 SD) is assumed. This results in a RDA for phosphorus of 1,250 mg (40.3 mmol)/day for girls and boys ages 9 through 18 years.

TABLE 5-6 Phosphorus Intakes Related to Specific Serum Inorganic Phosphorus Values in Adults

Serum P_i (mmol/liter)	Absorbed Intake (mmol/day)	Ingested Intake[a] (mmol/day)
0.87	11.6	18.6
1.00	23.9	38.2
1.15	43.2	69.2
1.40	71.0	113.6

[a] Ingested intake given as (absorbed intake)/0.625.

RDA for Boys	9 through 13 years	1,250 mg (40.3 mmol)/day
	14 through 18 years	1,250 mg (40.3 mmol)/day
RDA for Girls	9 through 13 years	1,250 mg (40.3 mmol)/day
	14 through 18 years	1,250 mg (40.3 mmol)/day

Ages 19 through 30 and 31 through 50 Years

Indicator Used to Set the EAR

Serum P_i. The relationship between serum P_i and absorbed intake, as presented in Figure 5-1, allows estimation of the intakes associated with P_i values within the range typically considered normal.

The extrapolation from absorbed intake to ingested intake shown in Table 5-6 is based on an absorption efficiency for phosphorus of 60 to 65 percent, the value typically observed in studies of adults on mixed diets (Heaney and Recker, 1982; Stanbury, 1971; Wilkinson, 1976). This absorption estimate for phosphorus is fairly robust, since variation in absorptive performance for phosphorus in adults is narrow (Heaney and Recker, 1982; Wilkinson, 1976).

The estimates of ingested intake in Table 5-6 apply to a typical, mixed diet. They will underestimate intakes needed to achieve a given serum P_i value if the dietary phosphorus consists heavily of phytate phosphorus. Thus, diets in which major fractions of the phosphorus intake are derived from unleavened cereal sources will require higher intakes to produce the curve of Figure 5-1 (which, as already noted, is for typical mixed diets), that is, the curve will be expanded to the right when the x-axis is expressed as ingested intake. This is shown by the lower dashed curve in Figure 5-1. Conversely, diets in which much of the phosphorus is derived, for example, from the phosphoric acid in certain carbonated beverages, and in which there is correspondingly little co-ingested calcium, may be expected to yield the curve of Figure 5-1 at lower phosphorus intakes; that is, the curve will shrink to the left—the upper dashed curve.

EAR Summary: Ages 19 through 30 and 31 through 50 Years

These latter considerations aside, using the lower end of the normal adult P_i range (0.87 mmol/liter [2.7 mg/dl]) yields an ingested intake value of ~580 mg (~19 mmol)/day, which may be the best available EAR for adults. By definition, roughly half of all adults would not be able to maintain a P_i of 0.87 mmol/liter (2.7 mg/dl) at this intake. (Importantly, while most adults have fasting serum P_i values above 1.0 mmol/liter [3.1 mg/dl], that fact cannot be used to establish the requirement, since intake in excess of the requirement will elevate the serum P_i.) If, alternatively, the middle of the normal range for serum P_i (1.15 mmol/liter [3.6 mg/dl]) is taken as the basis for the EAR, a much higher value, ~2,100 mg (~68 mmol)/day results. Since the slope of the curve of Figure 5-1 is very gradual above the renal threshold, intake estimates will be very sensitive to the value of serum P_i selected. Thus, the EAR for both men and women ages 19 through 50 is set at 580 mg (18.7 mmol)/day.

EAR for Men	**19 through 30 years**	**580 mg (18.7 mmol)/day**
	31 through 50 years	**580 mg (18.7 mmol)/day**
EAR for Women	**19 through 30 years**	**580 mg (18.7 mmol)/day**
	31 through 50 years	**580 mg (18.7 mmol)/day**

Utilizing the 1994 CSFII intake data, adjusted for day-to-day variations (Nusser et al., 1996), all males aged 19 through 50 years have phosphorus intakes above the EAR of 580 mg (18.7 mmol)/day (see Appendix D). The median intake for men, aged 19 through 30 years, is 1,613 mg (52.0 mmol)/day, and the first percentile of intake is 809 mg (26.1 mmol)/day. For men, aged 31 through 50 years, the median intake of phosphorus is 1,484 mg (47.9 mmol)/day, and the first percentile of intake is 705 mg (22.7 mmol)/day.

For women aged 19 through 30 years, the median phosphorus intake is 1,005 mg (32.4 mmol)/day, and the EAR of 580 mg (18.7 mmol)/day is at the first percentile of intake, 580 mg (18.7 mmol)/day. For women aged 31 through 50 years, the median phosphorus intake is 990 mg (31.9 mmol)/day. The EAR in this group of women is slightly below fifth percentile of intake, 593 mg (19.1 mmol)/day, based on the 1994 CSFII data.

Determination of the RDA: Ages 19 through 30 and 31 through 50 Years

The variance in requirements cannot be determined from the available data. Thus, a CV of 10 percent (1 SD) is assumed, resulting in an RDA of 700 mg (22.6 mmol)/day.

RDA for Men	19 through 30 years	700 mg (22.6 mmol)/day
	31 through 50 years	700 mg (22.6 mmol)/day
RDA for Women	19 through 30 years	700 mg (22.6 mmol)/day
	31 through 50 years	700 mg (22.6 mmol)/day

Ages 51 through 70 and > 70 Years

The data on which the foregoing phosphorus analyses were based were derived from adults of mixed ages, including 51 through 70 and > 70 years. Data specific to these ages are not available. Intestinal absorption efficiency for phosphorus is not known to change appreciably with age, and as noted above, changes in the renal clearance of phosphorus are not sufficient to alter the curve of Figure 5-1 until GFR is reduced by approximately 80 percent. Hence, it is reasonable to adopt the same phosphorus EAR for older adults as for younger adults.

EAR Summary: Ages 51 through 70 and > 70 Years

The EAR for both men and women ages 51 years and older is set at 580 mg (18.7 mmol)/day.

EAR for Men	51 through 70 years	580 mg (18.7 mmol)/day
	> 70 years	580 mg (18.7 mmol)/day
EAR for Women	51 through 70 years	580 mg (18.7 mmol)/day
	> 70 years	580 mg (18.7 mmol)/day

Utilizing the 1994 CSFII intake data, adjusted for day-to-day variations (Nusser et al., 1996), the median phosphorus intake for men, aged 51 through 70 years, is 1,274 mg (41.1 mmol)/day (see Appendix D). All of the men, aged 51 through 70 years, had phosphorus intakes in amounts above the EAR. The median intake for men, aged 71 years and older, is 1,176 mg (37.9 mmol)/day and the first percentile of intake is 559 mg (18.0 mmol)/day, which is close to their EAR of 580 mg (18.7 mmol)/day.

The median phosphorus intake for women aged 51 through 70 years is 966 mg (31.2 mmol)/day, based on the adjusted 1994 CSFII intake data. The EAR of 580 mg (18.7 mmol)/day for these women would fall close to the fifth percentile of intake, 599 mg (19.3 mmol)/day. The median phosphorus intake for women, aged 71 years and older, is 859 mg (27.7 mmol)/day, and the tenth percentile of phosphorus intake is 588 mg (19.0 mmol)/day, which is slightly above the EAR of 580 mg (18.7 mmol)/day.

Determination of the RDA: Ages 51 through 70 and >70 Years

The variance in requirements cannot be determined from the available data. Thus a CV of 10 percent (1 SD) is assumed, resulting in an RDA for phosphorus of 700 mg (22.6 mmol)/day for men and women ages 51 years and older.

RDA for Men	**51 through 70 years**	**700 mg (22.6 mmol)/day**
	> 70 years	**700 mg (22.6 mmol)/day**
RDA for Women	**51 through 70 years**	**700 mg (22.6 mmol)/day**
	> 70 years	**700 mg (22.6 mmol)/day**

Pregnancy

Indicator Used to Set the EAR

Phosphorus Content. Phosphorus content of the term infant at birth is 17.1 g (552 mmol), with 88.3 percent of phosphorus accounted for in bone and water (Fomon et al., 1982). The major physiological adaptations of the mother to meet the increased need for calcium to support fetal growth also should supply the fetus with a sufficient amount of phosphorus. The increased efficiency in intestinal absorption of calcium resulting from increased $1,25(OH)_2D$ concentrations also will lead to increased intestinal absorption of phosphorus.

Balance studies in 24 pregnant women demonstrated positive phosphorus balance, which increased with length of pregnancy (Heaney and Skillman, 1971). Net phosphorus absorption in these women averaged 70 percent, compared with absorption in the range of 60 to 65 percent typically found in nonpregnant adults (Heaney and Recker, 1982; Stanbury, 1971; Wilkinson, 1976). Daily fetal phosphorus requirements of about 62 mg (2 mmol) are needed to produce a term infant at birth with a phosphorus content of 17.1 g (552 mmol) (Fomon et al., 1982). The EAR for phosphorus in adults ages 19 through 30 years is approximately 580 mg (18.7 mmol)/day at an absorption of 60 percent (resulting in an absorbed phosphorus of 353 mg [11.4 mmol/day]). Assuming a 70 percent absorption of phosphorus during pregnancy (Heaney and Skillman, 1971), a similar EAR of 580 mg (18.7 mmol)/day would lead to an absorbed phosphorus of 412 mg (13.3 mmol)/day. This increase in absorbed phosphorus during pregnancy (59 mg [1.9 mmol/day]) approximately equals the estimated fetal phosphorus requirement of 62 mg (2 mmol)/day.

Serum phosphorus concentrations during pregnancy are within the normal range at mean daily intakes of approximately 1,550 mg (50 mmol) (95 percent CI range of 1,260 to 1,840 mg [40.6 to 59.4 mmol]) (Cross et al., 1995a). No studies have specifically investigated the effect of dietary intake of phosphorus on phosphorus balance during pregnancy.

EAR and RDA Summary for Pregnancy

No evidence at this time supports an increase of the EAR and RDA during pregnancy above the level recommended during the nonpregnant state. Intestinal absorption of phosphorus increases by about 10 percent during pregnancy (Heaney and Skillman, 1971). That change should be sufficient to provide the necessary phosphorus for fetal growth.

EAR for Pregnancy
14 through 18 years	1,055 mg (34.0 mmol)/day
19 through 30 years	580 mg (18.7 mmol)/day
31 through 50 years	580 mg (18.7 mmol)/day

RDA for Pregnancy
14 through 18 years	1,250 mg (40.3 mmol)/day
19 through 30 years	700 mg (22.6 mmol)/day
31 through 50 years	700 mg (22.6 mmol)/day

Utilizing the 1994 CSFII intake data for 33 pregnant women, adjusted for day-to-day variations (Nusser et al., 1996), the value derived for the EAR of 580 mg (18.7 mmol)/day for pregnant women ages 19 through 50 years represents a low dietary intake of phosphorus, as it falls below the first percentile of intake of 773 mg (24.9 mmol)/day (see Appendix D). The EAR of 1,055 mg (34 mmol) for pregnant women ages 14 through 18 years falls slightly above the fifth percentile of intake of 1,012 mg (32.6 mmol)/day.

Special Considerations

Adolescent Mothers and/or Multiple Fetuses. It is not known whether phosphorus requirements are increased in the adolescent mother and in mothers pregnant with more than one fetus. These conditions lead to increased maternal or fetal needs for phosphorus that may not be met by increased intestinal absorption. The mediating role of maintaining calcium homeostasis is also important in these situations: a diet insufficient in calcium may lead to increased PTH concentrations and decreased renal tubular reabsorption of phosphorus.

Lactation

Indicators Used to Set the EAR

Human Milk. Concentrations of phosphorus in human milk range from approximately 3.9 to 5.1 mmol/liter (12.1 to 15.8 mg/dl) and decrease as lactation progresses (Table 5-2). Assuming a milk production of 780 ml/day, a lactating woman may lose approximately 90 to 120 mg (2.9 to 3.9 mmol)/day of phosphorus in her milk. No studies have investigated the effect of varying phosphorus intake on phosphorus homeostasis during lactation.

Serum P_i. Despite the loss of phosphorus in milk, serum phosphorus concentrations in lactating women are in the high-normal or above-normal range, and they are higher in lactating women than in nonlactating women (Figure 5-2) (Byrne et al., 1987; Chan et al., 1982a; Cross et al, 1995a; Dobnig et al., 1995; Kalkwarf et al., 1996; Kent et al., 1990; Lopez et al., 1996; Specker et al., 1991a). This high serum phosphorus occurs at a time when there is an increase in bone resorption that appears to be related to non-dietary factors (see Chapter 4). The elevated serum phosphorus is due in whole or part to the fall in serum PTH which leads to high serum P_i.

EAR and RDA Summary for Lactation

Currently no evidence supports that phosphorus requirements are

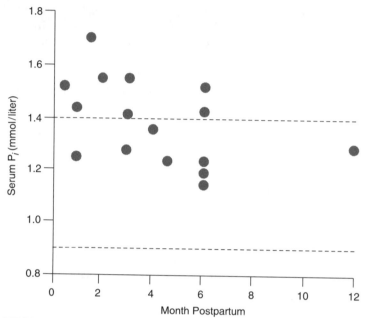

FIGURE 5-2 Serum phosphorus concentrations in lactating and non-lactating women. The dotted lines represent the normal range for non-lactating women. The circles represent the serum phosphorus levels of lactating women (Bryne et al., 1987; Chan et al., 1982b; Cross et al., 1995a; Dobnig et al., 1995; Kalkwarf et al., 1996; Kent et al., 1990; Lopez et al., 1996; Specker et al., 1991a).

increased during lactation. Apparently, increased bone resorption and decreased urinary excretion of phosphorus (Kent et al., 1990), which occur independent of dietary intake of phosphorus or calcium, provide the necessary phosphorus for milk production. Therefore, the EAR and RDA are estimated to be similar to that obtained for nonlactating women of their respective age groups.

EAR for Lactation
14 through 18 years	1,055 mg (34.0 mmol)/day
19 through 30 years	580 mg (18.7 mmol)/day
31 through 50 years	580 mg (18.7 mmol)/day

RDA for Lactation
14 through 18 years	1,250 mg (40.3 mmol)/day
19 through 30 years	700 mg (22.6 mmol)/day
31 through 50 years	700 mg (22.6 mmol)/day

Utilizing the 1994 CSFII intake data, adjusted for day-to-day variations (Nusser et al., 1996), the median intake of phosphorus for the 16 lactating women in the survey is 1,483 mg (47.8 mmol)/day and the lowest intake reported was at the first percentile of 1,113 mg (35.9 mmol)/day (see Appendix D). All women consumed above the phosphorus EAR of 580 to 1,055 mg (18.7 to 34 mmol)/day during lactation.

Special Considerations

Adolescent Mothers and Mothers Nursing Multiple Infants. As with calcium, phosphorus requirements may be increased in lactating adolescents and in mothers nursing multiple infants. Requirements during these periods may be higher because of the adolescent mother's own growth requirements and the requirement for increased milk production while nursing multiple infants. It is not known whether decreased urinary phosphorus and increased maternal bone resorption provides sufficient amounts of phosphorus to meet these increased needs.

TOLERABLE UPPER INTAKE LEVELS

Hazard Identification

As shown in Figure 5-1, serum P_i rises as total phosphorus intake increases. Excess phosphorus intake from any source is expressed as hyperphosphatemia, and essentially all the adverse effects of phosphorus excess are due to the elevated P_i in the ECF. The principal effects that have been attributed to hyperphosphatemia are: (1) adjustments in the hormonal control system regulating the calcium economy, (2) ectopic (metastatic) calcification, particularly of the kidney, (3) in some animal models, increased porosity of the skeleton, and (4) a suggestion that high phosphorus intakes could reduce calcium absorption by complexing calcium in the chyme. Concern about high phosphorus intake has been raised in recent years because of a probable population-level increase in phosphorus intake through such sources as cola beverages and food phosphate additives.

It has been reported that high intakes of polyphosphates, such as are found in food additives, can interfere with absorption of iron, copper, and zinc (Bour et al., 1984); however, described effects are small, and have not been consistent across studies (for example,

Snedeker et al., 1982). For this reason, as well as because trace mineral status may be low for many reasons, it was not considered feasible to use trace mineral status as an indicator of excess phosphorus intake. Nevertheless, given the trend toward increased use of phosphate additives in a variety of food products (Calvo and Heath, 1988; Calvo and Park, 1996), it would be well to be alert to the possibility of some interference in individuals with marginal trace mineral status.

Most of the studies that describe harmful effects of phosphorus intake used animal models. In extrapolating these data to humans, it is important to note that the phosphorus density of human diets represents the extreme low end of the continuum of standard diets for pets and laboratory animals. The median human dietary phosphorus density in the 1994 CSFII was very close to 62 mg (2.0 mmol)/100 kcal for all adults and for both sexes (Cleveland et al., 1996). By contrast, the diets of standard laboratory rats and mice have phosphorus densities ranging from 124 to 186 mg (4 to 6 mmol)/100 kcal. Cats and dogs have diets with densities close to 279 mg (9 mmol)/100 kcal, and laboratory primate diets average about 155 mg (5 mmol)/100 kcal.

Adjustments in Calcium-Regulating Hormones

As noted earlier, P_i is not, strictly speaking, regulated. Thus, a high phosphorus diet produces a higher level of plasma P_i, especially during the absorptive phase after eating. High P_i levels reduce urine calcium loss, reduce renal synthesis of $1,25(OH)_2D$, reduce serum ionized calcium, and lead to increases in PTH release (Portale et al., 1989; Wood et al., 1988). These effects reflect adjustments in the control system that regulates the calcium economy and are not in themselves necessarily adverse. As already noted, the reduction in $1,25(OH)_2D$ synthesis may slightly mitigate the hyperphosphatemia by a small reduction in phosphorus absorption from the intestine.

It is known that added dietary phosphate loads of 1.5 to 2.5 g of inorganic phosphorus (as phosphate) in humans lead acutely to very slight drops in ECF $[Ca^{2+}]$ and to correspondingly elevated PTH concentrations (Calvo and Heath, 1988; Silverberg et al., 1986). It has been proposed that these adjustments in circulating calcium regulating hormones (associated with any elevation of serum P_i, even though within the usual normal range) could have adverse effects on the skeleton (Calvo and Heath, 1988; Calvo et al., 1988, 1990; Krook et al., 1975). The increase in PTH is often presumed to be harmful to bone. The mild hypocalcemic effect seen with acute increases in phosphorus intake is often attributed to the formation of calcium phosphate ($CaHPO_4$) complexes in plasma, which is the presumed mechanism driving down $[Ca^{2+}]$ (Krook et al., 1975). However, it is doubtful that this is the correct explanation. As already noted, adult plasma is undersaturated with respect to $CaHPO_4 H_2O$, and the modest elevations in plasma P_i produced by a high phosphorus diet are probably not sufficient to alter plasma $[Ca^{2+}]$ directly. Moreover, causes of hypercalcemia, such as primary bone wasting and simple intravenous infusion of calcium, cause serum P_i to rise, not fall, as might be expected if concentrations of the two ions were reciprocally related to one another at normal concentrations (Howard et al., 1953). Rather, it is more likely that the initial fall in $[Ca^{2+}]$ following elevation of plasma P_i is produced by direct inhibition of PTH-mediated osteoclastic release of calcium from bone (Raisz and Niemann, 1969). Thus, rather than harmful, this inhibition of bone resorption and consequent increase in PTH may actually be beneficial to bone, since it amounts to a relative resistance to the bone-resorbing effects of PTH. This point had been made by an earlier expert panel (Chinn, 1981) and is supported by more recent evidence showing that, despite the elevated PTH, urine hydroxyproline (a measure of bone resorption) falls on high phosphorus intakes, as does urine calcium (Silverberg et al., 1986).

Diets high in phosphorus and low in calcium produce a sustained rise in PTH (Calvo et al., 1988, 1990); but diets low in calcium without extra phosphorus produce the same change (Barger-Lux et al., 1995), and for that reason it is unlikely that the high phosphorus feature of the altered intake is the culprit in the first instance. In addition, with respect to high phosphorus intakes, chronic administration of 2 g (65 mmol)/day phosphorus in men for at least 8 weeks produced no effect on calcium balance or calcium absorption relative to a diet containing only 806 mg (26 mmol) phosphorus (Spencer et al., 1965, 1978a). Calcium intake (low, normal, or high) had no influence on this lack of effect, underscoring the lack of physiological relevance of the dietary Ca:P ratio in adults. Further, calcium kinetic studies performed in adult women in whom phosphorus intake was doubled from 1.1 to 2.3 g (35.5 to 74.2 mmol), showed no effect whatsoever on bone turnover processes after 4 months of treatment (Heaney and Recker, 1987). A similar conclusion was reached more recently by Bizik et al. (1996), who doubled phosphorus intake (from 800 to 1,600 mg [26 to 52 mmol]/day) for 10 days in seven healthy young men (aged 22 to 31 years) and found no increase in urine deoxypyridinoline excretion (a marker of bone resorption). For all these reasons, it is doubtful whether phosphorus intakes, within the range currently thought to be experienced by the U.S. population and/or associated with serum P_i values in the normal range, adversely affect bone health.

Normal, healthy, term-born infants, like adults, can adjust to a relatively wide range of dietary Ca:P ratios as provided in contemporary infant formulas. However, as a result of developmental immaturity in renal handling of phosphorus by infants, ECF [Ca^{2+}] and P_i concentrations are closer to saturation in infancy, and infants are, therefore, more at risk of developing hypocalcemia as a consequence of hyperphosphatemia (DeVizia and Mansi, 1992). However, in the first month of life, some infants exhibit unusual sensitivity to phosphorus intakes above those associated with human milk. In the past, the clinical syndrome of late neonatal hypocalcemic tetany was observed when infants were fed whole evaporated cow milk with a very high phosphorus content (DeVizia and Mansi, 1992). Surprisingly, even with the introduction of modified cow milk formulas with phosphorus content reduced to one-half or less than that of evaporated whole milk, the syndrome of hypocalcemia has still been observed in young infants (Specker et al., 1991b; Venkataraman et al., 1985). However, the phosphorus content of such formulas is still substantially higher than that of human milk (Specker et al., 1991b). If such hyperphosphatemia is allowed to persist during early infancy, parathyroid hyperplasia, ectopic calcifications, and low serum calcitriol may occur (Portale et al., 1986). In such cases, the compensatory mechanisms for handling phosphate loads, mainly renal excretion, must be overwhelmed, leading to excessive phosphorus retention and the other metabolic consequences.

It has also been suggested that a high content of phosphorus and calcium in an infant's diet may be a predisposing factor for the development of retention acidosis (Manz, 1992). It is not possible to identify, in advance, infants at risk for these syndromes unless they have renal dysfunction. Based on the data of Specker et al. (1991b), the risk of hypocalcemia (serum calcium less than 1.1 mmol/liter [4.4 mg/dl]) is 30 out of 10,000 neonates fed such formulas. Human milk with its low phosphorus content is both safer and better suited to the growth needs of the infant than cow milk (Manz, 1992). Finally, one report associates high intakes of phosphoric acid-containing cola beverages with slight reductions of serum calcium in Mexican children (Mazariegos-Ramos et al., 1995), but it is not clear to what extent the effect is due to the acid load of the colas, the associated low intake of calcium-rich beverages, or the phosphorus itself.

Except as noted in very young infants, none of these adjustments in calcium-regulating hormones is clearly adverse in its own right, particularly if calcium intake is adequate. Hence these effects do not provide a useful basis for estimating the Tolerable Upper Intake Level (UL).

Metastatic Calcification

The most serious, clearly harmful effect of hyperphosphatemia is calcification of nonskeletal tissues. This occurs when the calcium and phosphorus concentrations of ECF exceed the limits of solubility for secondary calcium phosphate ($CaHPO_4$). This critical concentration is strongly dependent on amounts of other ions in the ECF, especially HCO_3^- citrate, H^+, and K^+, and so cannot be unambiguously defined. However, tissue calcification virtually never occurs at ECF calcium × phosphorus ion products less than ~4 (mmol/liter)^2 [~1(mg/dl)^2]. Although ECF in adults is normally less than half-saturated with respect to $CaHPO_4$, elevation of plasma P_i, if extreme, can bring the ECF to the point of saturation. Although both calcium and phosphate are involved in such ectopic mineralization, ECF calcium levels are tightly regulated and are usually affected little by even large variations in calcium intake. By contrast, the sensitivity of ECF P_i to joint effects of diet and renal clearance means that an elevation in ECF P_i will usually be the cause of supersaturation. When calcification involves the kidney, renal function can deteriorate rapidly, renal phosphorus clearance drops, and ECF P_i rises yet further, leading to a rapid downhill spiral.

Under saturated conditions, susceptible tissue matrices will begin to accumulate $CaHPO_4$ crystals, particularly if local pH rises above 7.4. Saturation of ECF with respect to calcium and phosphorus almost never occurs in individuals with normal renal function, mainly because urine phosphate excretion rises in direct proportion to dietary intake. As Figure 5-1 shows, the upper limit of the normal adult range for serum P_i typically occurs at absorbed intakes above 2.2 g (71 mmol)/day. At 62.5 percent absorption, that means ingested intakes above 3.4 g (110 mmol)/day. The 1994 CSFII data indicate that the reported intake at the ninety-fifth percentile was 2.5 g (81.7 mmol)/day in boys aged 14 through 18 years (see Appendix D). Hyperphosphatemia from dietary causes becomes a problem mainly in patients with end-stage renal disease or in such conditions as vitamin D intoxication. When functioning kidney tissue mass is reduced to less than ~20 percent of normal, the GFR becomes too low to clear typical absorbed loads of dietary phosphorus, and then even sharply reduced phosphorus diets may still be excessive as they lead to hyperphosphatemia.

Although metastatic calcification can occur in patients with end-stage renal disease in whom ECF P_i levels are not adequately controlled, it is not known to occur from dietary sources alone in persons with adequate renal function. For that reason, calcification in previously normal kidneys produced by high phosphorus intakes has been studied mainly in rats and mice (Craig, 1959; Hamuro et al., 1970; McFarlane, 1941; NRC, 1995). Production of calcification has required very high phosphate loads over and above the animals' already high basal phosphate intakes and in several reports has required partial reduction of renal tissue mass, as well.

Skeletal Porosity

Skeletal lesions associated with high phosphorus intakes have been described in rabbits (Jowsey and Balasubramaniam, 1972) and bulls (Krook et al., 1975). As with kidney toxicity, the bony lesions required extremely large phosphate intakes (in rabbits, about 40-fold typical human intakes on a body weight basis, and in bulls, feeding of a ration designed to support milk production in cows). None of these situations has any evident direct relevance to human nutrition or to human dietary intake of phosphate. Krook et al. (1975) also noted that bone loss develops in household pets and zoo animals fed human table scraps and meat. Despite acknowledging that such foods are poor in calcium, they attribute the bone loss to the high phosphorus content of such diets. Lacking evidence that phosphorus would produce this effect with diets adequate in calcium, this conclusion seems unwarranted. Finally, given the evidence cited above that high phosphorus intakes in humans do not lead to negative calcium balance or to increased bone resorption, it seems likely that the bone disease in other animals is more a consequence of low effective calcium intake than of high phosphorus intake per se.

Interference with Calcium Absorption

As noted, some concerns have been expressed that a high phosphorus intake could interfere with calcium nutrition by complexing calcium in the chyme and reducing its absorption (Calvo and Heath, 1988; Calvo and Park, 1996). Given the relative absorption efficiencies of calcium and phosphorus, there would not be a stoichiometric excess of phosphorus relative to calcium in the chyme until the Ca:P intake ratio fell below 0.375:1. However, even this is a purely theoretical concern. In the studies of Spencer et al. (1978a), in which inorganic neutral phosphate was added to the diet, and of Heaney and Recker (1982), who studied women on their habitual intakes of food phosphorus, even Ca:P ratios as low as 0.08:1 did not lower calcium absorption. Nevertheless, it must be noted that it is more difficult for the body to compensate for impaired calcium absorption at low dietary calcium intakes compared with higher intakes (Heaney, 1997). As prior expert panels have noted (Chinn, 1981), even the theoretical potential for interference with the calcium economy by high phosphorus intakes is effectively negated if calcium intake is adequate.

Dose-Response Assessment

Adults: Ages 19 through 70 Years

Data Selection. A UL can be defined as an intake associated with the upper boundary of adult normal values of serum P_i. No reports exist of untoward effects following high dietary phosphorus intakes in humans. Essentially all instances of dysfunction (and, hence, all instances of hyperphosphatemia) in humans occur for nondietary reasons (for example, end-stage renal disease, vitamin D intoxication). Therefore, data on the normal adult range for serum P_i are used as the basis for deriving a UL for adults.

Identification of a No-Observed-Adverse-Effect Level (NOAEL) (or Lowest-Observed-Adverse-Effect Level [LOAEL]) and Critical Endpoint. If the normal adult range for serum P_i is used as a first approach to estimating the UL, the upper boundary of adult normal values of serum P_i is reached at a daily phosphorus intake of 3.5 g (113 mmol) (Figure 5-1). There is no evidence that individuals consuming this intake may experience any untoward effects. As shown in Table 5-1, infants, children, and adolescents have higher upper limits for serum P_i than do adults, which indicates that their tissues tolerate the higher P_i levels well. Values of P_i above the nominal adult human normal range are also normally found in typical adult laboratory animals (for example, rats) and occur regularly in adult humans treated with the bisphosphonate, etidronate, used for the treatment of Paget's disease of the bone and osteoporosis (Recker et al., 1973). No suggestion of harm comes from any of these situations, indicating that the UL is substantially higher than that associated with the upper normal bound of serum P_i in adults.

    The higher values for serum P_i in infancy are manifestly tissue-safe levels, and if they are taken as an approximation of the upper normal human value (on the ground that there is no basis for assuming major differences in tissue susceptibility to metastatic mineralization at different ages), the corresponding ingested intake in an adult (assuming the relationship of Figure 5-1) would be over 10.2 g (330 mmol)/day.

Uncertainty Assessment. No benefit is evident from serum P_i values above the usual normal range in adults. Moreover, information is lacking concerning adverse effects in the zone between normal P_i and levels associated with ectopic mineralization. Therefore, in keeping with the pharmacokinetic practice where the relationship between intake and blood level is known (Petley et al., 1995), an uncertainty factor (UF) of 2.5 is chosen.

Derivation of the UL. A UL of ~4.0 g (~130 mmol)/day for adults is calculated by dividing a NOAEL of 10.2 g (330 mmol)/day by a UF of 2.5.

UL for Adults   19 through 70 years   4.0 g (130 mmol)/day

Infants: Ages 0 through 12 Months

As with adults, there are essentially no reports of adverse effects clearly attributable to high phosphorus intake of dietary origin in infants, children, or adolescents. Except for the sensitivity of very young infants noted above, there are no data relating to adverse effects of phosphorus intake for most of the first year of life. For that reason, it was determined that it was impossible to establish a specific UL for infants.

UL for Infants   0 through 12 months   Not possible to establish; source of intake should be from formula and food only

Toddlers and Children: Ages 1 through 8 Years

For toddlers and children, a UL of 3.0 g (96.8 mmol)/day is calculated by dividing the NOAEL for adults (10.2 g [330 mmol]/day by a UF of ~3.3 to account for potentially increased susceptibility due to smaller body size.

UL for Children   1 through 8 years   3.0 g (96.8 mmol)/day

Adolescents: Ages 9 through 18 Years

There is no evidence to suggest increased susceptibility to adverse effects during adolescence. Therefore, the same UL specified above for adults is selected for adolescents, 4.0 g (130 mmol)/day.

UL for Adolescents   9 through 18 years   4.0 g (130.0 mmol)/day

Older Adults: Ages > 70

Because of an increasing prevalence of impaired renal function after age 70, a larger UF of 3.3 seems prudent, and the UL for adults of this age is set at 3.0 g (96.8 mmol)/day.

UL for Older Adults   > 70 years   3.0 g (96.8 mmol)/day

Pregnancy and Lactation

During pregnancy, absorption efficiency for phosphorus rises by about 15 percent, and thus, the UL associated with the upper end of the normal range will be about 15 percent lower, that is, about 3.5 g (112.9 mmol)/day. During lactation, the phosphorus economy of a woman does not differ detectably from the nonlactating state. Hence the UL for this physiologic state is not different from the nonlactating state, 4.0 g (130 mmol)/day.

UL for Pregnancy   14 through 50 years   3.5 g (112.9 mmol)/day
UL for Lactation   14 through 50 years   4.0 g (130.0 mmol)/day

Special Considerations

It is recognized that population groups such as professional athletes, military trainees, or those whose level of energy expenditure exceeds 6,000 kcal/day, may have dietary phosphorus intakes whose distributions overlap these limits. In such individuals with phosphorus intakes above the UL, no harm is known to result.

Exposure Assessment

Utilizing the 1994 CSFII data, adjusted for one day food records (Nusser et al., 1996), the highest mean intake of phosphorus for any age and life stage group was reported for males aged 19 through 30 years: 1.7 g (53.5 mmol)/day. The highest reported intake at the ninety-fifth percentile was 2.5 g (81.7 mmol)/day in boys aged 14 through 18 years (see Appendix D), which is well below the UL of 4.0 g (130 mmol)/day. In 1986, approximately 10 percent of adults in the United States took a supplement containing phosphorus (Moss et al., 1989), and of those, the ninetieth percentile of supplemental phosphorus intake was 264 mg (8.5 mmol)/day. The ninety-fifth percentile intake for phosphorus supplements for adults was 448 mg (14.5 mmol)/day.

Risk Characterization

Phosphorus exposure data indicate that only a small percentage of the U.S. population is likely to exceed the UL. Because phosphorus supplements are not widely consumed, nor is the dosage high, total intake from diet plus supplements would infrequently exceed the UL.

RESEARCH RECOMMENDATIONS

• The model that relates absorbed phosphorus intake to serum phosphorus must be evaluated in clinical studies using oral phosphorus intakes, and investigated in children and adolescents as well as adults.

• Bone mineral mass as a function of dietary phosphorus intake should be investigated at all stages of the life cycle.

• The practical effect of phosphate-containing food additives on trace mineral status (iron, copper, and zinc) should be evaluated.

6

Magnesium

BACKGROUND INFORMATION

Overview

Total body magnesium (Mg) content is approximately 25 g (1,000 mmol), of which 50 to 60 percent resides in bone in the normal adult. One-third of skeletal magnesium is exchangeable, and it is this fraction that may serve as a reservoir for maintaining a normal extracellular magnesium concentration (Elin, 1987). Extracellular magnesium accounts for about 1 percent of total body magnesium. The normal serum magnesium concentration is 0.75 to 0.95 mmol/ liter (1.8 to 2.3 mg/dl).

Magnesium is a required cofactor for over 300 enzyme systems (Wacker and Parisi, 1968). It is required for both anaerobic and aerobic energy generation and for glycolysis, either indirectly as a part of the Mg-ATP complex or directly as an enzyme activator (Garfinkel and Garfinkel, 1985). Magnesium has also been shown to be required for mitochondria to carry out oxidative phosphorylation (Wacker and Parisi, 1968). The mitochondrial enzymes utilize the magnesium chelate of ATP and ADP as the actual substrates for phosphate transfer reactions.

Magnesium transport into or out of cells appears to require the presence of carrier-mediated transport systems (Gunther, 1993; Romani et al., 1993). The efflux of magnesium from the cell is coupled to sodium transport and requires energy. Magnesium influx also appears to be linked to sodium and bicarbonate transport but

190

by a different mechanism. The molecular characteristics of the magnesium transport proteins have not been described.

Magnesium transport in mammalian cells may be influenced by hormonal and pharmacological factors including β-agonists, growth factors, and insulin (Gunther, 1993; Hwang et al., 1993; Romani et al., 1993). It has been suggested that a hormonally regulated magnesium uptake system controls intracellular magnesium concentration in cellular compartments. The magnesium concentration in these compartments would then serve to regulate the activity of magnesium-sensitive enzymes.

Magnesium presence is important for maintaining an adequate supply of purine and pyrimidine nucleotides required for the increased DNA and RNA synthesis that occurs during cell proliferation (Rubin, 1975; Switzer, 1971). Replicating cells must be able to synthesize new protein, and this synthesis has been reported to be highly sensitive to magnesium depletion. Many hormones, neurotransmitters, and other cellular effectors regulate cellular activity via the adenylate cyclase system, and the activation of adenylate cyclase requires the presence of magnesium. There is also evidence for magnesium binding through which magnesium directly increases adenylate cyclase activity (Maguire, 1984).

Magnesium is necessary for sodium, potassium-ATPase activity, which is responsible for active transport of potassium (Dorup and Clausen, 1993). Magnesium regulates the outward movement of potassium in myocardial cells (Matsuda, 1991). The arrhythmogenic effect of magnesium deficiency may be related to magnesium's role in maintaining intracellular potassium.

Magnesium has been called "nature's physiological calcium channel blocker" (Iseri and French, 1984). During magnesium depletion, intracellular calcium rises. Since calcium plays an important role in skeletal and smooth muscle contraction, a state of magnesium depletion may result in muscle cramps, hypertension, and coronary and cerebral vasospasms. Magnesium depletion is found in a number of diseases of cardiovascular and neuromuscular function, in malabsorption syndromes, in diabetes mellitus, in renal wasting syndromes, and in alcoholism (Ma et al., 1995). These observations have led to studies regarding the role of inadequate magnesium intake in the development of disease, as opposed to abnormal handling of magnesium caused by the disease process. It is important to ensure that such evaluations are undertaken in apparently normal individuals for whom dietary intake is the primary independent variable.

Physiology of Absorption, Metabolism, and Excretion

In both children and adults, fractional intestinal magnesium absorption is inversely proportional to the amount of magnesium ingested (Kayne and Lee, 1993). In balance studies, under controlled dietary conditions in healthy older men, an average of 380 mg (15.8 mmol)/day of ingested magnesium resulted in net absorption of approximately 40 to 60 percent; true absorption ranged from 51 to 60 percent for various foodstuffs when subjects were on a constant diet (Schwartz et al, 1984). Net absorption has been estimated to be 15 to 36 percent at higher daily intakes (550 to 850 mg [22.9 to 35.4 mmol]) and with varying levels of dietary bran and oxalate (Schwartz et al., 1986). Magnesium is absorbed along the entire intestinal tract, but the sites of maximal magnesium absorption appear to be the distal jejunum and ileum (Kayne and Lee, 1993). Both an unsaturable passive and saturable active transport system for magnesium absorption may account for the higher fractional absorption at low dietary magnesium intakes (Fine et al., 1991a).

A principal factor that regulates intestinal magnesium transport has not been described. Vitamin D and its metabolites 25-hydroxyvitamin D (25(OH)D) and 1,25-dihydroxyvitamin D (1,25(OH)$_2$D) enhance intestinal magnesium absorption to a small extent (Hardwick et al., 1991; Krejs et al., 1983). Recently, a low magnesium diet in rats was shown to increase intestinal calbindin-D$_{9k}$. Although these preliminary data suggest a role for this vitamin D-dependent, calcium-binding protein in intestinal magnesium absorption, the severe magnesium deficiency imposed may have resulted in renal damage (not described) (Hemmingsen et al., 1994).

The kidney is the principal organ involved in magnesium homeostasis (Quamme and Dirks, 1986). The renal handling of magnesium in humans is a filtration-reabsorption process; there is no tubular secretion of magnesium. Approximately 65 percent of filtered magnesium is reabsorbed in the loop of Henle and 20 to 30 percent in the proximal convoluted tubule (Quamme and Dirks, 1986). Magnesium reabsorption in the proximal convoluted tubule appears to be passive; it follows changes in salt and water reabsorption and is associated with the rate of fluid flow. In the loop of Henle, there appears to be an additional active transport system: a decrease in magnesium reabsorption in this segment is independent of sodium chloride transport in either hypermagnesemia or hypercalcemia (Quamme, 1989). In vivo studies in animals and humans, however, have demonstrated a tubular maximum for magnesium that probably reflects a composite of these tubular reabsorptive processes (Quamme and Dirks, 1986).

During experimental magnesium depletion in humans, magnesium decreases in the urine to very low levels (< 20 mg [1 mmol]/day) within 3 to 4 days (Fitzgerald and Fourman, 1956; Heaton, 1969; Shils, 1969). Despite the close regulation of magnesium by the kidney, no one has described a hormone or factor that is responsible for renal magnesium homeostasis. Because patients with either primary hyper- or hypoparathyroidism usually have normal serum magnesium concentrations and a normal tubular maximum for magnesium, it is probable that parathyroid hormone (PTH) is not an important regulator of magnesium homeostasis (Rude et al., 1980). Glucagon, calcitonin, and ADH affect magnesium transport in the loop of Henle in a manner similar to PTH, but the physiological relevance of these actions is unknown (Quamme and Dirks, 1986). Little is known about the effect of vitamin D on renal magnesium handling.

Excessive alcohol intake has been shown to cause renal magnesium wasting, which, if a diet is marginal in magnesium content, could place an individual at risk for magnesium depletion. Indeed, nearly all chronic alcoholics have symptoms of magnesium depletion (Abbott et al., 1994). However, the evidence does not substantiate the suggestion that alcoholism is due to magnesium deficiency.

A growing list of medications has been found to result in increased renal magnesium excretion. Diuretics commonly used in the treatment of hypertension, heart failure, and other edematous states may cause hypermagnesuria (Ryan, 1987).

Factors Affecting the Magnesium Requirement

Bioavailability

As mentioned previously, net absorption of dietary magnesium in a typical diet is approximately 50 percent. High levels of dietary fiber from fruits, vegetables, and grains decrease magnesium absorption and/or retention (Siener and Hesse, 1995; Wisker et al., 1991). Men consuming 355 mg (14.8 mmol)/day of magnesium were in positive magnesium balance on a low-fiber (9 g/day) diet but in negative balance on a high-fiber (59 g/day) diet (Kelsay et al., 1979). Similar trends were observed in young women consuming 243 to 252 mg (10.0 to 10.5 mmol)/day of magnesium and receiving a lower fiber (23 g/day) versus higher fiber (39 g/day) diet (Wisker et al., 1991).

Nutrient-Nutrient Interactions

Phosphorus. Many foods high in fiber contain phytate, which may decrease intestinal magnesium absorption, probably by binding magnesium to phosphate groups on phytic acid (Brink and Beynen, 1992; Franz, 1989; Wisker et al., 1991). The ability of phosphate to bind magnesium may explain decreases in intestinal magnesium absorption seen in subjects on high phosphate diets (Franz, 1989; Hardwick et al., 1991; Reinhold et al., 1991).

Calcium. Most human studies of effects of dietary calcium on magnesium absorption have shown no effect (Fine et al., 1991a; Hardwick et al., 1991; Spencer et al., 1978b), but one has reported decreased magnesium absorption rates (Greger et al., 1981). Perfusion of the jejunum of normal subjects with 0 to 800 mg (0 to 20 mmol) calcium had no effect on magnesium absorption (Brannan et al., 1976). Increased calcium intake did not affect magnesium balance when as much as 2,000 mg (50 mmol)/day of calcium was given to adult men (Spencer et al., 1978b, 1994), or when an additional 1,000 mg (25 mmol)/day of calcium was given to adolescents (Andon et al., 1996). Magnesium intake ranging from 241 to 826 mg (10 to 34.4 mmol)/day did not alter calcium balance at either 241 mg (10 mmol) or 812 mg (20.3 mmol)/day of calcium (Spencer et al., 1994). However, intakes of calcium in excess of 2,600 mg (65 mmol)/day have been reported to decrease magnesium balance (Greger et al., 1981; Seelig, 1993). Several studies have found that high sodium and calcium intake may result in increased renal magnesium excretion (Kesteloot and Joossens, 1990; Martinez et al., 1985; Quamme and Dirks, 1986), which may be secondary to the interrelationship of the proximal tubular reabsorption of filtered sodium, calcium, and magnesium (Quamme and Dirks, 1986). Overall, at the dietary levels recommended in this report, the interaction of magnesium with calcium is not of concern.

Protein. Dietary protein may also influence intestinal magnesium absorption; magnesium absorption is lower when protein intake is less than 30 g/day (Hunt and Schofield, 1969). A higher protein intake (94 g/day) may increase renal magnesium excretion (Mahalko et al., 1983), presumably because an increased acid load increases urinary magnesium excretion (Wong et al., 1986). However, the increased urinary magnesium excretion did not change overall magnesium retention, which indicates an ability of subjects to adapt to this level of protein given the level of magnesium provided (258 mg [10.8 mmol]/ day). Other studies in adolescents have shown improved magnesium absorption and retention when protein intakes were higher (93 versus 43 g protein/day) (Schwartz et al., 1973).

Special Populations

Physical Activity. Dietary magnesium intake in athletes has been reported to be at or above recommended intakes (Clarkson and Haymes, 1995; Kleiner et al., 1994; Niekamp and Baer, 1995), presumably due to their higher food intake. Plasma/serum magnesium concentrations have been reported to fall with chronic endurance exercise activity, while red blood cell values appear to rise (Deuster and Singh, 1993). Although the decrease in plasma magnesium has been suggested to reflect magnesium depletion in athletes (Clarkson and Haymes, 1995), no clear demonstration of magnesium depletion directly related to exercise has been shown. Magnesium supplements did not enhance performance in a study of marathon runners (Terblanche et al., 1992).

Intake of Magnesium

The U.S. Department of Agriculture Continuing Survey of Food Intakes by Individuals (CSFII) in 1994, adjusted by the method of Nusser et al. (1996), indicated that the mean daily magnesium intake in males aged 9 and older was 323 mg (13.5 mmol) (fifth percentile = 177 mg [7.4 mmol]; fiftieth percentile = 310 mg [12.9 mmol]; ninety-fifth percentile = 516 mg [21.5 mmol]) (Cleveland et al., 1996) (see Appendix D for data tables). The mean daily intake for females aged 9 and older was 228 mg [9.5 mmol] (fifth percentile = 134 mg [5.6 mmol]; fiftieth percentile = 222 mg [9.3 mmol]; ninety-fifth percentile = 342 mg [14.3 mmol]). In both sexes, intake decreased at age 70 and older. These intakes were similar to those found in the National Health and Nutrition Examination Survey (NHANES) III from 1988–1991 (Alaimo et al., 1994). National survey data for Canada are not currently available. Other surveys have reported lower intakes in both men and women (Hallfrisch and Muller, 1993).

The NHANES III study demonstrated ethnic differences in intake. In that report, non-Hispanic black subjects were found to consume less than either non-Hispanic white or Hispanic subjects. Another study demonstrated that elderly Hispanic males consumed a mean of 237 ± 62 mg (9.9 ± 2.6 mmol)/day, while Hispanic females consumed a mean of 232 ± 71 mg (9.7 ± 3.0 mmol)/day (Plucke-baum and Chavez, 1994).

Food and Water Sources of Magnesium

Magnesium is ubiquitous in foods, but the magnesium content of foods varies substantially. Because chlorophyll is the magnesium chelate of porphyrin, green leafy vegetables are rich in magnesium. Foods such as unpolished grains and nuts also have high magnesium content, whereas meats, starches, and milk are more intermediate. Analyses from the 1989 Total Diet Study of the U.S. Food and Drug Administration indicated that approximately 45 percent of dietary magnesium was obtained from vegetables, fruits, grains, and nuts, whereas about 29 percent was obtained from milk, meat, and eggs (Pennington and Young, 1991). Refined foods generally have the lowest magnesium content. With the increased consumption of refined and/or processed foods, dietary magnesium intake in the United States appears to have decreased over the years (Marier, 1986). Total magnesium intake is usually dependent on caloric intake, which explains the higher intake levels seen in the young and in adult males and the lower levels seen in women and in the elderly.

Water is a variable source of intake; typically, water with increased "hardness" has a higher concentration of magnesium salts. Since this varies depending on the area from which water comes, much like fluoride, and the manner in which it is stored, magnesium intake from water is usually not estimated except in controlled diet studies. This omission may lead to underestimating total intake and its variability.

Intake from Supplements

Based on a national survey in 1986, 14 percent of men and 17 percent of women in the United States took supplements containing magnesium (Moss et al., 1989). Approximately 8 percent of young children (2 to 6 years of age) used magnesium-containing supplements. Women and men who use magnesium supplements took similar doses, about 100 mg (4.2 mmol)/day, although the ninety-fifth percentile of intake was somewhat higher for women, 400 mg (16.7 mmol)/day, than for men, who were taking 350 mg (14.6 mmol)/day. Children who took magnesium had a median daily intake of 23 mg (1 mmol) and a ninety-fifth percentile daily supplemental intake of 117 mg (4.9 mmol).

Effects of Inadequate Magnesium Intake

Severe magnesium depletion leads to specific biochemical abnormalities and clinical manifestations that can be easily detected. Hypocalcemia is a prominent manifestation of magnesium deficiency in humans (Rude et al., 1976). Magnesium deficiency must become moderate to severe before symptomatic hypocalcemia develops. Even mild degrees of magnesium depletion, however, may result in a significant fall in the serum calcium concentration, as demonstrated in a 3-week study of dietary-induced experimental human magnesium depletion (Fatemi et al., 1991).

Magnesium is also important in vitamin D metabolism and/or action. Patients with hypocalcemia and magnesium deficiency are resistant to pharmacological doses of vitamin D, 1α hydroxyvitamin D, and $1,25(OH)_2D$ (for a review, see Fatemi et al. [1991]).

Neuromuscular hyperexcitability is the initial problem cited in individuals who have or are developing magnesium deficiency (Rude and Singer, 1980). Latent tetany, as elicited by a positive Chvostek's and Trousseau's sign, or spontaneous carpal-pedal spasm may be present. Frank, generalized seizures may also occur. Although hypocalcemia may contribute to the neurological signs, hypomagnesemia without hypocalcemia may result in neuromuscular hyperexcitability.

There is emerging evidence that habitually low intakes of magnesium and resulting abnormal magnesium metabolism are associated with etiologic factors in various metabolic diseases. In considering data from such studies, it is important to separate the identification of associations between the effect of the disease on magnesium status from the effect of inadequate intake on magnesium status and subsequent risk of disease. The specific disease states in which magnesium status is implicated are discussed in the following sections.

Cardiovascular

In normal subjects, experimental magnesium depletion results in increased urinary thomboxane concentration, angiotensin II-induced plasma aldosterone levels, and blood pressure—indicating a potential effect of magnesium deficiency on vascular function (Nadler et al., 1993; Rude et al., 1989). Magnesium depletion is associated with cardiac complications, including electrocardiographic changes, arrhythmias, and increased sensitivity to cardiac glycosides (Rude, 1993). Atrial and ventricular premature systoles, atrial fibrillation, and ventricular tachycardia and fibrillation have been reported in hypomagnesemic patients (Hollifield, 1987; Rude, 1993). Significantly higher retention rates after magnesium load tests have been reported in patients with ischemic heart disease compared to normal controls (Rasmussen et al., 1988). This suggests that a low magnesium concentration may also play a role in cardiac ischemia. However, the extent to which the disease modifies the indicators of magnesium deficiency rather than the deficiency resulting in the disease manifestations varies with the symptom and the individual studied.

The development of atheromatous disease has been associated with magnesium in epidemiological observational studies. Areas with increased water hardness (which is due to high calcium and magnesium content) tend to have lower cardiovascular death rates (Altura et al., 1990; Hammer and Heyden, 1980; Leoni et al., 1985; Luoma et al., 1983; Neri and Johansen, 1978; Neri et al., 1985; Rubenowitz et al., 1996). Problems with evaluating epidemiological studies have been identified (Comstock, 1979), and some studies have not found such an association (Hammer and Heyden, 1980; Leoni et al., 1985). However, as presented by Tucker (1996) and Beaton (1996), a congruence of positive studies may suggest an association of dietary intake and disease. Animals on low magnesium diets develop arterial wall degeneration and calcification as well as hypertriglyceridemia, hypercholesterolemia, and atherosclerosis (Altura et al., 1990; Orimo and Ouchi, 1990). Controlled human studies that support this relationship are lacking.

Magnesium depletion in patients with cardiac diseases may be due to concomitant medications, such as diuretics, as well as to dietary magnesium depletion. Although cardiac arrhythmia may be associated with the primary cardiac disorders, magnesium depletion may further predispose to cardiac arrhythmias by decreasing intracellular potassium.

Accumulation of magnesium may reduce the morbidity and mortality of patients in the period following myocardial infarction. Two large, placebo-controlled, randomized, double-blind studies of patients with myocardial infarction have shown that intravenous magnesium therapy reduces the incidence of therapy-requiring arrhythmias to approximately one-half that seen in control patients (Antman, 1996; Seelig and Elin, 1996). In one study of patients with acute myocardial infarction, magnesium therapy given before thrombolytic therapy decreased mortality by 24 percent (Woods and Fletcher, 1994). Another large study of myocardial infarction did not find favorable effects of magnesium that was administered after thrombolytic therapy (ISIS-4, 1995). Debate currently centers over the time of administration of magnesium in terms of its favorable effects (for review see Antman [1996]). Evidence does not support the concept that the patients were magnesium deficient prior to onset of the acute attack, only that magnesium therapy was beneficial to outcome.

Blood Pressure

Epidemiologic evidence suggests that magnesium may play an important role in regulating blood pressure (Ascherio et al., 1992; Joffres et al., 1987; Ma et al., 1995; McCarron, 1983; Witteman et al., 1989). In these studies, populations that have low dietary intake of magnesium have been reported to have an increased incidence of hypertension. In one of the earlier studies, dietary intake of magnesium in 44 normotensive subjects was significantly greater than intake in 46 untreated hypertensive subjects (McCarron, 1983). In the Honolulu heart study, magnesium intake was the dietary variable that had the strongest association with blood pressure (Joffres et al., 1987). In another nutritional survey of 58,218 Caucasian women, those who reported intakes of less than 200 mg (8.33 mmol)/ day of magnesium had a significantly higher risk of developing hypertension than did women whose intakes were greater than 300 mg (12.5 mmol)/day. In a large prospective study of 30,681 men without diagnosed hypertension, dietary magnesium intake was inversely related to systolic and diastolic blood pressure and to change in blood pressure during a 4-year follow-up period (Ascherio et al., 1992). In this study, however, only dietary fiber had an independent inverse association. Another study of 15,248 subjects found that dietary magnesium intake was inversely associated with systolic and diastolic blood pressure (Ma et al., 1995).

Intervention studies with magnesium therapy for hypertensive patients have led to conflicting results. Several studies have shown a positive blood-pressure-lowering effect of magnesium supplements (Dyckner and Wester, 1983; Geleijnse et al., 1994; Motoyamo et al., 1989; Widman et al., 1993; Witteman et al., 1994); others have not (Cappuccio et al., 1985; Sacks et al., 1995; Wallach and Verch, 1986; Yamamoto et al., 1995; Zemel et al., 1990). Other dietary factors may also play a role. A recent study demonstrated that a diet of fruits and vegetables, which increased magnesium intakes from an average of 176 mg (7.3 mmol)/day to 423 mg (17.6 mmol)/day, significantly lowered blood pressure in adults who were not classified as hypertensive (systolic blood pressure < 140 mm Hg; diastolic blood pressure < 95 mm Hg) (Appel et al., 1997). The addition of nonfat dairy products to the high fruit and vegetable diet, which increased calcium intake as well, resulted in further lowering of blood pressure. Potassium intake was also greatly increased in both dietary regimens studied.

One study of hypertensive patients revealed low serum magnesium concentrations (Albert et al., 1958). No difference was detected in serum magnesium levels in other studies, however (Gadallah et al., 1991; Tillman and Semple, 1988). In patients with essential hypertension, free magnesium levels in erythrocytes were inversely related to both the systolic and diastolic blood pressure (Resnick et al., 1984). It is unclear whether the decrease in serum magnesium concentration was due to magnesium depletion or to pathophysiological events that lead to hypertension.

The possible relationship between hypertension and magnesium depletion is an important consideration, as the two coexist in a high proportion of individuals with diabetes and alcoholism (Resnick et al., 1991). However, the role of long-term dietary intake of magnesium in the prevalence of hypertension seen in the United States and Canada has not been established.

Skeletal Growth and Osteoporosis

Magnesium plays a major role in bone and mineral homeostasis and can also directly affect bone cell function as well as influence hydroxyapatite crystal formation and growth (Cohen, 1988).

Magnesium deficiency may be a risk factor for postmenopausal osteoporosis. Significant reductions in the serum magnesium and bone mineral content (BMC), but not red blood cell magnesium concentration or bone magnesium content, have been described in women with postmenopausal osteoporosis compared to age-matched controls (Reginster et al., 1989). No correlations were found in a 4-year clinical trial of magnesium intake and BMC in pre- and postmenopausal women consuming about 250 mg (10.4 mmol)/day of magnesium (Freudenheim et al., 1986), or in four of five skeletal sites measured in postmenopausal women also consuming an average of 253 mg ± 11 mg (10.5 ± 0.4 mmol)/day of magnesium (Angus et al., 1988).

In contrast, BMC of the radius in postmenopausal Japanese-American women was weakly positively correlated with magnesium intake (Yano et al., 1985), while elderly women who consumed less than 187 mg (7.8 mmol)/day had a significantly lower bone mineral density (BMD) compared with women whose average magnesium intake from diet was more than 187 mg (7.8 mmol)/day (Tucker et al., 1995).

Two studies are available on the effect of magnesium supplementation on osteoporosis. In women with documented osteoporosis, supplementation with 750 mg (31.3 mmol) of magnesium for the first 6 months followed by 250 mg (10.4 mmol) supplementation from the seventh to twenty-fourth month increased radial BMD after 12 months, but no further change was seen in BMD by the end of the second year (Stendig-Lindberg et al., 1993). Supplementation with 500 mg (20.8 mmol) of magnesium and 600 mg (15 mmol) of calcium in postmenopausal women who were receiving estrogen replacement therapy and daily multivitamin and mineral tablets resulted in increased calcaneous BMD in less than a year when compared with the postmenopausal women who received sex steroid therapy alone (Abraham and Grewal, 1990). These observations suggest that dietary magnesium may be related to osteoporosis and indicate a need for further investigation of the role of magnesium in bone metabolism (Sojka and Weaver, 1995).

Diabetes Mellitus

Magnesium depletion in a few studies has been shown to result in insulin resistance as well as impaired insulin secretion, and thereby may worsen control of diabetes (for review, see Paolisso et al. [1990]). An experimental magnesium depletion study was conducted to examine the development of insulin resistance. Normal male subjects were given a controlled diet for three weeks in a depletion metabolic study in which magnesium intake was 12 mg (0.5 mmol)/day. Intravenous glucose tolerance tests performed at the beginning and end of the 21-day depletion indicated a significant decrease in insulin sensitivity (Nadler et al., 1993). Such findings have raised the possibility that insulin resistance and abnormal glucose tolerance in individuals may be due to inadequate magnesium (Paolisso et al., 1992). Magnesium depletion in clinical observational studies has been defined by low serum magnesium concentrations as well as a reduction of total and/or ionized magnesium in red blood cells, platelets, lymphocytes, and skeletal muscle (Nadler et al., 1992), in spite of subjects consuming a level of magnesium similar to that in population studies (Schmidt et al., 1994).

Insulin resistance is commonly noted in the elderly (Fink et al., 1983; Rowe et al., 1983). Dietary magnesium supplements have been shown to improve glucose tolerance (Paolisso et al., 1992) and improve insulin response in elderly, non-insulin-dependent patients with diabetes (Paolisso et al., 1989). One possible cause for the magnesium depletion seen in diabetes is glycosuria-induced renal magnesium wasting (Rude, 1993). However, until magnesium de-pletion studies conducted in normal individuals can relate specific dietary intake levels with abnormal glucose tolerance testing or oth-er indicators of glucose metabolism, it is premature to consider the prevalence of diabetes mellitus as a functional indicator of adequa-cy for magnesium.

Increased Risk in the Elderly

Several studies have demonstrated that elderly people have rela-tively low dietary intakes of magnesium (Goren et al., 1993; Lowik et al., 1993). Their lower intake may be due to a variety of reasons, including poor appetite, loss of taste and smell, poorly fitting den-tures, and difficulty in shopping for and preparing meals (Moun-tokalakis, 1987). Meals in some long-term care facilities may pro-vide less than the recommended levels of magnesium (Lipski et al., 1993). In addition, magnesium metabolism may change with aging. As mentioned earlier, intestinal magnesium absorption tends to de-crease with aging, and urinary magnesium excretion increases (Low-ik et al., 1993; Martin, 1990). A suboptimal diet in magnesium may therefore place this population at risk for magnesium depletion.

ESTIMATING REQUIREMENTS FOR MAGNESIUM

Selection of Indicators for Estimating the Magnesium Requirement

Serum Magnesium

The serum magnesium concentration may not reflect intracellu-lar magnesium availability. Nevertheless, measurement of the se-rum magnesium concentration is the most available and commonly employed test to assess magnesium status. The serum magnesium level may be influenced by changes in serum albumin, other anion-ic ligands, and pH; however, correction for changes due to these factors is seldom made (Quamme, 1993). Normal values by age and gender have been derived from sampling the U.S. population in NHANES I (Lowenstein and Stanton, 1986). A serum magnesium concentration of less than 0.75 mmol/liter (1.8 mg/dl) is thought to indicate magnesium depletion (Elin, 1987).

Experimentally induced dietary magnesium depletion consistent-ly leads to decreased serum magnesium values in otherwise healthy humans. This suggests that, under these circumstances, serum mag-nesium is a sensitive indicator of magnesium status (Fatemi et al.,

1991). Hypomagnesemia (serum magnesium < 0.75 mmol/liter [1.8 mg/dl]) usually develops concurrently with moderate to severe magnesium depletion. However, in clinical studies in which concentrations of magnesium in blood cells, bone cells, or muscle cells are abnormally low (such as in diabetes mellitus, alcoholism, or malabsorption syndromes), serum magnesium values have been reported to be within the normal range (Abbott et al., 1994; Nadler et al., 1992; Rude and Olerich, 1996). These findings suggests that intracellular magnesium is a better guide to magnesium status in humans than is the concentration in serum (Reinhart, 1988; Ryzen et al. 1986). One recent longitudinal evaluation of 8,251 subjects who entered a study between 1971 and 1975 found 492 cardiovascular events when the subjects were reevaluated between 1982 and 1984 (Gartside and Glueck, 1995). Subjects with serum magnesium levels less than 0.81 mmol/liter (1.9 mg/dl) had greater risk of cardiovascular disease than did those with a serum magnesium level greater than 0.87 mmol/liter (2.1 mg/dl). Although both values were within what has been considered the normal range, 0.75 to 0.95 mmol/liter (1.8 to 2.3 mg/dl) (Elin, 1987), this variation in response questions the validity of serum magnesium levels as indicators of magnesium status (Gartside and Glueck, 1995). There are also reports that elderly subjects may have a decrease in magnesium status as determined by magnesium tolerance testing (see below) despite normal serum magnesium concentrations. Thus, serum magnesium concentration has not been validated as a reliable indicator of body magnesium status.

Plasma-Ionized Magnesium

Recently, ion-specific electrodes have become available for determining ionized magnesium in the plasma. Early results suggest that this may be a better index of magnesium status than the total serum magnesium concentration; however, further evaluation is necessary. Few studies have been conducted under varying conditions to assess its validity (Altura et al., 1992; Mimouni, 1996).

Intracellular Magnesium

The total magnesium contents of several tissues, including red blood cells, skeletal muscle, bone, and peripheral lymphocytes have been evaluated as indices of magnesium status. However, determination of intracellular magnesium concentration should be a more physiologically relevant measurement of magnesium status, as it is thought to play a critical role in enzyme activation within the cell. In general, poor correlation exists between the serum magnesium concentration and intracellular levels. Lymphocyte magnesium does not correlate well with serum or red blood cell magnesium levels (Elin and Hosseini, 1985; Ryzen et al., 1986) and serum magnesium concentration does not accurately reflect muscle magnesium content (Alfrey et al., 1974; Wester and Dyckner, 1980). In normal subjects lymphocyte and skeletal muscle magnesium did correlate well, however not in patients with congestive heart failure (Dyckner and Wester, 1985). Thus, further evaluation is needed before lymphocyte or muscle magnesium content can be utilized to assess magnesium status.

Red blood cell magnesium has been determined by nuclear magnetic resonance (Rude et al., 1991). The fluorescence probe has been utilized for determination of free magnesium in lymphocytes and platelets (Hua et al., 1995; Nadler et al., 1992). Red blood cell magnesium values fall within days following institution of a low-magnesium diet in normal subjects (Fatemi et al., 1991). The mean intracellular free magnesium was lower than normal in patients at high risk for magnesium depletion (for example, individuals with diabetes or alcoholism) (Hua et al., 1995; Nadler et al., 1992; Rude, 1991).

In one study, total red blood cell magnesium concentration was found to be lower in elderly subjects (77.8 ± 2.1 years), as compared with younger people (36.1 ± 0.4 years), when the mean magnesium consumption of both groups was 311 ± 21 mg (13.0 ± 0.9 mmol)/ day (Paolisso et al., 1992). However, the evidence was not judged sufficient to use red blood cell magnesium as an indicator of status.

Magnesium Balance Studies

The principal measure of adequate dietary magnesium in the past has been the dietary balance study (Greger and Baier, 1983; Hunt and Schofield, 1969; Mahalko et al., 1983; Schwartz et al., 1984, 1986). Most balance studies were performed at clinical research centers where the diet was constant and controlled. However, this technique still presents several problems, including the measurement of magnesium intake and urine and stool magnesium excretion. In addition, sweat and dermal losses of magnesium have not usually been considered.

In adults, balance studies should be performed at magnesium intakes just below and above those at which zero balance is achieved to obtain the approximately linear dependence of loss and retention near balance (Beaton, 1996). The intake associated with zero balance from each individual studied can then be grouped and the variability of requirements estimated (Beaton, 1996). Since magnesium intake is related to energy intake (Clarkson and Haymes, 1995; Niekamp and Baer, 1995), balance studies may report the findings in relation to estimated energy requirements if the data are to be applied to the general population. Magnesium may be obtained from food, water, nutrient supplements, or pharmalogical agents, but the bioavailability may differ.

Although numerous magnesium balance studies have been performed, not all met the requirements of a well-designed study. Some provided for a period of adaptation but did not include magnesium intakes, which would have allowed average requirements to be estimated. Balance studies performed prior to 1960 utilized less accurate means to measure magnesium as compared with atomic absorption spectrophotometry. The minimum criteria used here for inclusion of balance studies for the development of recommendations for magnesium requirements included either an adaptation period of at least 12 days or a determination of balance while the subjects consumed self-selected diets. The disadvantage of using self-selected diets is that only one level is being evaluated. If the individual is in balance or nearly so, it is not possible to discern if this is just an adaptation to that level or if it truly represents the minimal level of adequacy. Similarly, if only one level of intake is provided, no matter how accurate, it is not possible to get the dose response data necessary to estimate the requirement. At least two levels need to be evaluated: one below and one near the required level.

When a study is not carried out in a metabolic unit or under close supervision, data are generally lacking on magnesium intake from water. This omission precludes the use of many of the earlier studies conducted in free-living environments or current studies in which intakes were calculated rather than analyzed.

Estimates of Tissue Accretion During Growth

In the absence of data regarding specific requirements for magnesium for growth during various life stages, accretion rates of magnesium have been estimated (Nordin, 1976; Widdowson and Dickerson, 1964). The rates of tissue accretion during childhood are derived from analysis of cadavers, and the utility of these data is limited. In some cases using data from cadavers, the estimates of whole body mineral retention must be calculated based on measurements from regional sites (Fomon and Nelson, 1993). Fomon

and Nelson (1993) and Koo and Tsang (1997) used data from cadavers to estimate a net accretion of 10 mg (0.4 mmol)/day during
the second year of life. However, further information is needed
before this approach may be uniformly used to estimate magnesium needs throughout childhood.

The total magnesium content of an infant weighing 3.5 kg (7.7
lb) is approximately 220 mg (9.2 mmol)/kg or 760 mg (32 mmol).
Magnesium as a percentage of fat-free body mass increases during
gestation, but at birth the percentage is much less than that of an
adult (Widdowson and Dickerson, 1964). The content of magnesium in an adult man is estimated to total 27.4 g (1,141.7 mmol), or
about 390 mg (16.2 mmol)/kg (Widdowson and Dickerson, 1964).

In order to accumulate approximately 26.6 g (1,108.3 mmol) over
the 20 years of growth from infancy to adulthood, an average daily
accretion during this period of about 3.6 mg (0.2 mmol) would be
necessary. However, the growth rate is not linear with age. It has
been suggested that an adequate accretion rate (positive balance)
for girls 10 to 12 years of age and weighing about 40 kg (88 lb) is 8.5
mg (0.3 mmol)/day (Andon et al., 1996). For older children who
are heavier and experiencing greater growth in lean and bony tissue, a positive balance in the range of 10 mg (0.4 mmol)/day would
be appropriate.

Magnesium Tolerance Test

The magnesium tolerance test, which is based on the renal excretion of a parenterally administered magnesium load, has been used
for many years. It is considered by some to be an accurate means of
assessing magnesium status in adults, but not in infants and children (Gullestad et al., 1992; Ryzen et al., 1985). However, the sensitivity of this method in detecting magnesium depletion may be different between subjects with and without hypomagnesemia. In 15
hypomagnesemic subjects, 85 ± 3 percent of a parenterally administered magnesium load was retained, compared to only 14 ± 4 percent in 23 normal controls (Ryzen et al., 1985). In a group of 24
chronic alcoholics at risk of magnesium deficiency, retention of 51
± 5 percent was also significantly greater than the control group.
While the magnesium tolerance test has been shown in this and
other studies (Cohen and Laor, 1990; Costello et al., 1997; Gullestad et al., 1992) to detect magnesium depletion in both hypomagnesemic and normomagnesemic subjects at risk of magnesium
depletion, the test was not sensitive to detect treatment effects of
magnesium supplementation in otherwise healthy subjects (Costel-

lo et al., 1997). After 3 months of supplementation of 350 mg (14.5 mmol)/day of magnesium, the mean retention of 37 percent did not change significantly. Thus, the sensitivity of this method in normal subjects is not yet validated and so cannot be accepted as the primary indicator for assessing adequacy at this time.

One of the problems in using the magnesium tolerance test is that it requires normal renal handling of magnesium. Urinary magnesium loss (related to conditions such as diabetes or drug or alcohol use) may yield an inappropriate negative test. Moreover, impaired renal function may result in a false positive test (Martin, 1990). Age may also be a confounding variable, since older subjects (73 ± 6 years) have been reported to retain significantly more magnesium than younger subjects (33 ± 10 years), despite a comparable mean daily dietary magnesium intake of 5.1 mg (0.2 mmol)/kg of body weight (Gullestad et al., 1994). Supplements of 225 mg (9.4 mmol)/day of magnesium as magnesium lactate-citrate for 30 days to the elderly subjects turned the test results toward normal. Martin (1990) studied 30 elderly females (mean age of 82 years, range 72 to 93 years) who were stated to have "lower than recommended dietary magnesium intakes." Subjects with serum magnesium less than 0.59 ± 0.07 mmol/liter (1.4 ± 0.2 mg/dl) retained a higher percentage of the magnesium load (61 ± 12 percent) than subjects with mean serum magnesium levels of 0.72 ± 0.02 mmol/liter (1.7 ± 0.05 mg/dl) whose retention was 43 ± 16 percent. Both of these levels of retention, however, are high compared to that seen in younger age groups. Thus the influence of renal function in this test cannot be ignored. Of significant concern, even if this test is validated in future studies as a primary indicator of magnesium status, is the invasive procedure (intravenous administration) used.

Epidemiological Studies and Meta-analysis

As discussed in the previous section, epidemiologic studies have suggested that individuals or groups ingesting hard water that contains magnesium, consuming a diet higher in magnesium, or using magnesium supplements, have decreased morbidity from cardiovascular disease or less hypertension (Altura et al., 1990; Ascherio et al., 1992; Hammer and Heyden, 1980; Joffres et al., 1987; Leoni et al., 1985; Luoma et al., 1983; Ma et al., 1995; McCarron, 1983; Nadler et al., 1993; Neri and Johansen, 1978; Neri et al., 1985; Rubenowitz et al., 1996; Witteman et al., 1989). Low magnesium intake has also been linked to osteoporosis (Sojka and Weaver, 1995). Because of the difficulty of conclusively establishing that the lack of dietary magnesium was the primary causative factor in these chronic diseases, the basis for a claim is equivocal. Thus, based on the scientific literature currently available, these data can not serve as the indicators of adequacy in estimating magnesium requirements. However, as recently reviewed by Tucker (1996), the evidence from many studies, taken together, may lend confidence to the theory that dietary magnesium intake may indeed contribute to these disorders.

FINDINGS BY LIFE STAGE AND GENDER GROUP

Birth through 12 Months

No functional criteria of magnesium status have been demonstrated that reflect response to dietary intake in infants. Thus, recommended intakes of magnesium are based on an Adequate Intake (AI) that reflects the observed mean intake of infants fed principally with human milk.

Indicators Used to Set the AI

Human Milk. Human milk is recognized as the optimal milk source for infants throughout at least the first year of life and recommended as the sole nutritional milk source for infants during the first 4 to 6 months of life (IOM, 1991). Therefore, determination of the AI for magnesium for infants is based on data from infants fed human milk as the principal fluid during periods 0 through 6 and 7 through 12 months of age. The AI is set at the mean value for observed intakes as determined from studies in which intake of human milk was measured by test weighing volume, and intake of food was determined by dietary records for 3 days or more.

Balance Studies. The limited data on magnesium balance in infants were considered supportive evidence for the derived AI. Many of the magnesium balance studies involving human milk-fed infants have been performed on premature infants or infants in the first weeks of life. Net retention of magnesium in the studies of premature infants was 10 to 15 mg (0.4 to 0.6 mmol)/day with 45 percent absorption (Atkinson et al., 1987; Schanler et al., 1985). This level of retention was similar to that reported earlier in 10 breast-fed infants at 5 to 7 days of age, with repeat balance studies performed in three of these infants again at 4 to 6 weeks of age (Widdowson, 1965).

Differences in magnesium needs between infants fed human milk and those fed infant formula are described in the "Special Considerations" section.

AI Summary: Ages 0 through 6 Months

Based on data from a summary of recent studies in North America and the United Kingdom (Atkinson et al., 1995), the concentration of magnesium in human milk is about 34 mg (1.4 mmol)/liter, and the concentration remains relatively constant over the first year of lactation (Allen et al., 1991; Dewey et al., 1984). The AI is set based on a reported average intake of human milk of 780 ml/day (Allen et al., 1991; Butte et al., 1984; Heinig et al., 1993) and the average milk magnesium concentration of 34 mg (1.4 mmol)/liter. This gives an AI of 30 mg (1.3 mmol)/day. The balance data cited above support an AI of 30 mg (1.3 mmol)/day for this age range, as it would allow infants to maintain a positive magnesium balance of at least 10 mg (0.4 mmol)/day during early infancy.

AI Summary: Ages 7 through 12 Months

During the second 6 months of life, solid foods become a more important part of the infant diet and add a significant but poorly defined amount of magnesium. The absorption of magnesium from solid foods and the effects of solid foods on absorption of magnesium from human milk are unknown. To set an AI for infants from 7 through 12 months of age, the average magnesium intake from solid foods—55 mg (2.2 mmol)/day—for 9- to 12-month-old formula-fed infants (Specker et al., 1997) was used. This approach assumes that infants who are fed human milk have intakes of solid food similar to those fed formulas.

Based on the data of Heinig et al. (1993), the mean volume of human milk consumed between 7 and 11 months of age would be 600 ml/day. Thus, magnesium intake from human milk with an average magnesium concentration of 34 mg (1.4 mmol)/liter would be about 20 mg (0.8 mmol)/day. Summing the intake from human milk and from solid food, the AI for magnesium for infants 7 through 12 months of age is set at 75 mg (3.1 mmol)/day.

AI for Infants	0 through 6 months	30 mg (1.1 mmol)/day
	7 through 12 months	75 mg (3.1 mmol)/day

Special Considerations

Infant Formulas. Commercial infant formulas that are cow milk-based are generally higher in magnesium concentration, 40 to 50 mg (1.7 to 2.1 mmol)/liter, than human milk. Soy-based formulas may have even higher concentrations of magnesium, 50 to 80 mg (2.1 to 3.3 mmol)/liter (Fomon and Nelson, 1993; Greer, 1989). In a large series of studies (>300 balances), Fomon and Nelson (1993) reported approximately 40 percent net absorption of magnesium in infants fed soy or cow milk-based formulas with a net retention of 10 mg (0.4 mmol)/day based on total intakes of 53 to 59 mg (2.2 to 2.5 mmol)/day of magnesium.

Higher absorption values of 57 to 71 percent of magnesium intake from standard cow milk-based infant formulas have been reported (Kobayashi et al., 1975; Moya et al., 1992). A dietary fractional absorption rate of 64 ± 4 percent was reported in three infants aged 4 to 10 months. Magnesium intakes of the infants exceeded 150 mg (6.3 mmol)/day in the latter study.

Direct assessment of an AI for magnesium for formula-fed infants is not possible due to the lack of data comparing magnesium absorption from human milk and from infant formulas. Based on the current U.S. practices of infant formula manufacturers, the increase of 20 percent above the level of magnesium intake of human milk-fed infants allows for the possibility of a lower bioavailability of magnesium from formulas. This leads to an estimated intake of 35 mg (1.5 mmol)/day (human milk + 20 percent) for formula-fed infants. Similar absorption of magnesium from soy versus routine formulas (Fomon and Nelson, 1993) does not indicate a greater need for magnesium in soy formula-fed infants, but the practice of increasing magnesium intake in soy formulas relative to cow-milk formulas is widely followed by formula manufacturers.

Ages 1 through 3, 4 through 8, 9 through 13, and
14 through 18 Years

Indicators Used to Set the EAR

A possible approach to determining human magnesium requirements is to estimate the intake required to achieve a level of retention associated with a beneficial outcome. Although magnesium retention during growth should be positive, the desirable extent of retention for magnesium is unknown. As discussed earlier, there are inadequate data upon which to attribute a specific benefit to maximal retention of magnesium. This is unlike calcium, for which maximal retention can be associated with benefit to bone mass accretion. Since the criterion of maximal retention could not be used for magnesium, magnesium balance data were used as the basis for establishing Estimated Average Requirements (EARs) for these age groups.

As mentioned previously, an adequate accretion rate (positive balance) for girls 10 to 12 years of age and weighing about 40 kg (88 lb) may be 8.5 mg (0.3 mmol)/day (Andon et al., 1996). It is probable that for older children, who are heavier and experiencing greater growth in lean and bony tissue, a positive balance in the range of 10 mg (0.4 mmol)/day of magnesium would be appropriate. This would allow for the greater need for magnesium during the specific periods of faster growth during older childhood. In the absence of more definitive goals, a daily positive balance of 8 to 10 mg (0.3 to 0.4 mmol) of magnesium seems to be a reasonable goal upon which to base an EAR for growing children and adolescents.

Balance Studies. For children under 10 years of age, there is only one report of a balance study published since 1960 (Schofield and Morrell, 1960). For children between 10 and 15 years of age, seven studies were available for consideration (see Table 6-1). The amount of magnesium lost via other routes (dermal, sweat, menses, and other losses) was not measured or estimated in the calculations of any of these studies. Other balance studies performed in children prior to 1960 (see review by Seelig [1981]) were not considered because information regarding absorption over a range of intakes was not provided and results reported may not be reliable using the analytical methodology available at that time.

Given the information provided in the available balance studies, expression of magnesium requirements for children is probably more accurate on the basis of intake per day, rather than per unit of body weight or per amount of lean tissue. When expressed on a mg/kg/day basis, magnesium requirements determined by balance studies in subjects who were obese were much lower than those in subjects of normal weight (Jones et al., 1967), as fat contains less magnesium than other tissues and body fat increases with age. Expressing EARs and Recommended Dietary Allowances (RDAs) per kg ideal body weight or lean body mass would be more accurate than per kg total weight. However, since most reports of balance studies do not provide individual intake and body weight or height data, it is seldom possible to determine the response of individuals to specific levels of magnesium consumed on either an ideal or actual body weight basis. Future experiments might address requirements in relation to energy needs (Shils and Rude, 1996).

Because of the lack of studies in younger children, the data from children 10 to 15 years old (see Table 6-1) were extrapolated using reference body weights. Interpretation of the available balance data are confounded by the lack of information provided on individual body weights, varying age and weight ranges studied within and between studies, and variations in dietary protein (both in amount and source) and calcium (see "Calcium" and "Protein" below). In reviewing the details of the studies summarized in Table 6-1, it appears that, provided the diet has adequate protein for 9 through 13 year olds, group mean positive magnesium balance in the range of 10 mg (0.41 mmol)/day is achieved at intakes of approximately 5 mg (0.21 mmol)/kg/day. In the recent short-term study using multitracer stable isotope technique to assess magnesium balance in 13 adolescent girls (Abrams et al., 1997), the mean magnesium balance was slightly negative (–0.9 ± 41 mg [0.04 ± 1.7 mmol]/day) at comparatively high levels of average intake (6.4 mg [0.27 mmol]/kg/day of magnesium). Some of this may have been due to the amount of calcium in the diet (1,310 mg [33 mmol]/day); however, another recent study using multitracer stable isotopes (Sojka et al., 1997), did not show a significant difference in magnesium balance with two levels of dietary calcium (see "Calcium" below).

In the one balance study in which children 7 to 9 years old were evaluated, positive magnesium balance was achieved on daily dietary magnesium intakes that ranged from 121 to 232 mg (5.0 to 9.7 mmol)/day (Schofield and Morrell, 1960); a magnesium intake of 5 mg (0.21 mmol)/kg/day appeared to meet some but not all of the younger children's needs. Taken together with the data on older children, the available balance studies suggest that at a magnesium intake of 5 mg/kg body weight/day, some but not all children would be in magnesium balance. The extent to which this represents 50 percent of children in these age groups and pubertal stages meeting their needs is difficult to predict because of the confounding variables of other dietary components. For establishing the EARs for magnesium for children ages 1 through 3 and 4 through 8, for which balance studies are unavailable, the value of 5 mg/kg/day is adopted.

Additional Factors Considered for the Above Studies

Calcium. As stated earlier, increasing calcium intake may have a negative effect on magnesium balance (Greger et al., 1981). In two recent studies in this age group, however, little effect was noted. Compared with a calcium intake of 667 mg (16.7 mmol)/day, intakes of 1,667 mg (41.7 mmol)/day (the additional 1,000 mg [25 mmol] from two divided doses of a supplement) did not decrease magnesium retention in girls aged 10 to 12 years (Andon et al., 1996). In a magnesium kinetic study in which five girls aged 12 to 14 years were given two stable isotopes of magnesium at two levels of calcium, 800 mg (20 mmol) and 1,800 mg (45 mmol), no significant differences were seen in the magnesium balances measured or in the percentage of magnesium absorbed (Sojka et al., 1997). The calcium contents of the diets provided in the other two balance studies of adolescents were 1,200 mg (30 mmol) (which included supplements) (Schwartz et al., 1973) and 1,060 to 1,080 mg (26.5 to 27 mmol) from foods (Greger et al., 1978). Supplementation with 900 mg (22.5 mmol) of calcium to a controlled, food-based diet containing 300 to 350 mg (12.5 to 14.6 mmol) and 697 mg (17.4 mmol) calcium/day did not affect overall magnesium retention in eight adult male subjects (Lewis et al., 1989).

Protein. Magnesium requirements are influenced by the level of dietary protein, apparently in part related to effects on urinary magnesium excretion (Lakshmanan et al., 1984; Mahalko et al., 1983; Wisker et al., 1991). Magnesium intakes in male adolescents on lower protein intakes (50 g/day) were inadequate, but with higher protein diets (94 g/day), balances became positive (Schwartz et al., 1973). Some have suggested that the effect of protein may differ for animal and vegetable sources. However, in one study of adolescent girls, little difference was noted in this age group when soy was substituted for animal protein at a level of 30 percent of the total protein that was fed at a level of 46 to 49 g/day (Greger et al., 1978). The influence of protein intake on magnesium requirements needs additional study.

EAR Summary: Ages 1 through 3 and 4 through 8 Years

In the absence of adequate balance or usual accretion data in children aged 1 through 8 years, it is necessary to interpolate data from other age groups based on changes in body weight and linear growth.

TABLE 6-1 Magnesium (Mg) Balance Studies in Adolescents Aged 9 through 18 Years

Study, Year	n	Age (y)	Weight (kg)	Adaptation period (d)	Balance period (d)	Average Daily Mg Intake	Balance	Comments
Females								
Andon et al., 1996	13	10.5–12.5	39 ± 5	7	7	176 mg (4.45 mg/kg)	19 ± 25 mg/d	Intake >5.0 mg/kg/d resulted in positive balance in all subjects.
	13		42 ± 8	7	7	176 mg (4.45 mg/kg)	22 ± 15 mg/d	Half of subjects on 1,667 mg Ca/d; half on 1667 mg Ca/d.
Greger et al., 1978	5	12.5–14.5	34.5–58.5	9	21	190 ± 29 mg	−6.8 ± 10.4 mg/d	At intakes of 4.0 mg/kg/d, only 2 of the 26 girls were in positive balance.
	5			9	21	195 ± 29 mg	−6.8 ± 10.4 mg/d	At intakes of 4.0 mg/kg/d, only 2 of the 26 girls were in positive balance.
	4			9	21	195 ± 29 mg	−1.8 ± 2.2 mg/d	
Greger et al., 1979	11	12.5–14.2	52.5 ± 13.6	5	9	Avg. 276 mg	15 ± 18 mg/d	Diet contained 1,049 mg calcium; 11.3 mg zinc.
				5	9		2 ± 36 mg/d	Diet contained 1,049 mg calcium; 14.5 mg zinc.

Reference								
Abrams et al., 1997	13	12.3 ± 1.6	48 ± 17.7	14	10	19–321 mg (6.4 ± 1.2 mg/kg/d)	−0.9 ± 41.2 mg/d	Six of 13 in negative balance; adapted to 1,310 mg calcium intake before entry.
Sojka et al., 1997	5	12–14	54.6	7	14	264–346 mg (305 ± 30 mg)	13 ± 35 mg/d	Diet contained 61 g protein; 823 mg calcium.
				7	14	272–294 mg (286 ± 9 mg)	−34 ± 48 mg/d	Diet contained 61 g protein; 1,824 mg calcium.
Males								
Schwartz et al., 1973	6	13.8–15	40.5–70.5*	15	15 2x/2 y	240 mg (4.3 + 0.21 mg/kg)	−0.62 ± .07 mg/kg/d	43 g/d protein.
					15 2x/2 y	240 mg (4.1 ± 0.16 mg/kg)	0.19 ± 0.08 mg/kg/d	93 g/d protein.
					15 2x/2 y	740 mg (13.1 ± 0.51 mg/kg)	1.25 ± 0.26 mg/kg/d	43 g/d protein.
					15 2x/2 y	740 mg (14.5 ± 0.61 mg/kg)	0.88 ± 0.48 mg/kg/d	93 g/d protein.
Abrams et al., 1997	12	10.9 ± 1.1	35.7 ± 7.0	14	10	194–321 (6.4 ± 1.2 mg/kg/d)	15.6 ± 36.8 mg/d	Five of 12 in negative balance; adapted to 1,310 mg calcium before entry.

* Weights at end of first balance study.

Based on studies in adolescents (Abrams et al., 1997; Andon et al., 1996; Greger et al., 1978, 1979; Schwartz et al., 1973) and the one study in 7- to 9- year-old children (Schofield and Morrell, 1960), a magnesium intake of 5 mg (0.21 mmol)/kg/day appears to have met some but not all the needs of those evaluated. This is the basis for the EAR for children ages 1 through 3 years and 4 through 8 years. For children ages 1 through 3 years with a reference weight of 13 kg (Table 1-3), the EAR is 65 mg (2.7 mmol)/day. For children ages 4 through 8 years with a reference weight of 22 kg, the EAR is 110 mg (4.6 mmol)/day. It is recognized that further studies specific to this age group are needed before more precise EARs can be assigned or distinctions made between males and females or between children of different racial or ethnic groups.

EAR for Children   1 through 3 years   65 mg (2.7 mmol)/day
4 through 8 years   110 mg (4.6 mmol)/day

Based on the 1994 CSFII magnesium intake data, adjusted for day-to-day variation (Nusser et al., 1996), the first percentile of intake for children ages 1 through 3 years is 80 mg (3.3 mmol) (see Appendix D), which is above the EAR of 65 mg (2.7 mmol)/day. The median intake for magnesium for this age group is 180 mg (7.5 mmol). For children ages 4 through 8 years, the first percentile of intake is 103 mg (4.3 mmol)/day, slightly below the EAR of 110 mg (4.6 mmol)/day. The median magnesium intake is 206 mg (8.6 mmol)/day.

Determination of the RDA: Ages 1 through 3 and 4 through 8 Years

The variance in requirements cannot be determined from the available data. Thus, a coefficient of variation (CV) of 10 percent is assumed, which results in an RDA for magnesium of 80 mg (3.3 mmol)/day for children ages 1 through 3 years, and an RDA of 130 mg (5.4 mmol)/day for children ages 4 through 8 years.

RDA for Children   1 through 3 years   80 mg (3.3 mmol)/day
4 through 8 years   130 mg (5.4 mmol)/day

EAR Summary: Ages 9 through 13 Years, Boys

The Abrams et al. (1997) study provides some data for boys ages 9 through 13 years that leads to the conclusion that boys, not yet into maximal growth at this age, appear to require about the same amount of magnesium as girls per kg per day. Thus, the EAR is estimated to be 5 mg (0.21 mmol)/kg/day for boys ages 9 through 13 years. Based on a reference weight of 40 kg (Table 1-3) for boys ages 9 through 13 years, their EAR is 200 mg (8.3 mmol)/day.

EAR for Boys   9 through 13 years   200 mg (8.3 mmol)/day

Based on the 1994 CSFII magnesium intake data adjusted for day-to-day variation (Nusser et al., 1996), the tenth percentile of intake for boys ages 9 through 13 years is 181 mg (7.5 mmol)/day, and the twenty-fifth percentile intake is 216 mg (9 mmol)/day (see Appendix D). Thus the EAR of 200 mg (8.3 mmol)/day for boys ages 9 through 13 years would fall between the tenth and twenty-fifth percentile of intake in this age category.

EAR Summary: Ages 9 through 13 Years, Girls

Because the protein intake of the younger girls in the Andon et al. (1996) study was not indicated, it is possible that one of the reasons that most of the girls were in positive magnesium balance on the 176 mg (7.3 mmol)/day intake was their higher intake of dietary protein. The second possible reason is their younger age and body size. In the absence of additional data and assuming a protein intake of 50 g/day, the EAR for girls ages 9 through 13 years is 5 mg (0.21 mmol)/kg/day, based primarily on the Andon et al. (1996) study, in which all girls who consumed this level or less were in positive balance. Their average weights were 41 kg (90 lb), and few had yet started menarche. In the Greger et al. study (1979), the average weight was 52.5 kg (115.7 lb), and 6 of the 11 girls had already started menarche. Their requirements reflect a greater lean body mass. Thus, based on the reference weight of 40 kg (Table 1-3) for girls ages 9 through 13 years, their EAR is 200 mg (8.3 mmol)/day.

EAR for Girls   9 through 13 years   200 mg (8.3 mmol)/day

Based on the 1994 CSFII intake data and adjusted for day-to-day variation (Nusser et al., 1996), the twenty-fifth percentile magnesium intake for girls ages 9 through 13 years is 194 mg (8.1 mmol), and the median intake is 224 mg (9.3 mmol)/day (see Appendix D). Thus, the magnesium EAR of 200 mg (8.1 mmol)/day would be between the twenty-fifth percentile and the median intake for girls ages 9 through 13 years.

Determination of the RDA for Magnesium: Ages 9 through 13 Years

The variance in requirements cannot be determined from the data available. Thus, a CV of approximately 10 percent is assumed for each EAR. This results in an RDA of 240 mg (10 mmol)/day for both boys and girls ages 9 through 13 years.

RDA for Boys   **9 through 13 years**   **240 mg (10 mmol)/day**
RDA for Girls   **9 through 13 years**   **240 mg (10 mmol)/day**

EAR Summary: Ages 14 through 18 Years

Given the available data, it seems appropriate to conclude that for older adolescents, the average magnesium requirement is greater than 5 mg (0.21 mmol)/kg/day. The average *additional* magnesium intake necessary to result in a net retention of about 8 mg (0.33 mmol)/day is about 16 mg (0.67 mmol) or 0.3 mg (0.12 mmol)/kg/day for a 55 kg adolescent based on an assumed absorption rate of 40 percent (range 30 to 50 percent) (Abrams et al., 1997). Less than 5 mg (0.21 mmol)/kg/day of magnesium resulted in negative balances in all boys when they consumed the lower protein intake in the Schwartz et al. (1973) study and in most of the older girls in the Greger et al. (1978) study. In the 2-year Schwartz et al. (1973) study, even for subjects on the high protein diet, average magnesium retention was 6 and 15 mg (0.25 and 0.63 mmol)/day for each year, respectively, at the 240 mg (10 mmol)/day intake level. Thus, the EAR is estimated to be 5.3 mg (0.22 mmol)/kg/day in 14- through 18-year-old boys and girls, given that the highest average level provided in any of the five long-term balance studies (Andon et al., 1996; Greger et al., 1978, 1979; Schwartz et al., 1973, Sojka et al., 1997) was 5.6 mg (0.23 mmol)/kg/day. This resulted in slightly negative nitrogen balances in the older children studied (Greger et al., 1978; Schwartz et al., 1973). An average intake of 6.4 mg (0.27 mmol)/kg/day resulted in net positive magnesium retention in the more recent stable isotope study of Abrams et al. (1997). Thus, for boys ages 14 through 18 years, with reference weight 64 kg (Table 1-3), the EAR for magnesium is 340 mg (14.2 mmol)/day, and for girls in this age range with reference weight of 57 kg, the EAR is 300 mg (12.5 mmol)/day.

EAR for Boys   **14 through 18 years**   **340 mg (14.2 mmol)/day**
EAR for Girls   **14 through 18 years**   **300 mg (12.5 mmol)/day**

Based on the 1994 CSFII intake data, adjusted for day-to-day variation (Nusser et al., 1996), the magnesium EAR of 345 mg (14.4 mmol)/day for boys ages 14 through 18 years is above the median intake of 301 mg (12.5 mmol)/day and below the seventy-fifth percentile of intake, 372 mg (15.5 mmol)/day (see Appendix D). For girls in this age range, the EAR for magnesium of 300 mg (12.5 mmol)/day is just above the ninetieth percentile of intake, 296 mg (12.3 mmol)/day.

Determination of the RDA: Ages 14 through 18 Years

The variance in requirements cannot be determined from the available data. Thus, a CV of approximately 10 percent is assumed for each EAR. This results in an RDA for magnesium of 410 mg (17.1 mmol)/day for boys ages 14 through 18 years and an RDA for magnesium of 360 mg (15.0 mmol)/day for girls ages 14 through 18 years when rounded.

RDA for Boys   **14 through 18 years**   **410 mg (17.1 mmol)/day**
RDA for Girls   **14 through 18 years**   **360 mg (15.0 mmol)/day**

Ages 19 through 30 Years

Indicators Used to Set the EAR for Men

Balance Studies. The results of studies that have looked at magnesium balance in men and women aged 19 through 30 years in various situations are included in Table 6-2. As with the balance studies conducted in adolescents, no estimates or measurements of other losses of magnesium (due to dermal, sweat, etc.) are included. Since few references are available to estimate these losses, gross balances are presented. In the controlled diet study (Greger and Baier, 1983), which was designed to look at the influence of aluminum on mineral balances, men (25 ± 3 years) were in positive balance on average intakes of 447 mg (18.6 mmol) from food and dietary supplements. This represents 6.4 mg (0.27 mmol)/kg/day for these subjects, but may overestimate requirements as only one level was given.

Another controlled study, this one designed to look at the effect of bran on mineral requirements, was conducted in seven men aged

TABLE 6-2 Magnesium (Mg) Balance Studies in Men and Women Aged 19 through 30 Years

Study, Year	n	Age (y)	Adaptation Period (d)	Balance Period (d)	Average Daily Mg Intake	Balance (mg/d)	Comments
Males							
Greger and Baier, 1983	8	25 ± 3	12	6	Avg. 447 mg (6.4 mg/kg)	−1 ± 8	6.4 mg/kg maintained balance but adaptation period was too short.
Lakshmanan et al., 1984	9	20–35	N/A	Four 1-wk periods over 1 y	Self-selected; 190–595 mg (avg. 333 ± 120 mg) (avg. 4.3 mg/kg)	−19 ± 48	Self-selected intakes (ranging from 204 to 595 mg) sufficient to maintain balance in 4 of 9 subjects.
Schwartz et al., 1986	7	22–32	28	21	Avg. 719 ± 105 mg	27 ± 19	Intakes greater than 597 mg/d were sufficient to maintain balance in all but one subject (who received 788 mg/d).
Females							
Lakshmanan et al., 1984	8	20–35	N/A	Four 1-wk periods over 1 y	Self-selected; 132–350 mg (avg. 239 ± 80 mg) (avg. 4.2 mg/kg)	−25 ± 40	Three of the 8 subjects in balance on average intakes self-selected (ranging from 213 to 304 mg).
Wisker et al., 1991	12	22–28	14 14 14	7 7 7	252 mg 243 mg 245 mg	7 ± 5 −12 ± 5 5 ± 2	22.5 g/d fiber 71.8 g/d protein. 38.6 g/d fiber 55.7 g/d protein. 38.6 g/d fiber 73.8 g/d protein.

22 to 32 years (Schwartz et al., 1986); dietary magnesium intake was 719 ± 105 mg (30 ± 4.4 mmol)/day. With one exception, all subjects were in magnesium equilibrium or positive balance after 48 days. These levels were thus not low enough to accurately estimate average requirements. In a year-long study of men aged 20 to 35 years, subjects kept daily food records for 1 year, and 1-week balance studies were conducted four times. The subjects continued to select their own diet but provided food and beverage samples for analysis (Lakshmanan et al., 1984). The assumption in this study was that each subject's average of the four weekly balances over the year would be representative of his typical intake and requirement. The average magnesium intake of 333 ± 120 mg (13.9 ± 5 mmol)/day resulted in a slight overall average negative balance. Again, since multiple levels were not evaluated, it is difficult to ascertain actual requirements from these data; however it appears that five of the nine subjects consuming this average intake of 333 mg (13.9 mmol)/day of magnesium were probably meeting their needs.

Indicators Used to Set the EAR for Women

Balance Studies. The results of two balance studies for women in this age range are also summarized in Table 6-2. The year-long study by Lakshmanan and coworkers (1984) included young women (20 to 35 years) on self-selected diets, with duplicates of week-long intakes analyzed four times during the year. The average magnesium intake of this age group of women was 239 ± 80 mg (10 ± 3.3 mmol); this intake resulted in positive magnesium balance or equilibrium in three of the eight subjects. A controlled food intake study in Germany tested a low-phytate barley fiber added to two levels of dietary protein to determine the effects of the fiber and protein on mineral balances (Wisker et al., 1991). Magnesium intake of 243 to 252 mg (10.1 to 10.5 mmol)/day (reported to be on the average 4.3 mg [0.18 mmol]/kg/day) in women resulted in the 12 subjects being close to equilibrium on the low-fiber, high-protein diet but not as close on the high-fiber, low-protein diet.

EAR Summary: Ages 19 through 30 Years, Men

Based primarily on the study of Lakshmanan et al. (1984) and the others cited above, the EAR for magnesium for males ages 19 through 30 years is estimated to be 330 mg (13.8 mmol)/day. This is based on the assumption that the best current indicator of adequacy, given the lack of supporting data for other outcomes, is for an individual to maintain total body magnesium over time as opposed to being in negative magnesium balance. The absence of confirmatory research providing causal relationships in human studies between magnesium intake and risk of cardiovascular disease precludes use of markers for cardiovascular disease in this age group at this time. This EAR also reflects the lack of data to support the concept that there is a need for continued accretion of magnesium during this life stage.

EAR for Men   19 through 30 years   330 mg (13.8 mmol)/day

Based on the 1994 CSFII intake data and adjusted for day-to-day variation (Nusser et al., 1996), the median magnesium intake for men ages 19 to 30 years is 331 (13.8 mmol)/day (see Appendix D), which is approximately the same magnesium intake as the EAR of 330 mg (13.8 mmol)/day.

EAR Summary: Ages 19 through 30 Years, Women

Based on the studies described above, and primarily on the overall negative balances of the Lakshmanan et al. (1984) study, which found average magnesium intakes of 239 mg (10 mmol)/day, the EAR for women ages 19 through 30 years is estimated to be above 239 mg (10.0 mmol)/day. The Wisker et al. (1991) study had somewhat more positive balances on a slightly higher overall intake of 255 mg (10.6 mmol)/day. This EAR is also based on the assumption that the best current indicator of adequacy, given the lack of supporting data for other outcomes, is for an individual to maintain total body magnesium over time as opposed to being in negative magnesium balance. This EAR also reflects the lack of data that there is a specific need for accretion of magnesium during this period.

EAR for Women   19 through 30 years 255 mg (10.6 mmol)/day

Based on the 1994 CSFII intake data and adjusted for day-to-day variation (Nusser et al., 1996), the median magnesium intake for women ages 19 through 30 years is 205 mg (8.5 mmol)/day, and the seventy-fifth percentile of magnesium intake is 250 mg (10.4 mmol)/day (see Appendix D), which is slightly below the EAR of 255 mg (10.6 mmol)/day.

Determination of the RDA: Ages 19 through 30 Years

The variance in requirements cannot be determined from the data available for either men or women. Thus, a CV of 10 percent is assumed in both cases. This results in an RDA for magnesium in men ages 19 through 30 years of 400 mg (16.7 mmol)/day, and for women ages 19 through 30 years of 310 mg (12.9 mmol)/day.

RDA for Men   **19 through 30 years 400 mg (16.7 mmol)/day**
RDA for Women **19 through 30 years 310 mg (12.9 mmol)/day**

Ages 31 through 50 Years

Indicators Used to Set the EAR in Men

Balance Studies. The results of five balance studies in men aged 31 through 50 years, which met the criteria for inclusion, are shown in Table 6-3. Two controlled-intake studies which looked at the influence of dietary oxalate and fiber on mineral balances, included magnesium balances for men aged 34 to 58 years who were consuming either high-fiber (Kelsay et al., 1979) or high-oxalate (Kelsay and Prather, 1983) diets. Intakes ranged from 308 to 356 mg (12.8 to 14.8 mmol)/day. On a low, nondigestible fiber diet (4.9 g/day), average magnesium balance was positive; but the magnesium intake was not sufficient on the high-fiber or high-oxalate diets to maintain magnesium balance. Magnesium balance in male subjects aged 19 to 64 years given lower magnesium intakes (229 or 258 mg [9.5 or 10.8 mmol]) at two levels of dietary protein has also been estimated (Mahalko et al., 1983). Average magnesium balance at either protein level was at equilibrium for this wider-age-range group, indicating that, at least based on crude magnesium balance, dietary intake was near adequacy overall. However, in another study, magnesium intakes of 240 to 264 mg (10 to 11 mmol)/day resulted in net negative balances (–23 mg [1 mmol]/day and –26 mg [1.1 mmol]/day) in the five subjects studied (Spencer et al., 1994). Magnesium intakes of 789 to 826 mg (32.9 to 34.4 mmol)/day resulted in positive balances in these same subjects. Finally, in a year-long study of magnesium intakes by individuals on self-selected diets with periodic measurements of balance, average intake of seven male subjects aged 35 to 53 years, was 310 ± 88 mg (12.9 ± 3.7 mmol)/day (Lakshmanan et al., 1984). The individual averages of the four 1-week balance periods during the year resulted in a group mean negative magnesium balance, although three subjects had average

TABLE 6-3 Magnesium (Mg) Balance Studies in Men and Women Aged 31 through 50 Years

Study, Year	n	Age (y)	Adap-tation Period (d)	Balance Period (d)	Average Daily Mg Intake (mean ± SEM)	Balance (mg/d) (mean ± SEM)	Comments
Males							
Kelsay et al., 1979	12	37–58	19	7	356 ± 10 mg	28 ± 17	4.9 g fiber from fruit and vegetable juices; Mg and iron added to be equivalent to higher fiber test diet.
			19	7	322 ± 12 mg	−32 ± 10	23.8 g fiber from fruits and vegetables.
Kelsay and Prather, 1983	12	34–58	21	7	308 ± 10 mg	20 ± 14	4.9 ± 0.4 g fiber including spinach.
			21	7	350 ± 7 mg	−10 ± 13	26.5 ± 0.6 g fiber with spinach.
			21	7	356 ± 10 mg	18 ± 13	24.0 ± 0.6 g fiber with cauliflower substituted for spinach.
Mahalko et al., 1983	10	19–64	16	12 (6 2x)	229 ± 24 mg[a]	13 ± 30[a]	65 g/d protein.
				12	258 ± 24 mg[a]	17 ± 36[a]	94 g/d protein.

Reference	n	Age		Duration	Intake	Balance[a]	Comments
Spencer et al., 1994	5	38–75	28	40	264 ± 26 mg	−23 ± 21	241 mg/d Ca.
				32	240 ± 24 mg	−26 ± 14	812 mg/d Ca.
				28	826 ± 37 mg	23 ± 24	241 mg/d Ca.
				39	798 ± 28 mg	48 ± 24	812 mg/d Ca.
Lakshmanan, 1984	7	35–53	N/A	Four 1-wk periods over 1 y	Self-selected; 157–418 mg	−48 ± 59	Three in equilibrium (intakes ranging from 286 to 418 mg); 4 subjects in average negative balance (intakes ranging from 157 to 344 mg) on self-selected average intakes.
Females							
Lakshmanan, 1984	10	35–53	N/A	Four 1-wk periods over 1 y	Self-selected; 164–301 mg (avg 231 ± 46 mg) (avg 4.2 mg/kg)	−25 ± 37	Four in positive balance or at equilibrium with intakes ranging from 182 to 258 mg; 6 were in negative balance with intakes ranging from 164 to 301 mg on self-selected average intakes.

[a] Mean ± SD.

positive balances or were in equilibrium and four were in negative balance.

Indicators Used to Set the EAR in Women

Balance Studies. The only study in females for this age group was part of the year-long study of dietary intakes of men and women, which included an estimation of magnesium balance in 10 women aged 25 to 53 years (Lakshmanan et al., 1984). The average magnesium intake was 231 ± 80 mg (9.6 ± 3.3 mmol)/day. Four subjects were in positive or zero balance, while six were in negative balance, which suggests that 231 mg (9.6 mmol)/day is probably less than is necessary to prevent magnesium loss in 50 percent of women ages 31 through 50 years. Thus, the average requirement for women ages 31 through 50 years appears to be somewhat higher than 231 mgs (9.6 mmol)/day.

EAR Summary: Ages 31 through 50 years, Men

Based on the studies described above, the average requirement for males ages 31 through 50 years does not appear to differ substantially from that of men ages 19 through 30 years. However, there are more instances of negative balance in the intake range of 300 to 350 mg (12.5 to 14.6 mmol)/day in the older subjects studied. The EAR is thus set at 350 mg (14.6 mmol)/day, with the expectation that with age, consumption of diets with higher fiber content increases. Since the two studies in which lower magnesium levels were consumed resulted in predominantly negative balances (Mahalko et al., 1983; Spencer et al., 1994), the data of the Lakshmanan et al. study (1984) raise a concern: the self-selected magnesium intake of the older men was more than 10 percent below that of the younger men in the same study.

This EAR is also based on the assumption that the best current indicator of adequacy, given lack of supporting data for other outcomes, is for an individual to maintain total body magnesium over time as opposed to being in negative magnesium balance. The observed change from average negative magnesium retention to positive retention or vice versa caused by changes in other factors in the diet (for example, fiber, protein) rather than the level of magnesium consumed provides two perspectives: (1) it gives some assurance that the dietary level being evaluated is within the range of the average requirement, and (2) it gives an indication of the many factors that affect magnesium requirements as evaluated by balance studies. Thus, it is the combination of balance studies that provides some assurance that the estimates of average requirements derived are of value as dietary reference intakes.

EAR for Men   31 through 50 years   350 mg (14.6 mmol)/day

Based on the 1994 CSFII magnesium intake data and adjusted for day-to-day variation (Nusser et al., 1996), the EAR of 350 mg (14.6 mmol)/day for men ages 31 through 50 years falls between the median magnesium intake of 327 mg (13.6 mmol)/day and the seventy-fifth percentile of magnesium intake of 397 mg (16.5 mmol)/day (see Appendix D).

EAR Summary: Ages 31 through 50 Years, Women

Based on the one study described above in which women aged 25 to 53 years were predominantly in negative magnesium balance at an average intake of 231 mg (9.6 mmol)/day (Lakshmanan et al., 1984), and comparing the information on younger women and on men, the EAR for women ages 31 through 50 years is estimated to be 265 mg (11.0 mmol)/day. This is quite close to the EAR for younger women, which was based on data from the same study. However, two pieces of evidence lead to the conclusion that the EAR is somewhat greater for this age group. Since renal function is critical to maintenance of magnesium status, and it has been shown to decline with age, it follows that an increased EAR is warranted. Also, a higher percentage of the older women were in negative balance compared to the younger women. This was also demonstrated when comparing the older men (31 through 50 years) with the younger men (19 through 30 years). This EAR is based on the assumption that the best current indicator of adequacy, given lack of supporting data for other outcomes, is for an individual to maintain total body magnesium over time.

EAR for Women 31 through 50 years   265 mg (11.0 mmol)/day

Based on the 1994 CSFII intake data and adjusted for day-to-day variation (Nusser et al., 1996), the median magnesium intake of women aged 31 through 50 years is 229 mg (9.5 mmol)/day (see Appendix D). This is below the EAR of 265 mg (11.0 mmol). The seventy-fifth percentile of intake is 277 mg (11.5 mmol)/day, which is above the EAR.

Determination of the RDA: Ages 31 through 50 Years

The variance in requirements cannot be determined from the available data for either men or women. Thus, a CV of 10 percent is assumed for both cases. This results in an RDA for men ages 31 through 50 years for magnesium of 420 mg (17.5 mmol) and for women, 320 mg (13.3 mmol)/day.

RDA for Men   **31 through 50 years**   **420 mg (17.5 mmol)/day**
RDA for Women 31 through 50 years   **320 mg (13.3 mmol)/day**

Ages 51 through 70 Years

Indicators Used to Set the EAR for Men

Balance Studies. The results of five balance studies for men aged 51 through 70 years are shown in Table 6-4. Balance studies cited in Table 6-3 (aged 31 through 50 years) by Kelsay et al. (1979), Kelsay and Prather (1983), Mahalko et al. (1983), and Spencer et al. (1994) included some male subjects in this age range, so these data are also included in this age group. Schwartz et al. (1984) assessed magnesium balance in eight males, mean age 53 ± 5 years and mean weight 67 ± 14 kg (148 ± 31 lb). A positive magnesium balance was found in the men who consumed an average intake of 381 mg (15.9 mmol)/day of magnesium (5.9 mg or 0.25 mmol/kg/day on the average).

Indicators Used to Set the EAR for Women

No studies have been reported for women in this age group.

EAR Summary: Ages 51 through 70 Years, Men

A mean daily magnesium intake of 381 mg (15.9 mmol) maintained balance in all eight subjects in the Schwartz et al. (1984) study, following a 30-day adaptation period. This would indicate that, in the absence of other studies that might demonstrate different results, the EAR should be less than 380 mg (15.8 mmol) in order to prevent magnesium loss. This study, along with those discussed above in the other adult age groups, indicates that the EAR can be expected to be somewhere between 330 and 380 mg (13.8 and 15.8 mmol)/day. Given the lower body weights in the Schwartz et al. (1984) study compared with those in the younger age groups, the magnesium intakes per kg body weight are greater (approxi-

TABLE 6-4 Magnesium (Mg) Balance Studies in Men and Women Aged 51 through 70 Years

Author, Year	n	Age (y)	Adaptation Period (d)	Balance Period (d)	Average Daily Mg Intake (mean ± SEM)	Balance (mg/d) (mean ± SEM)	Comments
Males							
Kelsay et al., 1979	12	37–58	19	7	356 ± 10 mg	28 ± 17	4.9 g fiber from fruit and vegetable juices; Mg and iron added to be equivalent to higher fiber test diet.
			19	7	322 ± 12 mg	−32 ± 10	23.8 g fiber from fruits and vegetables.
Kelsay and Prather, 1983	12	34–58	21	7	308 ± 10 mg	20 ± 14	4.9 ± 0.4 g fiber including spinach.
			21	7	350 ± 7 mg	−10 ± 13	26.5 ± 0.6 g fiber with spinach.
			21	7	356 ± 10 mg	18 ± 13	24.0 ± 0.6 g fiber with cauliflower substituted for spinach.
Mahalko et al., 1983	10	19–64	16	12 (6 2x)	229 ± 24 mg[b]	13 ± 30[b]	65 g/d protein.
				12	258 ± 24 mg[b]	17 ± 36[b]	94 g/d protein.
Spencer et al., 1994	5	38–75	28	40	264 ± 26 mg	−23 ± 21	241 mg/d Ca.
				32	240 ± 24 mg	−26 ± 14	812 mg/d Ca.
				28	826 ± 37 mg	23 ± 24	241 mg/d Ca.
				39	798 ± 28 mg	48 ± 24	812 mg/d Ca.
Schwartz et al., 1984	8	53 ± 5	30	6	381 ± 36 mg (5.7 mg/kg)	25 ± 15	Balance was positive in all subjects.
Females[a]							

[a] No studies have been reported in females in this age group.
[b] Mean ± SD.

mately 5.9 mg [0.25 mmol]/kg/day). Because the data for the age group 31 through 50 years reflect more instances of negative balance when dietary magnesium intakes were in the range of 300 to 350 mg (12.5 to 14.6 mmol)/day, it is appropriate to estimate the EAR to be 350 mg (14.6 mmol)/day, particularly in light of the importance of renal function to maintaining magnesium homeostasis. This EAR is based on the assumption that the best current indicator of adequacy, given lack of supporting data for other outcomes, is to maintain total body magnesium over time.

EAR for Men   51 through 70 years   350 mg (14.6 mmol)/day

Based on the 1994 CSFII intake data and adjusted for day-to-day variation (Nusser et al., 1996), the median intake of magnesium for men aged 51 through 70 years is 295 mg (12.3 mmol)/day, and the seventy-fifth percentile of intake is 362 mg (15.1 mmol)/day (see Appendix D), which is slightly above the EAR of 350 mg (14.6 mmol)/day.

EAR Summary: Ages 51 to 70 Years, Women

Because there are no studies in women in this age group, the EAR is based on the one study described in women aged 31 through 50 and on comparisons of the information in younger women and in men. There is no basis on which to change the EAR for this age group from that for women ages 31 through 50 years, which is estimated to be 265 mg (11.0 mmol)/day, other than a concern about the possible decline in renal function associated with aging. However, since an adjustment for declining renal function was included in the estimate of the 31- through 50-year-old women, no further adjustment is needed for this age group. Thus, the EAR is also 265 mg (11.0 mmol)/day for women ages 51 through 70 years. This EAR is also based on the assumption that the best current indicator of adequacy, given lack of supporting data for other outcomes, is to maintain total body magnesium over time.

EAR for Women 51 through 70 years   265 mg (11.0 mmol)/day

Based on the 1994 CSFII intake data and adjusted for day-to-day variation (Nusser et al., 1996), the median intake of magnesium for women aged 51 through 70 years is 230 mg (9.6 mmol)/day, and the seventy-fifth percentile of intake is 276 mg (11.5 mmol)/day (see Appendix D), which is slightly above the EAR of 265 mg (11.0 mmol)/day for women in this age range.

Determination of the RDA: Ages 51 through 70 Years

The variance in requirements cannot be determined from the data available for either men or women ages 51 through 70 years. Thus, a CV of 10 percent is assumed for both cases. This results in an RDA for men ages 51 through 70 years of approximately 420 mg (17.5 mmol)/day, and for women, 320 mg (13.3 mmol)/day.

RDA for Men   **51 through 70 years**   **420 mg (17.5 mmol)/day**
RDA for Women   **51 through 70 years**   **320 mg (13.3 mmol)/day**

Ages >70 Years

Indicators Used to Set the EAR

Studies in this age group have aggregated data from both men and women, and therefore the requirements will be considered together. The greater numbers of individuals with chronic diseases in this population, and the comparative lack of research studies carried out in healthy free-living individuals in this age category, make estimation of requirements problematic.

Balance Studies. No magnesium balance studies that meet the criteria previously described have been reported in subjects over 70 years of age.

Magnesium Tolerance Tests. One study with 36 healthy elderly subjects (8 males and 28 females) 65 years of age and older (average age 73 ± 6 years), used magnesium tolerance testing as the indicator of adequacy (Gullestad et al., 1994). The self-selected dietary magnesium intake was estimated from food frequency questionnaires to be 380 ± 94 mg (15.8 ± 3.9 mmol)/day in the males and 300 ± 61 mg (12.5 ± 2.5 mmol)/day in the females. When corrected for body weight, this intake was similar in both sexes, 5.1 mg (0.21 mmol)/kg/day. Magnesium retention from the load given was 28 ± 16 percent in the elderly and was significantly greater than the 3.6 percent retention in a reference group of 53 subjects aged 55 ± 12 years. However, no correlation was seen between estimated magnesium intake and magnesium retention from the load given. These data do not provide convincing evidence on which to base an estimated requirement.

Intracellular Studies. Intracellular magnesium was assessed in two studies in elderly subjects. Total red blood cell magnesium was measured in 381 institutionalized, elderly subjects aged 80 ± 9.5 years (Touitou et al., 1987). The mean dietary magnesium intake was 240 mg (10 mmol)/day. Abnormally low blood cell magnesium was found in 21 percent of the subjects (about 10 percent had low plasma magnesium concentrations as well). A large number of these subjects had conditions and/or had been on medications that contributed to the apparent poor magnesium status. After excluding these factors, the prevalence of low red blood cell magnesium in the remaining 198 subjects was not significantly different (19 percent). Again, no correlation was found between dietary intake and red blood cell magnesium values. In another study, red blood cell magnesium values in 12 nonobese elderly subjects (6 males, 6 females) aged 78 ± 2 years were compared with those of 25 young healthy subjects (13 males, 12 females) aged 36 ± 0.4 years (Paolisso et al., 1992). Self-selected dietary magnesium intakes of both groups were estimated to be 311 ± 21 mg (13.0 ± 0.9 mmol)/day. Red blood cell magnesium levels in the elderly were 1.86 mmol/liter (4.5 mg/dl), which was significantly less than that of the control subjects, with average levels of 2.18 mmol/liter (5.2 mg/dl). Magnesium therapy in the elderly resulted in a rise in red blood cell magnesium and an increase in insulin secretion and action, which suggests that the low red blood cell magnesium was physiologically relevant in this population.

EAR Summary: Ages > 70 Years

Because no balance studies meeting appropriate criteria are available, other possible indicators of magnesium requirements for this age group were reviewed. However, no conclusive studies were found. The methods used in the studies of magnesium tolerance testing and intracellular magnesium discussed above have yet to be validated sufficiently to serve as the basis for estimating average requirements.

The reported magnesium intakes from the three available studies using these methodologies, however, are consistent with balance studies in younger age groups. The study by Gullestad et al. (1994), using magnesium tolerance testing, found an estimated average dietary magnesium intake in males of 380 mg (15.8 mmol)/day and 300 mg (12.5 mmol)/day in females. The study of intracellular magnesium by Touitou and coworkers (1987) suggests that the average requirement would be approximately 240 mg [10 mmol]/day). The study by Paolisso and colleagues (1992) found that in elderly subjects, an average dietary magnesium intake of 311 mg (13.0 mmol)/day was accompanied by a lower mean red blood cell magnesium concentration, which was not found in younger controls.

Given the uncertainty in the above methods, and the lack of balance data in healthy, elderly individuals to support the intake levels that may appear to be warranted based on the above analysis, estimates of magnesium requirements are suggested to remain at the level established for the other older adult age groups. These estimates would be within the range identified above as estimating the average requirement for elderly. It must be remembered, though, that urinary magnesium excretion has been shown to increase with age (Lowik et al., 1993, Martin, 1990), indicating a decrease in renal function.

EAR for Men	**> 70 years**	**350 mg (14.6 mmol)/day**
EAR for Women	**> 70 years**	**265 mg (11.0 mmol)/day**

Based on the 1994 CSFII intake data and adjusted for day-to-day variation (Nusser et al., 1996), the median magnesium intake for men aged > 70 years is 274 mg (11.4 mmol)/day (see Appendix D). The EAR of 350 mg (14.6 mmol)/day falls between the seventy-fifth percentile of magnesium intake of 334 mg (13.9 mmol)/day and the ninetieth percentile of intake of 394 mg (16.4 mmol)/day. For women in this same age range, the median magnesium intake is 205 mg (8.5 mmol)/day. As for men ages > 70 years, the magnesium EAR for women of 265 mg (11.0 mmol)/day falls between the seventy-fifth percentile of intake of 248 mg (10.3 mmol)/day and the ninetieth percentile of intake of 290 mg (12.1 mmol)/day.

Determination of the RDA for Magnesium: Ages > 70 Years

The variance in requirements could not be determined from the available data for either men or women ages > 70 years. Thus, a CV of 10 percent is assumed for the > 70 years age group. This results in an RDA for men ages > 70 years for magnesium of approximately 420 mg (17.5 mmol)/day and for women ages > 70 years of 320 mg (13.3 mmol)/day.

RDA for Men	**> 70 years**	**420 mg (17.5 mmol)/day**
RDA for Women	**> 70 years**	**320 mg (13.3 mmol/day**

Pregnancy

Indicators Used to Set the EAR

Serum Magnesium Concentrations. Because serum magnesium concentration is reduced during pregnancy (Kurzel, 1991; Weissberg et al., 1992), the use of magnesium sulfate as a tocolytic agent has led some investigators to study the possible role of magnesium status in determining pregnancy and infant outcome, including the incidence of preterm labor and pregnancy-induced hypertension and fetal growth retardation, mental retardation, and cerebral palsy in the newborn (Conradt et al., 1984; Rudnicki et al., 1991; Schendel et al., 1996). However, the reduction in serum magnesium concentration during pregnancy is thought to be due, in part, to hemodilution, and this decrease parallels the decrease seen in serum protein (Seydoux et al., 1992). Serum ionized magnesium has also been reported to decrease late in pregnancy (Bardicef et al., 1995; Handwerker et al., 1996). Therefore, serum magnesium concentrations do not appear to be adequate indicators of magnesium status.

Intracellular Magnesium. Inconsistent findings have been reported on changes in lymphocyte magnesium concentrations during pregnancy. Some investigators report no change (Seydoux et al., 1992), while others find intracellular magnesium depletion (Bardicef et al., 1995). Such indicators of magnesium status have not been adequately assessed during pregnancy and thus are not used here as the basis for determining requirements.

Balance Studies. Few magnesium balance studies have been performed in pregnant subjects. One study of 48 magnesium balances conducted in 10 subjects for 7-day periods at various stages of pregnancy has been reported (Ashe et al., 1979). The balances, which were not carried out in a metabolic unit setting, demonstrated an average negative magnesium balance of –40 mg (–1.7 mmol)/day on a mean daily magnesium intake of 269 ± 55 mg (11.2 ± 2.3 mmol) (Ashe et al., 1979).

Magnesium Tolerance Tests. Parenteral magnesium load tests in postpartum American and Thai women have been conducted to evaluate the methodology (Caddell et al., 1973, 1975). In 185 American women, the mean magnesium retention was 51 percent. Higher magnesium retention was associated with lower serum magnesium concentrations as well as with diets low in magnesium-rich foods (Caddell et al., 1975). In Thai women, who consumed a diet containing more magnesium-rich foods, a mean retention of 23 percent was observed (Caddell et al., 1973).

Pregnancy Outcome. Several cross-sectional studies have investigated whether magnesium status is altered in women with gestational diabetes, preterm labor, pregnancy-induced hypertension, or preeclampsia (Bardicef et al., 1995; Kurzel, 1991; Seydoux et al., 1992; Weissberg et al., 1992). The results of these studies are not consistent, possibly due to the control groups that were used or the inability to distinguish whether altered magnesium status precedes the outcome or the outcome influences magnesium status.

In one cross-sectional study, lower serum magnesium concentrations were observed in women during preterm labor ($n = 71$) compared with normal pregnant women in labor ($n = 128$) (Kurzel, 1991). Although this study found no difference in serum magnesium concentrations between the two groups, others have observed reduced serum magnesium during labor (Weissberg et al., 1992). Therefore, it is not clear whether hypomagnesemia induces uterine irritability and leads to preterm labor or whether labor results in a reduction in serum magnesium concentration.

Longitudinal studies have an advantage over cross-sectional studies in that changes in magnesium intake or status can be determined prior to knowing the final outcome of pregnancy. A prospective observational study of 965 women who were followed from 30 weeks gestation found no effect of magnesium intake on birthweight, as determined by a self-administered questionnaire and a structured interview (Skajaa et al., 1991). The mean reported daily magnesium intake was relatively high at 445 mg (18.5 mmol) for the entire population, with a 95 percent range of 256 to 631 mg (10.7 to 26.3 mmol). The subgroups of women who gave birth to a small-for-gestational age infant, had preterm labor, or who later developed preeclampsia all had similar mean magnesium intakes and serum magnesium concentrations during their third trimester compared with women who had normal pregnancies. There were no differences in tissue magnesium concentrations determined from either abdominal rectus or myometrial muscle biopsies among women delivering by cesarean section because of intrauterine growth retardation ($n = 5$), preeclampsia ($n = 12$), or labor difficul-

TABLE 6-5 Magnesium (Mg) Supplementation Trials During Pregnancy

Criteria	Magnesium Dose (mg/d)	Mg Supplement		Placebo		Significance (p value)
		n	%	n	%	
Serum Magnesium						
Sibai et al., 1989	365	105	1.68 mg/dl[a]	112	1.56 mg/dl[a]	<0.01
Preeclampsia						
Sibai et al., 1989	365	4/185	2.2	7/189	3.7	NS
Spatling and Spatling, 1988	365	2/278	0.7	2/290	1.0	NS
Preterm Labor						
Sibai et al., 1989	365	13/185	7.0	14/189	7.4	NS
Spatling and Spatling, 1988	365	12/278	4.3	26/290	9.0	<0.05
Preterm Delivery						
Sibai et al., 1989	365	19/185	10.2	18/189	9.5	NS
Spatling and Spatling, 1988	365	4/278	1.4	8/290	2.8	NS
Kuti et al., 1981	127–202	2/111	1.8	50/365	7.9	<0.05
Intrauterine Growth Retardation						
Sibai et al., 1989	365	9/187	4.9	12/190	6.3	NS
Spatling and Spatling, 1988	365	5/278	1.8	6/290	2.1	NS
Kuti et al., 1981	127–202	1/111	1.0	2/635	0.3	NS
Infants Admitted to Special Care Unit						
Sibai et al., 1989	365	14/187	7.5	13/190	6.8	NS
Spatling and Spatling, 1988	365	20/278	7.2	36/290	12.4	<0.01

[a] Mean serum magnesium level.

NS = non-significant.

ties ($n = 14$). The results of this study appear to indicate that intrauterine growth retardation, preterm labor, and preeclampsia are not associated with daily magnesium intakes around 445 mg (18.5 mmol) or with serum magnesium concentrations at approximately 30 weeks gestation; and in a small number of women with adverse outcomes, tissue concentrations of magnesium were not abnormal at the time of delivery (Skajaa et al., 1991).

A retrospective study by Conradt and coworkers (1984) found that magnesium supplementation had a beneficial effect on pregnancy outcome. Pregnancy outcomes were studied during a period when the practice of magnesium supplementation changed. Women with high-risk pregnancies were routinely supplemented with 36 to 72 mg (1.5 to 3 mmol)/day magnesium throughout the study ($n = 660$), whereas during the previous 2 years women were routinely supplemented with 360 to 480 mg (15 to 20 mmol)/day magnesium ($n = 264$). Unfortunately, the study groups were not randomized, and baseline estimates of magnesium intakes were not determined. Pregnancy outcomes among these two groups were compared with outcomes among high-risk women not receiving magnesium supplements ($n = 4,023$). The results showed that women receiving either level of magnesium did not develop pregnancy-induced hypertension and preeclampsia; among those not receiving supplements, 97 cases (2 percent) occurred. Women with the higher intake of magnesium had a lower incidence of intrauterine growth retardation than did women with the lower intake.

Three prospective trials of magnesium supplementation during pregnancy have been conducted (Table 6-5). One study was a double-blind, randomized, controlled trial (Sibai et al., 1989), one was a quasi-randomized trial (group assignment determined by mother's date of birth) (Spatling and Spatling, 1988), and the randomization method of the other was not clear (Kuti et al., 1981). In the first two studies, women were supplemented with magnesium aspartate-hydrochloride containing 365 mg (15.2 mmol)/day of magnesium. In the third study, women were supplemented with magnesium citrate, which provided a daily magnesium average intake of 170 to 340 mg (7.1 to 14.2 mmol). Women were categorized into three levels of total magnesium consumed throughout the pregnancy. Daily magnesium intake from supplements was estimated to be 127 to 202 mg (5.3 to 8.4 mmol) for the category with the highest level of magnesium consumed (Table 6-5).

Baseline magnesium intake was not reported in any of the studies. The mean daily magnesium intake for women in Hungary at the time the study by Kuti and coworkers (1981) was conducted was 330 mg (13.8 mmol). Daily magnesium intakes by pregnant women in the United States, where the study by Sibai and coworkers was completed, ranged from 158 to 259 mg (6.6 to 10.8 mmol) (Franz, 1987). Based on these baseline estimates of dietary magnesium intake and the amounts provided in the above trials, total magnesium intakes in the supplemented groups would have ranged from 420 to 625 mg (17.5 to 26 mmol). The results of magnesium supplementation trials indicate that the incidence of preeclampsia and intrauterine growth retardation was not affected by magnesium supplementation in two studies, the incidence of preterm delivery decreased in only one of three studies, and preterm labor was less frequent in one of two studies (see Table 6-5).

Accretion Rate during Pregnancy. The increase in body weight caused by lean tissue accretion during pregnancy is expected to result in a greater requirement for magnesium if there are no pregnancy-induced increases in intestinal absorption and renal reabsorption. Data are not available on accretion of magnesium in lean tissue during pregnancy, but this accretion can be estimated (see following section). Given that fat-free body mass contains about 470 mg (19.6 mmol) of magnesium/kg (Widdowson and Dickerson, 1964), it is possible to determine the amount necessary for accretion for an appropriate weight gain.

EAR Summary for Pregnancy

Inconsistent findings on the effect of magnesium supplementation on pregnancy outcome make it difficult to determine whether magnesium intakes greater than those recommended for non-pregnant women are beneficial. In addition, there are no data indicating that magnesium is conserved during pregnancy or intestinal absorption is increased. The gain in weight associated with pregnancy alone may result in a greater requirement for magnesium.

The EAR for pregnancy is set at an additional 35 mg (1.5 mmol)/day. This additional requirement is based on the following assumptions:

• Appropriate added lean body mass (LBM) is 6 to 9 kg with a midpoint of 7.5 kg (IOM, 1991).
• The magnesium content of 1 kg of LBM is 470 mg (19.6 mmol) (Widdowson and Dickerson, 1964).
• The adjustment factor for a bioavailability of 40 percent (Abrams et al., 1997) is 2.5.

Calculation: (7.5 kg /270 days) × 470 mg/kg × 2.5 = 33 mg/day (rounded up to 35) This value is to be added to the EAR for the woman's age group.

EAR for Pregnancy   All ages   + 35 mg (1.5 mmol)/day

Based on the 1994 CSFII intake data for 33 pregnant women and adjusted for day-to-day variation (Nusser et al., 1996), the median magnesium intake of pregnant women is 292 mg (12.2 mmol)/day, and the seventy-fifth percentile of intake is 332 mg (13.8 mmol)/day (see Appendix D). The EAR of 290 mg (12.1 mmol)/day for pregnant women ages 19 through 30 years and the EAR of 300 mg (12.7 mmol)/day for pregnant women ages 31 through 50 would fall close to the median of magnesium intake. The seventy-fifth percentile of intake, 332 mg (15.3 mmol)/day, is near the magnesium EAR of 335 mg (15.2 mmol)/day for pregnant women ages 14 through 18 years.

Determination of the RDA: Pregnancy

The variance in requirements cannot be determined from the available data for pregnant women. Thus a CV of 10 percent is assumed. This results in an increase in the RDA for pregnancy for magnesium as follows:

EAR for Pregnancy
14 through 18 years	335 mg (14.0 mmol)/day
19 through 30 years	290 mg (12.7 mmol)/day
31 through 50 years	300 mg (12.7 mmol)/day

RDA for Pregnancy
14 through 18 years	400 mg (16.7 mmol)/day
19 through 30 years	350 mg (15.0 mmol)/day
31 through 50 years	360 mg (15.0 mmol)/day

Special Considerations

Diabetes Mellitus. Infants of mothers with Type I insulin-dependent diabetes mellitus are at risk of hypocalcemia and hypomagnesemia, possibly due to magnesium deficiency in the mother (Mimouni et al., 1986; Tsang et al., 1976). Lower intracellular magnesium concentrations have been recently reported in women with gestational diabetes (Bardicef et al., 1995). It is not known whether this is a sequellae of the condition or a factor in its causation.

Pregnant Adolescents, Multiparous Births. A prospective study of 53 nulliparous teenagers found no difference in serum or erythrocyte magnesium concentrations between those pregnant adolescents who developed pregnancy-induced hypertension and those who had normal term deliveries, with both groups having decreasing concentrations of magnesium over gestation (Boston et al., 1989). However, Caddell and coworkers (1975) found a greater renal retention of a parenteral load of magnesium in pregnant adolescents and women with twin pregnancies, suggesting that magnesium requirements during these periods may be increased.

Lactation

Indicators Used to Set the EAR

Human Milk Content. The concentration of magnesium in human milk averages between 25 to 35 mg (1.0 to 1.5 mmol)/liter and is not influenced by the mother's magnesium intake (Moser et al., 1983, 1988). Assuming a milk production of 780 ml/day, a lactating woman may secrete from 9 to 26 mg (0.4 to 1.1 mmol)/day of magnesium in her milk (Allen et al., 1991).

Despite the secretion of magnesium in milk during lactation, plasma and erthyrocyte magnesium concentrations do not differ between lactating and nonlactating women at daily magnesium intakes of approximately 250 mg (10.4 mmol) (Moser et al., 1983), and milk concentrations do not change throughout lactation (Dewey et al., 1984; Moser et al., 1983; Rajalakshmi and Srikantia, 1980).

Balance Studies. A magnesium balance study in six lactating women, six nonlactating postpartum women, and seven women who were never pregnant found lower urinary magnesium concentrations in lactating women compared with women who were never pregnant (Dengel et al., 1994). A positive magnesium balance of 20 mg (0.84 mmol)/day was reported in lactating women consuming a daily magnesium intake of 217 mg (9 mmol). However, there was only a 5-day adaptation period, and although the women appeared to conserve magnesium, the small number of subjects may have lead to an insufficient ability to detect a difference. Whether the increased bone resorption that occurs during lactation contributes to the magnesium pool available for milk production, or whether renal conservation is sufficient to meet the increased need, is unknown. Urinary magnesium concentrations in the lactating women were similar to those of nonlactating postpartum women; however, the 24-hour urinary magnesium losses in these lactating women were similar to urinary losses in women determined to be magnesium depleted based on the results of magnesium loading tests (Caddell et al., 1975). Although this study found lower urinary magnesium excretion in lactating women consuming an estimated daily average magnesium intake of 217 mg (9 mmol), another study found no difference in urinary magnesium concentrations between lactating and never-pregnant women who consumed higher average daily intakes of magnesium, around 270 mg (11.3 mmol) (Klein et al., 1995).

EAR and RDA Summary for Lactation

Currently, no consistent evidence exists to support an increased requirement for dietary magnesium during lactation. It appears that decreased urinary excretion of magnesium and increased bone resorption during lactation may provide the necessary magnesium for milk production. Therefore, the EAR and RDA are estimated to be the same as that obtained for nonlactating women of similar age and body weight.

EAR for Lactation

14 through 18 years	300 mg (12.5 mmol)/day
19 through 30 years	255 mg (11.3 mmol)/day
31 through 50 years	265 mg (11.3 mmol)/day

RDA for Lactation

14 through 18 years	360 mg (15.0 mmol)/day
19 through 30 years	310 mg (13.3 mmol)/day
31 through 50 years	320 mg (13.3 mmol)/day

Based on the 1994 CSFII intake data and adjusted for day-to-day variation (Nusser et al., 1996), the median intake of magnesium in 16 lactating women is 316 mg (13.2 mmol)/day; the fifth percentile of intake for the 16 women (of unspecified age) was 267 mg (11.1 mmol)/day (see Appendix D), which is slightly above the magnesium EAR for lactating women 19 through 30 years and close to the magnesium EAR of 265 mg (11.3 mmol)/day for lactating women ages 31 through 50 years. The twenty-fifth percentile intake is 296 mg (12.3 mmol)/day, which is slightly below the EAR of 300 mg (13.8 mmol)/day for lactating women ages 14 through 18 years.

Special Considerations

Mothers Nursing Multiple Infants. Increased intakes of magnesium during lactation, as with calcium, should be considered in mothers nursing multiple infants concurrently. Magnesium requirements may be higher due to the increased milk production of a mother while nursing multiple infants. It is not known whether decreased urinary magnesium and increased maternal bone resorption provide sufficient amounts of magnesium to meet these increased needs.

TOLERABLE UPPER INTAKE LEVELS

Hazard Identification

Magnesium, when ingested as a naturally occurring substance in foods, has not been demonstrated to exert any adverse effects. However, adverse effects of excess magnesium intake have been observed with intakes from nonfood sources such as various magnesium salts used for pharmacologic purposes. Thus, a Tolerable Upper Intake Level (UL) cannot be based on magnesium obtained from foods. All reports of adverse effects of excess magnesium intake concern magnesium taken in addition to that consumed from food sources. Therefore, for the purposes of this review, magnesium intake that could result in adverse effects was from that obtained from its pharmacological use.

The primary initial manifestation of excessive magnesium intake from nonfood sources is diarrhea (Mordes and Wacker, 1978; Rude and Singer, 1980). Magnesium has a well-known cathartic effect and is used pharmacologically for that purpose (Fine et al., 1991b). The diarrheal effect produced by pharmacological use of various magnesium salts is an osmotic effect (Fine et al., 1991b) and may be accompanied by other mild gastrointestinal effects such as nausea and abdominal cramping (Bashir et al., 1993; Marken et al., 1989; Ricci et al., 1991). Osmotic diarrhea has not been reported with normal dietary intakes of magnesium. Magnesium ingested as a component of food or food fortificants has not been reported to cause this mild, osmotic diarrhea even when large amounts are ingested.

Magnesium is absorbed much more efficiently from the normal concentrations found in the diet than it is from the higher doses found in nonfood sources (Fine et al., 1991a). The presence of food likely counteracts the osmotic effect of the magnesium salts in the gut lumen (Fine et al., 1991a). In normal individuals, the kidney seems to maintain magnesium homeostasis over a rather wide range of magnesium intakes. Thus, hypermagnesemia has not been documented following the intake of high levels of dietary magnesium in the absence of either intestinal or renal disease (Mordes and Wacker, 1978).

Hypermagnesemia can occur in individuals with impaired renal function and is most commonly associated with the combination of impaired renal function and excessive intake of nonfood magnesium (for example, as antacids) (Mordes and Wacker, 1978; Randall et al., 1964). Hypermagnesemia resulting from impaired renal function and/or intravenous administration of magnesium can result in more serious neurological and cardiac symptoms, but elevated serum magnesium concentrations greater than 2 to 3.5 mmol/liter (4.8 to 8.4 mg/dl) must be attained before onset of these symptoms (Rude and Singer, 1980). Intakes of nonfood magnesium have rarely been reported to cause symptomatic hypermagnesemia in individuals with normal renal function.

Although magnesium supplements are used (see Table 2-2), comparatively few serious adverse reactions are reported until high doses are ingested (see data following). However, some individuals in the population may be at risk of a mild, reversible adverse effect (diarrhea) even at doses from nonfood sources that are easily tolerated by others. Thus, diarrhea was chosen as the most sensitive toxic manifestation of excess magnesium intake from nonfood sources.

It is not known if all magnesium salts behave similarly in the induction of osmotic diarrhea. In the absence of evidence to the contrary, it seems prudent to assume that all dissociable magnesium salts share this property. Reports of diarrhea associated with magnesium frequently involve preparations that include aluminum, and therefore a specific magnesium-associated effect cannot be ascertained.

Large pharmacological doses of magnesium can clearly result in more serious adverse reactions. An 8-week-old infant suffered metabolic alkalosis, diarrhea, and dehydration after receiving large amounts of magnesium oxide powder on each of two successive days (Bodanszky and Leleiko, 1985). Urakabe et al. (1975) reported that a female adult suffered from metabolic alkalosis and hypokalemia from the repeated daily ingestion of 30 g (1,250 mmol) of magnesium oxide. Several cases of paralytic ileus were encountered in adult patients who had taken large, cathartic doses of magnesium: in one case, two bottles of magnesium citrate and several doses of milk of magnesia, and in the other case, several doses of magnesium sulfate in a patient with mild renal impairment (Golzarian et al., 1994). Cardiorespiratory arrest was encountered in a suicidal patient given 465 g (19.1 mol) of magnesium sulfate as a cathartic to counteract an intentional drug overdose (Smilkstein et al., 1988). Deaths from very large exposures to magnesium in the form of magnesium sulfate or magnesium oxide have been reported following cardiac arrest, especially in individuals with renal insufficiency (Randall et al., 1964; Thatcher and Rock, 1928).

Dose-Response Assessment

Adolescents and Adults: Ages > 8 Years

Data Selection. A review of the scientific literature revealed relatively few reports that were useful in establishing a UL for magnesium. Because magnesium has not been shown to produce any toxic effects when ingested as a naturally occurring substance in foods, a UL cannot be established for dietary magnesium at this time. In addition, studies involving intravenous administration of comparatively large doses of magnesium used in the treatment of preterm labor, pregnancy-induced hypertension, or other clinical conditions were not considered applicable for the derivation of ULs. Based on limited data described below, a UL can be established for magnesium from nonfood sources.

Identification of a NOAEL (or LOAEL) and Critical Endpoint. As the primary initial manifestation of excessive magnesium intake, diarrhea was selected as the critical endpoint. The few studies that report mild diarrhea and other gastrointestinal symptoms from uses of magnesium salts were reviewed to identify a No-Observed-Adverse-Effect Level (NOAEL) (or Lowest-Observed-Adverse-Effect-Level [LOAEL]). Gastrointestinal symptoms, including diarrhea, developed in 6 of 21 patients (51- to 70-year-old males and females) receiving long-term magnesium chloride therapy at levels of 360 mg (15 mmol) of magnesium (Bashir et al., 1993). Gastrointestinal manifestations developed in 5 of 25 pregnant women being given 384 mg (16 mmol) of daily magnesium as magnesium chloride supplements for the prevention of preterm delivery, although one patient receiving the placebo treatment also developed diarrhea (Ricci et al., 1991). Diarrhea was also noted in 18 of 50 healthy white and black men and women (aged 31 through 50 years) who were ingesting 470 mg (19.6 mmol) of magnesium as magnesium oxide daily (Marken et al., 1989). Levels of fecal output of soluble magnesium and fecal magnesium concentration were elevated in individuals with diarrhea induced by 168 to 2,320 mg (7 to 97 mmol) of magnesium as magnesium hydroxide (Fine et al., 1991b).

However, other studies using similar or even higher levels of supplemental magnesium reported no diarrhea or other gastrointestinal complaints. Healthy 18- to 38-year-old males given diets enriched with magnesium oxide at levels up to 452 mg (18.9 mmol) daily for 6 days did not report the occurrence of any gastrointestinal symptoms (Altura et al., 1994). This study of the effect of magnesium-enriched diets on absorption involved the fortification of foods with magnesium, which may have different effects from the administration of magnesium supplements outside the normal diet. Furthermore, no diarrhea was reported in patients of varying ages receiving an average of 576 mg (24 mmol)/day of supplemental magnesium as magnesium oxide in a metabolic balance study for 28 days (Spencer et al., 1994). Diarrhea or other gastrointestinal complaints were not observed in patients receiving up to 1,200 mg (50 mmol) of magnesium in the form of an aluminum-magnesium-hydroxycarbonate antacid over a 6-week trial period (Nagy et al., 1988). In a longer-term study, a group of postmenopausal women received daily supplements of 226 to 678 mg (9.4 to 28.3 mmol) of magnesium as magnesium hydroxide for 6 months followed by 226 mg (9.4 mmol) of magnesium for 18 months without any observations of gastrointestinal complaints (Stendig-Lindberg et al., 1993). Diabetics were supplemented with 400 mg (16.7 mmol) of magnesium daily for 8 weeks in the form of magnesium oxide or magnesium chloride without any gastrointestinal complications (Nadler et al., 1992). Elderly subjects supplemented with 372 mg (15.5 mmol) of magnesium daily over a 4-week period did not report any diarrheal effects or other gastrointestinal complaints (Paolisso et al., 1992).

The LOAEL identified for magnesium-induced diarrhea in adults is 360 mg (15 mmol)/day of magnesium from nonfood sources based on the results of Bashir et al. (1993). Studies by Fine et al. (1991b), Marken et al. (1989), and Ricci et al. (1991) provide evidence to support the use of this dose as the LOAEL.

Uncertainty Assessment. Due to the very mild, reversible nature of osmotic diarrhea caused by ingestion of magnesium salts, an uncertainty factor (UF) of approximately 1.0 was selected. Unlike possible adverse effects of other nutrients, osmotic diarrhea is quite apparent to the individual and thus is not a symptom that is masked until serious consequences result.

Derivation of the UL. Because excessive magnesium intake from nonfood sources causes adverse effects, the UL will be established for magnesium from nonfood sources. The UL for magnesium for adolescents and adults is established at 350 mg (14.6 mmol)/day, based on a LOAEL of 360 mg (15 mmol)/day and a UF very close to 1.0. Although a few studies have noted mild diarrhea and other mild gastrointestinal complaints in a small percentage of patients at levels of 360 to 380 mg (15.0 to 15.8 mmol)/day, it is noteworthy that many other individuals have not encountered such effects even when receiving substantially more than this UL of supplementary magnesium, as indicated previously.

UL for Adolescents and Adults > 8 years   350 mg (14.6 mmol) of supplementary magnesium

Infants: Ages 0 through 12 Months

No specific toxicity data exist on which to establish a UL for infants, toddlers, and children. The lack of any available data regarding the effects of magnesium supplements in infants makes it impossible to establish a specific UL for infants. Thus, it is important to get magnesium via food sources only in this age group.

UL for Infants   0 through 12 months   Not possible to establish for supplementary magnesium

Children: Ages 1 through 8 Years

It is assumed that children are as susceptible to the osmotic effects of nonfood sources of magnesium as are adults. Thus, adjusting the value for adults on a body-weight basis established a UL for children at a magnesium intake of 5 mg/kg/day (0.2 mmol/kg/day) (see Table 1-3 for reference weights).

UL for Children   1 through 3 years   65 mg (2.7 mmol) of supplementary magnesium
**   4 through 8 years   110 mg (4.6 mmol) of supplementary magnesium**

Pregnancy and Lactation

No evidence suggests increased susceptibility to adverse effects of supplemental magnesium during pregnancy and lactation. Therefore, the UL for pregnant and lactating women is set at 350 mg (14.6 mmol)/day—the same value as used for other adults.

UL for Pregnancy 14 through 50 years   **350 mg (14.6 mmol) of supplementary magnesium**

UL for Lactation   14 through 50 years   **350 mg (14.6 mmol) of supplementary magnesium**

Special Considerations

Individuals with impaired renal function are at greater risk of magnesium toxicity. However, as noted above, magnesium levels obtained from food are insufficient to cause adverse reactions even in these individuals. Patients with certain clinical conditions (for example, neonatal tetany, hyperuricemia, hyperlipidemia, lithium toxicity, hyperthyroidism, pancreatitis, hepatitis, phlebitis, coronary artery disease, arrhythmia, and digitalis intoxication [Mordes and Wacker, 1978]) may benefit from the prescribed use of magnesium in quantities exceeding the UL in the clinical setting.

Exposure Assessment

In 1986, the most recent year that data were available to estimate nonfood nutrient supplement intakes, approximately 15 percent of adults in the United States reported taking a supplement containing magnesium (although it is unclear whether supplements were taken on a daily basis) (Moss et al., 1989). Of those, the ninetieth percentile of daily supplemental magnesium intake was 200 mg (9.1 mmol) for men and 240 mg (10 mmol) for women; the ninety-fifth percentile was 350 mg (14.4 mmol) for men and 400 mg (16.6 mmol) for women. Thus, approximately 5 percent of the men and over 5 percent of the women who used magnesium supplements exceeded the UL of 350 mg (14.6 mmol)/day in 1986.

Children's intakes from nonfood nutrient supplements were estimated to be much lower. The ninetieth percentile of intake for children 2 to 6 years of age who used magnesium supplements in 1986 was 70 mg (2.9 mmol)/day, which is approximately the UL for a 2-year-old child weighing 14 kg; the ninety-fifth percentile of intake from supplements was 117 mg (4.9 mmol)/day, or approximately the UL (115 mg [4.8 mmol]/day) for a 6-year-old child weighing 23 kg. Assuming older children were taking the higher doses, it appears that about 5 percent of the users in this study were exceeding the UL.

Risk Characterization

Using data from 1986, almost 1 percent of all adults in the United States took a nonfood magnesium supplement that exceeded the reference UL of 350 mg (14.6 mmol)/day in the 2-week period preceding the survey (Moss et al., 1989). It is important to note that many of the individuals whose intakes of supplemental magnesium exceeded the UL may be self-selected as not experiencing diarrhea, but this is uncertain. More recent data on estimates of supplement intakes of a national sample have not been published, but it is unlikely that usage has declined.

The data on supplement use in 1986 also indicate that at least 5 percent of young children who used magnesium supplements exceeded the UL for magnesium, 5 mg (0.2 mmol)/kg/day. However, because less than 10 percent of the children had taken a magnesium supplement in the past 2 weeks, less than 1 percent of all children would be at risk of adverse effects. These estimates assume that older children (with a higher UL) are taking the higher doses; the percentage at risk would be higher if dosage were not related to age (and, therefore, to body size). More information on supplement use by specific ages is needed.

RESEARCH RECOMMENDATIONS

The ability to determine reference dietary intakes for magnesium is, as indicated throughout this chapter, hampered by available data. Areas of investigation that are particularly needed include the following:

• Reliable data on population intakes of magnesium are required based on dietary surveys that include estimates of intakes from food, water, and supplements in healthy populations in all life stages.

• Biochemical indicators that provide an accurate and specific marker(s) of magnesium status must be investigated in order to assess their ability to predict functional outcomes that indicate adequate magnesium status over prolonged periods.

• Basic studies need to be initiated in healthy individuals, including experimental magnesium depletion studies that measure changes in various body magnesium pools.

• Magnesium balance studies may be one indicator utilized. If so, strict adherence to criteria suggested in the chapter would improve their application to dietary recommendations. Moreover, a determination of the most valid units to use in expressing estimates of requirements (body weight, fat-free mass, or total body unit) is needed.

• Investigations are needed to assess the inter-relationships between dietary magnesium intakes, indicators of magnesium status, and possible health outcomes that may be affected by inadequate magnesium intakes, such as hypertension, hyperlipidemia, atherosclerotic vascular disease, altered bone turnover, and osteoporosis.

• Based on the evidence of abnormal magnesium status and health outcomes (as noted above), intervention studies to improve magnesium status and to assess its impact on specific health outcomes would be appropriate.

• The toxicity of pharmacological doses of magnesium requires investigation.

7

Vitamin D

BACKGROUND INFORMATION

Overview

Vitamin D (calciferol), which comprises a group of fat soluble seco-sterols that are found in very few foods naturally, is photosynthesized in the skin of vertebrates by the action of solar ultraviolet B radiation (Holick, 1994). Vitamin D comes in many forms, but the two major physiologically relevant ones are vitamin D_2 (ergocalciferol) and vitamin D_3 (cholecalciferol) (Fieser and Fieser, 1959). Vitamin D_2 originates from the yeast and plant sterol, ergosterol; vitamin D_3 originates from 7-dehydrocholesterol, a precursor of cholesterol, when synthesized in the skin (Figure 7-1). Major metabolic steps involved with the metabolism D_2 are similar to those of the metabolism of D_3. Vitamin D without a subscript represents either D_2 or D_3 or both and is biologically inert, requiring two obligate hydroxylations to form its biologically active hormone, 1,25-dihydroxyvitamin D ($1,25(OH)_2D$) (DeLuca, 1988; Reichel et al., 1989).

Vitamin D's major biologic function in humans is to maintain serum calcium and phosphorus concentrations within the normal range by enhancing the efficiency of the small intestine to absorb these minerals from the diet (DeLuca, 1988; Reichel et al., 1989) (Figure 7-2). $1,25(OH)_2D$ enhances the efficiency of intestinal calcium absorption along the entire small intestine, but primarily in the duodenum and jejunum. $1,25(OH)_2D_3$ also enhances dietary phosphorus absorption along the entire small intestine (Chen et

250

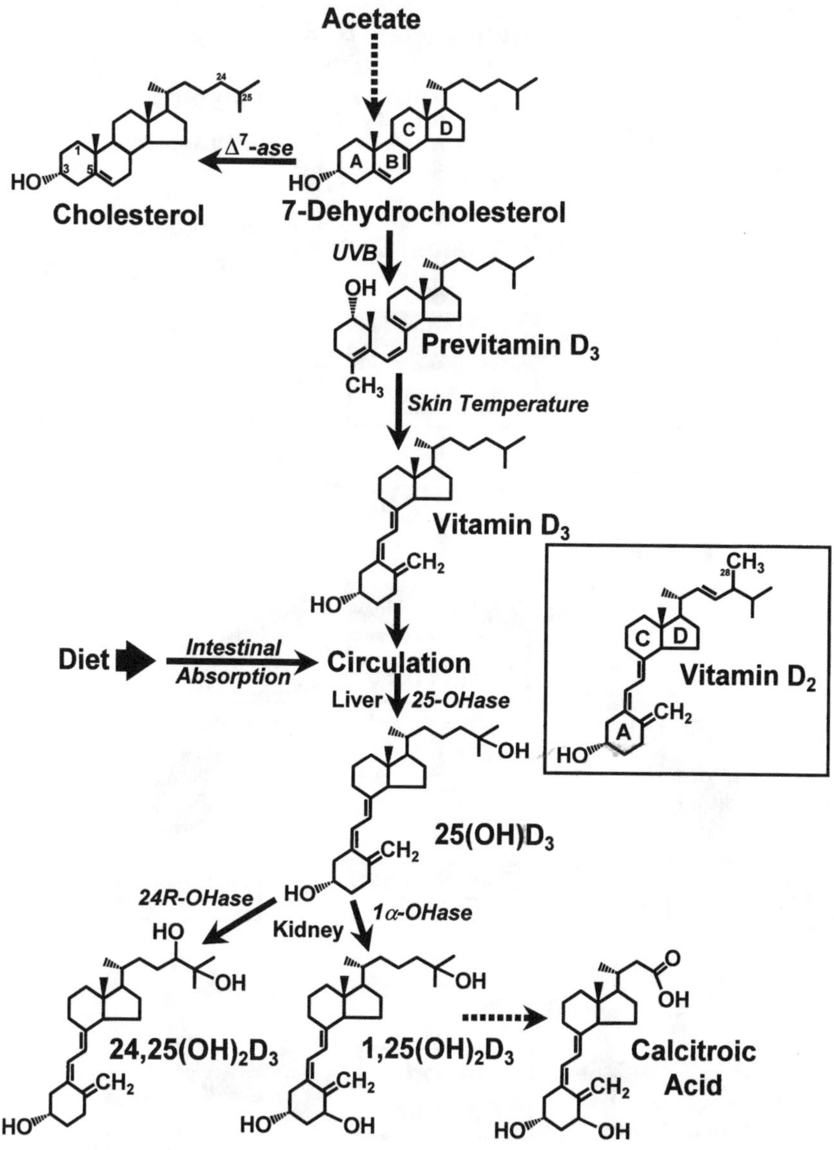

FIGURE 7-1 The photochemical, thermal, and metabolic pathways for vitamin D_3. Specific enzymes abbreviated as follows: Δ^7ase,7-dehydrocholesterol reductase; 25-OHase, vitamin D-25-hydroxylase; 1α-OHase, 25-OH-D-1α-hydroxylase; 24R-OHase, 25(OH)D-24-hydroxylase. Inset: the structure of vitamin D_2. Reproduced with permission, Holick (1996).

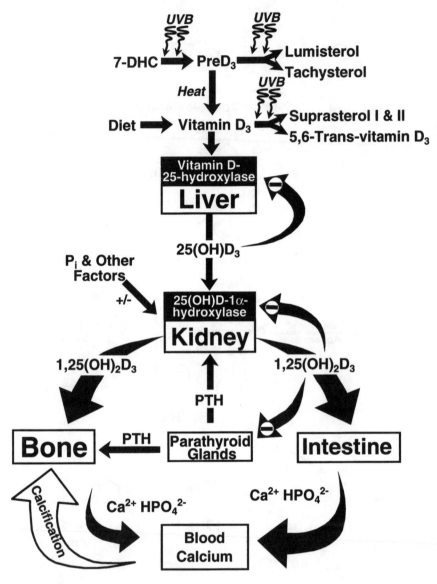

FIGURE 7-2 Photosynthesis of vitamin D_3 and the metabolism of vitamin D_3 to $25(OH)D_3$ and $1,25(OH)_2D_3$. Once formed, $1,25(OH)_2D_3$ carries out the biologic functions of vitamin D_3 on the intestine and bone. Parathyroid hormone (PTH) promotes the synthesis of $1,25(OH)_2D_3$, which, in turn, stimulates intestinal calcium transport and bone calcium mobilization, and regulates the synthesis of PTH by negative feedback. Reproduced with permission, Holick (1996).

al., 1974), but its major influence is in the jejunum and ileum. When dietary calcium intake is inadequate to satisfy the body's calcium requirement, $1,25(OH)_2D$, along with parathyroid hormone (PTH), mobilizes monocytic stem cells in the bone marrow to become mature osteoclasts (Holick, 1995; Merke et al., 1986). The osteoclasts, in turn, are stimulated by a variety of cytokines and other factors to increase the mobilization of calcium stores from the bone (Figure 7-2). Thus, vitamin D maintains the blood calcium and phosphorus at supersaturating concentrations that are deposited in the bone as calcium hydroxyapatite.

A multitude of other tissues and cells in the body can recognize $1,25(OH)_2D$ (Stumpf et al., 1979). Although the exact physiologic function of $1,25(OH)_2D$ in the brain, heart, pancreas, mononuclear cells, activated lymphocytes, and skin remains unknown, its major biologic function has been identified as a potent antiproliferative and prodifferentiation hormone (Abe et al., 1981; Colston et al., 1981; Eisman et al., 1981; Smith et al., 1987). There is little evidence that vitamin D deficiency leads to major disorders in these organ and cellular systems.

Physiology of Absorption, Metabolism, and Excretion

Because dietary vitamin D is fat soluble once it is ingested, it is incorporated into the chylomicron fraction and absorbed through the lymphatic system (Holick, 1995). It is estimated that approximately 80 percent of the ingested vitamin D enters the body via this mechanism. Vitamin D is principally absorbed in the small intestine.

Vitamin D is principally excreted in the bile. Although some of it is reabsorbed in the small intestine (Nagubandi et al., 1980), the enterohepatic circulation of vitamin D is not considered to be an important mechanism for its conservation (Fraser, 1983). However, since vitamin D is metabolized to more water-soluble compounds, a variety of vitamin D metabolites, most notably calcitroic acid, are excreted by the kidney into the urine (Esvelt and DeLuca, 1981).

Once vitamin D enters the circulation from the skin or from the lymph via the thoracic duct, it accumulates in the liver within a few hours. In the liver, vitamin D undergoes hydroxylation at the 25-carbon position in the mitochondria, and soon thereafter, it appears in the circulation as 25-hydroxyvitamin D (25(OH)D) (DeLuca, 1984) (Figures 7-1 and 7-2). The circulating concentration of 25(OH)D is a good reflection of cumulative effects of exposure to sunlight and dietary intake of vitamin D (Haddad and Hahn, 1973; Holick, 1995; Lund and Sorensen, 1979). In the liver, vitamin D-25-

hydroxylase is regulated by vitamin D and its metabolites, and therefore, the increase in circulating concentration of 25(OH)D after exposure to sunlight or ingestion of vitamin D is relatively modest compared with cumulative production or intake of vitamin D (Holick and Clark, 1978). The appearance in the blood of the parent compound, vitamin D, is short-lived as it is either stored in the fat or metabolized in the liver (Mawer et al., 1972). The half-life of 25(OH)D in the human circulation is approximately 10 days to 3 weeks (Mawer et al., 1971; Vicchio et al., 1993). Administration of 25(OH)D results in approximately two to five times more activity than giving vitamin D itself in curing rickets and in inducing intestinal calcium absorption and mobilization of calcium from bones in rats. However, at physiologic concentrations, it is biologically inert in affecting these functions (DeLuca, 1984).

In order to have biologic activity at physiologic concentrations, 25(OH)D must be hydroxylated in the kidney on the 1-carbon position to form $1,25(OH)_2D$ (Holick et al., 1971; Lawson et al., 1971) (Figures 7-1 and 7-2). It is $1,25(OH)_2D$ that is thought to be the biologically active form of vitamin D and that is responsible for most, if not all, of its biologic functions (DeLuca, 1988; Fraser, 1980; Reichel et al., 1989). The production of $1,25(OH)_2D$ in the kidney is tightly regulated, principally through the action of PTH in response to serum calcium and phosphorus levels (DeLuca, 1984; Portale, 1984; Reichel et al., 1989) (Figure 7-2). The half-life of $1,25(OH)_2D$ in the circulation of humans is approximately 4 to 6 hours (Kumar, 1986). Because of the tight regulation of the production of $1,25(OH)_2D$ and its relatively short serum half-life, it has not proven to be a valuable marker for vitamin D deficiency, adequacy, or excess.

$25(OH)D$ and $1,25(OH)_2D$ may undergo a hydroxylation on the 24-carbon to form their 24-hydroxy counterparts, 24,25-dihydroxyvitamin D $(24,25(OH)_2D)$ (Figure 7-1) and 1,24,25-trihydroxyvitamin D (DeLuca, 1984; Holick, 1995). It is believed that the 24-carbon hydroxylation is the initial step in the metabolic degradation of 25(OH)D and $1,25(OH)_2D$ (DeLuca, 1988). The final degradative product of $1,25(OH)_2D_3$ is calcitroic acid, which is excreted by the kidney into the urine (Esvelt and DeLuca, 1981) (Figure 7-1).

Although the kidney supplies the body with $1,25(OH)_2D$ to regulate calcium and bone metabolism, it is recognized that activated macrophages, some lymphoma cells, and cultured skin and bone cells also make $1,25(OH)_2D$ (Adams et al., 1990; Holick, 1995; Pillai et al., 1987). Although the physiologic importance of locally produced $1,25(OH)_2D$ is not well understood, the excessive unregulated production of $1,25(OH)_2D$ by activated macrophages and lymphoma cells is responsible for the hypercalciuria associated with chronic granulomatous disorders and the hypercalcemia seen with lymphoma (Adams, 1989; Davies et al., 1994).

Factors Affecting the Vitamin D Requirement

Special Populations

Elderly. Aging significantly decreases the capacity of human skin to produce vitamin D_3 (MacLaughlin and Holick, 1985). In adults over age 65 years, there is a fourfold decrease in the capacity to produce vitamin D_3 when compared with younger adults aged 20 to 30 years (Holick et al., 1989; Need et al., 1993). Although one study suggested that there may be a defect in intestinal calcium absorption of tracer quantities of vitamin D_3 in the elderly (Barragry et al., 1978), two other studies demonstrated that aging does not significantly affect absorption of pharmacologic doses of vitamin D (Clemens et al., 1986; Holick, 1986). It is not known whether the absorption of physiologic amounts of vitamin D is altered in the elderly.

Malabsorption Disorders. Patients suffering from various intestinal malabsorption syndromes such as severe liver failure, Crohn's disease, Whipple's disease, and sprue often suffer from vitamin D deficiency because of their inability to absorb dietary vitamin D (Lo et al., 1985). Thus, patients who are unable to secrete adequate amounts of bile or who have a disease of the small intestine are more prone to develop vitamin D deficiency owing to their inability to absorb this fat-soluble vitamin.

Sources of Vitamin D

Vitamin D intake from food and nutrient supplements is expressed in either international units (IU) or micrograms (µg). One IU of vitamin D is defined as the activity of 0.025 µg of cholecalciferol in bioassays with rats and chicks. Thus, the biological activity of 1 µg of vitamin D is 40 IU. The activity of 25(OH)D is 5 times more potent than cholecalciferol; thus, 1 IU = 0.005 µg 25(OH)D.

Sunlight

Throughout the world, the major source of vitamin D for humans is the exposure of the skin to sunlight (Holick, 1994). During sun exposure, the ultraviolet B photons with energies between 290 and 315 nm are absorbed by the cutaneous 7-dehydrocholesterol to form the split (seco) sterol previtamin D_3 (Holick et al., 1980; MacLaughlin et al., 1982). This photosynthesis of vitamin D occurs in most plants and animals (Holick et al., 1989).

However, a variety of factors limit the cutaneous production of vitamin D_3. Excessive exposure to sunlight causes a photodegradation of previtamin D_3 and vitamin D_3 to ensure that vitamin D_3 intoxication cannot occur (Holick, 1994; Holick et al., 1981; Webb et al., 1989) (Figure 7-2). An increase in skin melanin pigmentation or the topical application of a sunscreen will absorb solar ultraviolet B photons and thereby significantly reduce the production of vitamin D_3 in the skin (Clemens et al., 1982; Matsuoka et al., 1987). Latitude, time of day, and season of the year have a dramatic influence on the cutaneous production of vitamin D_3. Above and below latitudes of approximately $40°$ N and $40°$ S, respectively, vitamin D_3 synthesis in the skin is absent during most of the three to four winter months (Ladizesky et al., 1995; Webb et al., 1988). The far northern and southern latitudes extend this period for up to 6 months (Holick, 1994; Oliveri et al., 1993).

Dietary Intake

Accurate estimates of vitamin D intakes in the United States are not available, in part because the vitamin D composition of fortified foods is highly variable (Chen et al., 1993; Holick et al., 1992) and because the U.S. intake surveys do not include estimates of vitamin D intake. Using food consumption data from the second National Health and Nutrition Examination Survey (NHANES II), median vitamin D intakes from food by young women were estimated to be 2.9 µg (114 IU)/day, with a range of 0 to 49 µg (0 to 1,960 IU)/day (Murphy and Calloway, 1986). A similar median vitamin D intake, 2.3 µg (90 IU)/ day, was estimated for a sample of older women (Krall et al., 1989).

Food Sources

In nature, very few foods contain vitamin D. Those that do include some fish liver oils, the flesh of fatty fish, the liver and fat from aquatic mammals such as seals and polar bears, and eggs from hens that have been fed vitamin D (Holick, 1994; Jeans, 1950). Almost all of the human intake of vitamin D from foods comes from fortified milk products and other fortified foods such as breakfast cereals. The vitamin D content of unfortified foods is generally low, with the exception of fish, many of which contain 5 to 15 µg (200 to

600 IU)/100 g; Atlantic herring contain up to as much as 40 µg (1,600 IU)/100 g (USDA, 1991).

After vitamin D was recognized as being critically important for the prevention of rickets, the United States, Canada, and many other countries instituted a policy of fortifying some foods with vitamin D (Steenbock and Black, 1924). Milk was chosen as the principal dietary component to be fortified with either vitamin D_2 or vitamin D_3. In other countries, some cereals, margarine, and breads also have small quantities of added vitamin D (Lips et al., 1996). In the United States and Canada, all milk, irrespective of its fat content, is fortified with 10 µg (400 IU)/quart and 9.6 µg (385 IU)/liter, respectively, of vitamin D. However, during the past decade, three surveys in which the vitamin D content in milk was analyzed revealed that up to 70 percent of milk sampled throughout the United States and Canada did not contain vitamin D in the range of 8 to 12 µg (320 to 480 IU)/quart (the 20 percent variation allowed by current labeling standards). Furthermore, 62 percent of 42 various milk samples contained less than 8 µg (320 IU)/quart of vitamin D, and 14 percent of skim milk samples had no detectable vitamin D (Chen et al., 1993; Holick et al., 1992; Tanner et al., 1988). All proprietary infant formulas must also contain vitamin D in the amount of 10 µg (400 IU)/liter. However, these products have also been found to have wide variability in their vitamin D content (Holick et al., 1992).

Intake from Dietary Supplements

In the one available study of dietary supplement intake in the United States, use of vitamin D supplements in the previous 2 weeks in 1986 was reported for over one-third of the children 2 to 6 years of age, over one-fourth of the women, and almost 20 percent of the men (Moss et al., 1989). For supplement users, the median dose was the same for men, women, and children: 10 µg (400 IU)/day. However, the ninety-fifth percentile was the same as the median for the children (still 10 µg [400 IU]/day), indicating little variation in the upper range for young children, while the ninety-fifth percentile for adults was considerably higher: 20 µg (800 IU)/day for men and 17.2 µg (686 IU)/day for women.

Effects of Vitamin D Deficiency

Vitamin D deficiency is characterized by inadequate mineralization or demineralization of the skeleton. In children, vitamin

D deficiency results in inadequate mineralization of the skeleton causing rickets, which is characterized by widening at the end of the long bones, rachitic rosary, deformations in the skeleton including frontal bossing, and outward or inward deformities of the lower limbs causing bowed legs and knocked knees, respectively (Goldring et al., 1995). In adults, vitamin D deficiency leads to a mineralization defect in the skeleton causing osteomalacia. In addition, the secondary hyperparathyroidism associated with vitamin D deficiency enhances mobilization of calcium from the skeleton, resulting in porotic bone (Favus and Christakos, 1996).

Any alteration in the cutaneous production of vitamin D_3, the absorption of vitamin D in the intestine, or the metabolism of vitamin D to its active form, $1,25(OH)_2D$, can lead to a vitamin D-deficient state (Demay, 1995; Holick, 1995). In addition, an alteration in the recognition of $1,25(OH)_2D$ by its receptor can also cause vitamin D deficiency, metabolic bone disease, and accompanying biochemical abnormalities (Demay, 1995).

Vitamin D deficiency causes a decrease in ionized calcium in blood, which in turn leads to an increase in the production and secretion of PTH (Fraser, 1980; Holick, 1995). PTH stimulates the mobilization of calcium from the skeleton, conserves renal loss of calcium, and causes increased renal excretion of phosphorus leading to a normal fasting serum calcium with a low or low-normal serum phosphorus (Holick, 1995). Thus, vitamin D deficiency is characterized biochemically by either a normal or low-normal serum calcium with a low-normal or low-fasting serum phosphorus and an elevated serum PTH. Serum alkaline phosphatase is usually elevated in vitamin D deficiency states (Goldring et al., 1995). The elevated PTH leads to an increase in the destruction of the skeletal tissue in order to release calcium into the blood. The bone collagen by-products, including hydroxyproline, pyridinoline, deoxypyridinoline, and N-telopeptide, are excreted into the urine and are usually elevated (Kamel et al., 1994).

It is well recognized that vitamin D deficiency causes abnormalities in calcium and bone metabolism. The possibility that vitamin D deficiency is associated with an increased risk of colon, breast, and prostate cancer was suggested in epidemiologic surveys of people living at higher latitudes (Garland et al., 1985, 1990; Schwartz and Hulka, 1990). At this time, it is premature to categorically suggest that vitamin D deficiency increases cancer risk. Prospective studies need to be carried out to test the hypothesis.

ESTIMATING REQUIREMENTS FOR VITAMIN D

Selection of Indicators for Estimating the Vitamin D Requirement

Serum 25(OH)D

The serum 25(OH)D concentration is the best indicator for determining adequacy of vitamin D intake of an individual since it represents a summation of the total cutaneous production of vitamin D and the oral ingestion of either vitamin D_2 or vitamin D_3 (Haddad and Hahn, 1973; Holick, 1995). Thus, serum 25(OH)D will be used as the primary indicator of vitamin D adequacy.

The normal range of serum 25(OH)D concentration is the mean serum 25(OH)D ± 2 standard deviations (SD) from a group of healthy individuals. The lower limit of the normal range can be as low as 20 nmol/liter (8 ng/ml) and as high as 37.5 nmol/liter (15 ng/ml) depending on the geographic location where the blood samples were obtained. For example, the lower and upper limits of the normal range of 25(OH)D in California will be higher than those limits in Boston (Clemens and Adams, 1996). Two pathologic indicators, radiologic evidence of rickets (Demay, 1995) and biochemical abnormalities associated with metabolic bone disease, including elevations in alkaline phosphatase and PTH concentrations in the circulation (Demay, 1995), have been correlated with serum 25(OH)D. A 25(OH)D concentration below 27.5 nmol/liter (11 ng/ml) is considered to be consistent with vitamin D deficiency in infants, neonates, and young children (Specker et al., 1992) and is therefore used as the key indicator for determining the vitamin D reference value.

Little information is available about the level of 25(OH)D that is essential for maintaining normal calcium metabolism and peak bone mass in older children and in young and middle-aged adults. For the elderly, there is mounting scientific evidence to support their increased requirement for dietary vitamin D in order to maintain normal calcium metabolism and maximize bone health (Dawson-Hughes et al., 1991; Krall et al., 1989; Lips et al., 1988). Therefore, the serum 25(OH)D concentration was utilized to evaluate vitamin D deficiency in this age group, but it was not the only indicator used to determine the vitamin D reference value for the elderly.

Serum PTH concentrations are inversely related to 25(OH)D serum levels (Krall et al., 1989; Kruse et al., 1984; Lips et al., 1988; Webb et al., 1990; Zeghoud et al., 1997). Therefore, the serum PTH concentration, in conjunction with 25(OH)D, has proven to be a valuable indicator of vitamin D status.

The few studies conducted in African Americans and Mexican Americans suggest that these population groups have lower circulating concentrations of 25(OH)D and higher serum concentrations of PTH and 1,25(OH)$_2$D when compared with Caucasians (Bell et al., 1985; Reasner et al., 1990). It is likely that increased melanin pigmentation (which decreases the cutaneous production of vitamin D) and the lack of dietary vitamin D (due to a high incidence of lactose intolerance) are the contributing causes for this.

Serum Vitamin D

The serum concentration of vitamin D is not indicative of vitamin D status. As stated previously, its half-life is relatively short, and the blood concentrations can range from 0 to greater than 250 nmol/liter (0 to 100 ng/ml) depending on an individual's recent ingestion of vitamin D and exposure to sunlight.

Serum 1,25(OH)$_2$D

Similarly, the serum 1,25(OH)$_2$D level is not a good indicator of vitamin D. This hormone's serum concentrations are tightly regulated by a variety of factors, including circulating levels of serum calcium, phosphorus, parathyroid hormone, and other hormones (Fraser, 1980; Holick, 1995).

Evaluation of Skeletal Health

The ultimate effect of vitamin D on human health is maintenance of a healthy skeleton. Thus, in reviewing the literature for determining vitamin D status, one of the indicators that has proven to be valuable is an evaluation of skeletal health. In neonates and children, bone development and the prevention of rickets, either in combination with serum 25(OH)D and PTH concentrations, or by itself, are good indicators of vitamin D status (Gultekin et al., 1987; Koo et al., 1995; Kruse et al., 1984; Markested et al., 1986; Meulmeester et al., 1990). For adults, bone mineral content (BMC), bone mineral density (BMD), and fracture risk, in combination with serum 25(OH)D and PTH concentrations, have proven to be the most valuable indicators of vitamin D status (Brazier et al., 1995; Dawson-

Hughes et al., 1991, 1995; Lamberg-Allardt et al., 1989, 1993; Sorva et al., 1991; Webb et al., 1990).

Recommendations for Adequate Intake

The recommendation for how much vitamin D is required to maintain adequate calcium metabolism and good bone health for all ages may be considered the easiest, as well as at times the most difficult, to determine. Humans of all ages, races, and both sexes can obtain all of their body's requirement for vitamin D through exposure to an adequate amount of sunlight. However, the sunlight-mediated synthesis of vitamin D in the skin is profoundly affected by a wide variety of factors, including degree of skin pigmentation, latitude, time of day, season of the year, weather conditions, and the amount of body surface covered with clothing or sunscreen (Holick, 1994). Therefore, it is very difficult to determine an accurate value for an Estimated Average Requirement (EAR) as most of the studies are subject to one or more of these variables, especially exposure to sunlight, which is difficult to quantitate.

Vitamin D is a hormone, and therefore, when considering the requirements for vitamin D, EARs would represent gross estimates of the need for the active hormone. The only studies that provide an approximation of how much vitamin D is required to maintain an individual's serum 25(OH)D concentration above that associated with abnormalities in BMD are ones that have been conducted in the winter at far northern and southern latitudes where exposure to sunlight does not produce any significant quantities of vitamin D (Ladizesky et al., 1995; Markestad and Elzouki, 1991). However, these studies still do not account for subjects' exposure to sunlight in the spring, summer, and fall when the cutaneous synthesis of vitamin D occurs and it is stored in the body fat for use in the winter.

Another limitation of the reported studies is the assumption made regarding the vitamin D content of various foods. Despite government mandates for vitamin D fortification of milk in both the United States and Canada, actual analysis has shown this fortification to be highly variable (Chen et al., 1993; Holick et al., 1992; Tanner et al., 1988). Furthermore, the amount of vitamin D found naturally in foods, such as fish liver oils, fatty fish, and egg yolks, is very dependent on the time of the year these foods are harvested. Studies that report the dietary intake of vitamin D based on the expected amount of vitamin D fortification of milk, margarine, cereals, and breads are highly suspect because the analysis of the vitamin D content in the foods at the time of the studies may have been either inadequate or not determined (Chen et al., 1993; Holick et al., 1992; Tanner et al., 1988). Although dietary intake studies rarely conduct simultaneous analysis of the chemical composition of food, it is assumed that the data in the food composition database are adequate.

Infants aged 0 to 6 months who are born in the late fall in far northern and southern latitudes can only obtain vitamin D from their own stores, which have resulted from transplacental transfer in utero, or from that provided by the diet, including mother's breast milk, infant formula, or supplements. Because human milk has very little vitamin D, breast-fed infants who are not exposed to sunlight are unlikely to obtain adequate amounts of vitamin D from mother's milk to satisfy their needs beyond early infancy (Nakao, 1988; Specker et al., 1985b). Therefore, an Adequate Intake (AI) for infants ages 0 through 12 months is based on the lowest dietary intake of vitamin D that has been associated with a mean serum 25(OH)D concentration greater than 2.2 IU (11 mg)/liter (the lower limit of normal). Further, it is assumes no exogenous source of vitamin D from sunlight exposure.

Children aged 1 through 18 years and most adults obtain some of their vitamin D requirement from sunlight exposure. Since the issue of sunlight exposure confounds the literature, intake data are not available to determine an EAR, a true estimated average requirement, that can be strongly supported as a value at which half of the population group for which it is derived would be at increased risk of inadequate serum 25(OH)D. In addition, no studies have evaluated how much vitamin D is required to maintain normal blood levels of 25(OH)D and PTH in children or adults who have been deprived of sunlight and dietary vitamin D for a period of more than 6 months. Because sufficient scientific data are not available to estimate an EAR, an AI will be the reference value developed for vitamin D. The AI represents the intake that is considered likely to maintain adequate serum 25(OH)D for individuals in the population group who have limited but uncertain sun exposure and stores, multiplied by a safety factor of 100 percent for those unable to obtain sunlight. When consumed by an individual, the AI is sufficient to minimize the risk of low serum 25 (OH)D and may actually represent an overestimate of true biological need.

The recommended AI assumes that no vitamin D is available from sun-mediated cutaneous synthesis. This synthesis is especially important for calcium metabolism and bone health for the very young and for older adults. It is well documented that infants and young children who live in far northern latitudes are at high risk for developing rickets (Lebrun et al., 1993). At the other end of the age spectrum, older adults are more prone to developing vitamin D deficiency (Holick et al., 1989; Need et al., 1993). Indeed, vitamin D deficiency is now a significant concern in adults over the age of 50 years who live in the northern industrialized cities of the world (Dawson-Hughes et al., 1991; Gloth et al., 1995; Lips et al., 1988).

FINDINGS BY LIFE STAGE AND GENDER GROUP

Ages 0 through 6 Months

Indicators Used to Estimate the AI

Human Milk. The vitamin D available to the infant during the first 6 months of life depends initially on the vitamin D status of the mother during pregnancy and later on the infant's exposure to sunlight and diet. Conservative estimates of the length of time a human milk-fed infant in the Midwest must be exposed to sunlight to maintain serum concentrations above the lower limit of normal are 2 hours/week with only the face exposed to sunlight or 30 minutes/week with just a diaper on (Specker et al., 1985b). Human milk contains low amounts of vitamin D, and colostrum averages 397 ± 216 ng (15.9 ± 8.6 IU)/liter of vitamin D (Nakao, 1988). In a population of 25 Caucasian and African American women who had a mean vitamin D intake of 11.4 µg (457 IU)/day, milk concentrations of vitamin D and 25(OH)D were 315 ng (12.6 IU)/liter and 188 ng (37.6 IU)/liter respectively, with a total of 51 IU/liter of biologic activity (1 IU of vitamin D = 25 ng and 1 IU of 25(OH)D = 5 ng). Women consuming 15 to 17.5 µg (600 to 700 IU)/day of vitamin D had total milk vitamin D concentrations ranging from 120 to 3,400 ng (5 to 136 IU)/liter with a predicted mean of 645 ng (26 IU)/liter (Specker et al., 1985b). Although maternal vitamin D intake is associated with the vitamin D content of human milk, the latter is not correlated with the infant's serum 25(OH)D concentrations, due to the overwhelming effect of sunlight exposure on the infant's vitamin D status (Ala-Houhala, 1985; Ala-Houhala et al., 1986; Feliciano et al., 1994; Hillman, 1990; Markestad and Elzouki, 1991).

Serum 25(OH)D, Linear Growth, and Bone Mass. Although an individual's serum 25(OH)D concentration is the best biochemical marker of vitamin D status, functional indicators of bone length and reduced bone mass (rickets in the extreme form) serve as useful evaluative outcomes of deficiency. Vitamin D intakes between 8.5 and 15 µg (340 and 600 IU)/day would have the maximum effect on linear growth (Feliciano et al., 1994; Fomon et al., 1966; Jeans and Stearns, 1938; Stearns, 1968). At intakes greater than 45 µg (1,800 IU)/day, linear growth may be reduced (Jeans and Stearns, 1938).

A recent study in Chinese infants (Specker et al., 1992) demonstrated that both latitude and intake of vitamin D over a relatively narrow range affect infant vitamin D status. Although there was no evidence of rickets in any of the infants from northern China (40 to 47° N), vitamin D supplements of 2.5 or 5 µg (100 or 200 IU)/day resulted in 17 of 47 and 11 of 37 infants, respectively, having serum 25(OH)D concentrations less than 27.5 nmol/liter (11 ng/ml) by 6 months of age. For infants supplemented with 10 µg (400 IU)/day, only 2 of 33 had deficient vitamin D status. In contrast, Chinese infants from two southern cities (22° N and 30° N) maintained normal vitamin D status even on 2.5 µg (100 IU)/day of vitamin D.

Seasonal variation in vitamin D status of infants is also apparent. In studies from the United States (Greer et al., 1982a; Specker and Tsang, 1987) and Norway (Markestad and Elzouki, 1991), serum 25(OH)D concentrations in human milk-fed infants not receiving vitamin D supplements decreased in winter due to less sunlight exposure. However, this decrease did not occur in infants receiving a vitamin D supplement of 10 µg (400 IU)/day beginning at 3 weeks of age (Greer et al., 1982a). The impact of the seasonal reduction in vitamin D status on bone mineral mass has not been clearly delineated. In Greer's (1982) study, BMC of the placebo group was significantly less than the vitamin D-supplemented group at 12 weeks, but this difference was no longer significant by 26 weeks of age. However, there were no differences in the mean serum calcium, alkaline phosphatase, or PTH levels between the placebo and vitamin D-supplemented groups.

AI Summary: Ages 0 through 6 Months

With habitual small doses of sunshine, breast- or formula-fed infants do not require supplemental vitamin D. For infants who live in far northern latitudes or who are restricted in exposure to sunlight, a minimal intake of 2.5 µg (100 IU)/day of vitamin D will likely prevent rickets (Glaser et al., 1949; Specker et al., 1992). However, at this intake and in the absence of sunlight, many infants will have serum 25(OH)D concentrations within the range often observed in cases of rickets (Specker et al., 1992). For this reason, and assuming that infants are not obtaining any vitamin D from sunlight, an AI of at least 5 µg (200 IU)/day is recommended.

AI for Infants   0 through 6 months   5.0 µg (200 IU)/day

Special Considerations

Infant Formula. Dietary needs for vitamin D are similar for infants fed formula or human milk. Koo et al. (1995) studied infants of very low birth weight who were fed high-calcium and high-phosphorus infant formulas. They found that an average intake of vitamin D as low as 4 µg (160 IU)/day in the experimental formula maintained normal and stable vitamin D status, physical growth, biochemical and hormonal indices of bone mineral metabolism, and skeletal radiographs. In another study of exclusively formula-fed Norwegian infants who received 7.5 µg (300 IU)/day of vitamin D, all infants attained a serum 25(OH)D concentration above 27.5 nmol/liter (11 ng/ml) (Markestad and Elzouki, 1991). This result was similar to the concentrations attained by infants studied at the end of the summer who were fed human milk.

From a physiological perspective, whether infants are fed human milk or formula, their needs for dietary vitamin D when not exposed to sunlight are the same. Thus, vitamin D intake of formula-fed infants not exposed to sunlight should be at least 5 µg (200 IU)/day. However, 10 µg (400 IU)/day, the current amount included in 1 liter of standard infant formula or 1 quart of commercial cow milk, would not be excessive.

Ages 7 through 12 Months

Indicator Used to Estimate the AI

Serum 25(OH)D. Studies from three countries provide evidence for the lower range of intake of vitamin D that will support normal serum 25(OH)D concentration in infants between 7 and 12 months of age. In Norway, Markestad and Elzouki (1991) reported that in the winter, older infants who had received a vitamin preparation containing on average 5 µg (200 IU)/day of vitamin D achieved serum 25(OH)D levels that were intermediate between those of the infants studied at the end of summer and formula-fed infants. In the United States, Greer et al. (1982a) followed groups of infants who were fed human milk and exposed on average to 35 minutes/day of sunshine. Those who received either a placebo or 10 µg (400 IU)/day of vitamin D had similar serum 25(OH)D concentrations at 1 year of age. Similarly, in Hong Kong, Leung et al. (1989) followed 150 formula-fed infants who had a mean intake of 8.6, 3.9, and 3.8 µg (345, 154, and 153 IU)/day of vitamin D at 6, 12, and 18 months, respectively. They observed that none of the infants at 18 months had a serum 25(OH)D level less than 25 nmol/liter (10 ng/ml) and that the mean values in May and June were higher than in January through April.

AI Summary: Ages 7 through 12 Months

In the absence of any sunlight exposure, an AI of 5 µg (200 IU)/day will result in few infants ages 7 through 12 months with serum 25(OH)D concentrations less than 27.5 nmol/liter (11 ng/ml). This is based on the observation that, in the absence of sun-mediated vitamin D synthesis, approximately 5 µg (200 IU)/day of vitamin D maintained 25(OH)D levels in the normal range, but below circulating concentrations attained by infants in the summer. However, an intake of 10 µg (400 IU), which is supplied by 1 liter of most infant formulas or 1 quart of milk, would not be excessive.

AI for Infants   7 through 12 months 5 µg (200 IU)/day

Ages 1 through 3 and 4 through 8 Years

Indicator Used to Estimate the AI

Serum 25(OH)D. Essentially no scientific literature exists that systematically evaluates the influence of different amounts of vitamin D intake on either BMC, bone radiography, or serum 25(OH)D in children aged 1 through 3 and 4 through 8. Although vitamin D intake was not reported, Meulmeester et al. (1990) measured circulating concentrations of 25(OH)D and PTH in 8-year-old children in an observational study and found that the serum PTH increased when the 25(OH)D levels were below 20 nmol/liter (8 ng/ml). Because serum 25(OH)D concentrations in children correlate well with cumulative exposure to sunlight or dietary intake of vitamin D, this biochemical marker is appropriate for assessment of vitamin D needs of growing children. The major limiting factor in interpreting relevant studies in this age group is the inconsistency in control of sun exposure when measuring dietary intake as the intervention and vice versa. Often, relative sun exposure has to be presumed from the country where the study was conducted.

When sun exposure is consistently adequate throughout the year, as it is presumed to be in South Africa, 1- to 8-year-old children of mixed race showed no evidence of vitamin D deficiency (serum 25(OH)D > 77.5 nmol/liter [31 ng/ml]) (Pettifor et al., 1978b). Unfortunately, dietary intake was not evaluated. When vitamin D intakes were less than 2.5 µg (100 IU)/day (mean intakes 0.6 ± 1.8 µg or 25 ± 70 IU/day) in vegetarian children younger than 6 years living in Boston, 4 out of 70 children in this 3-year longitudinal study developed radiologic evidence of vitamin D deficiency (Dwyer et al., 1979).

In the absence of age-specific data, additional observations in slightly older children were considered. In a longitudinal study in Norway, where sun exposure is presumed to vary over the year, an intake of vitamin D of about 2.5 µg (100 IU)/day from fortified margarine maintained normal vitamin D status in children aged 8 to 18 years (Aksnes and Aarskog, 1982). In 6- to 17-year-old Indian children in Turkey, a daily average intake (calculated from a 1-week diet history) of 2.0 ± 0.4 µg (78.6 ± 17.9 IU) compared with 1.1 ± 0.3 µg (45.3 ± 10.8 IU) vitamin D, appeared to support a better serum 25(OH)D status in most children in this observational study (Gultekin et al., 1987). In neither study was sun exposure measured. Taken together, these studies suggest that a dietary vitamin D intake of 1.9 to 2.5 µg (75 to 100 IU)/day may be adequate when skin synthesis of vitamin D is limited by sun exposure or skin pigmentation.

Children aged 2 to 8 years obtain most of their vitamin D from exposure to sunlight (Ala-Houhala et al., 1984; Gultekin et al., 1987; Meulmeester et al., 1990; Oliveri et al., 1993; Pettifor et al., 1978a; Riancho et al., 1989; Taylor and Norman, 1984) and therefore do not normally need to ingest vitamin D. However for children who live in far northern latitudes such as in northern Canada and Alaska, vitamin D supplementation may be necessary.

AI Summary: Ages 1 through 3 and 4 through 8 Years

There are no data on how much vitamin D is required to prevent vitamin D deficiency in children aged 1 through 8 years. Extrapolating from available data in slightly older children (Aksnes and Aarskog, 1982; Gultekin et al., 1987) and from different continents for children who are not exposed to adequate sunlight, most children who had a mean dietary intake of 1.9 to 2.5 µg (75 to 100 IU)/day (Gultekin et al., 1987) showed no evidence of vitamin D deficiency and had normal serum 25(OH)D values. To cover the needs of almost all children ages 1 though 8, regardless of exposure to sunlight, the above value is doubled for an AI of 5 µg (200 IU)

AI for Children   **1 through 3 years**   **5.0 µg (200 IU)/day**
AI for Children   **4 through 8 years**   **5.0 µg (200 IU)/day**

Ages 9 through 13 and 14 through 18 Years

Indicator Used to Estimate the AI

Serum 25(OH)D. During puberty, the metabolism of 25(OH)D to 1,25(OH)$_2$D increases (Aksnes and Aarskog, 1982). The increased blood concentrations of 1,25(OH)$_2$D enhance intestinal calcium absorption to provide adequate calcium for the rapidly growing skeleton. However, there is no scientific evidence that demonstrates an increased requirement for vitamin D. In boys and girls aged 8 to 18 years, who are estimated to ingest 2.5 µg (100 IU)/day of vitamin D from margarine, the mean 25(OH)D concentration in the children in late March was 55 ± 2.5 nmol/liter (22 ± 1 ng/ml) (Aksnes and Aarskog, 1982).

In the few studies available, children during the pubertal years maintained a normal serum 25(OH)D level with dietary vitamin D intakes of 2.5 to 10 µg (100 to 400 IU)/day. Aksnes and Aarskog (1982) had the same result in Scandinavian children aged 8 to 18 years consuming 2.5 µg (100 IU)/day from margarine or 10 µg (400 IU)/day from supplements during the winter months. At intakes less than 2.5 µg (100 IU)/day, Turkish children aged 12 to 17 years had mean serum 25(OH)D concentrations that were consistent with vitamin D deficiency (< 27.5 nmol/liter [< 11 ng/ml]) (Gultekin et al., 1987). In those with mean intakes of 2.0 ± 0.5 µg (79 ± 18 IU)/day of vitamin D, serum 25(OH)D levels were 32.75 ± 2.75 nmol/liter (13.1 ± 1.1 ng/ml) for boys and 14.5 ± 1.75 nmol/liter (5.8 ± 0.7 ng/ml) for girls. With regular sun exposure, there would not be a dietary need for vitamin D (Ala-Houhala et al., 1984; Gultekin et al., 1987; Pettifor et al., 1978a; Riancho et al., 1989; Taylor and Norman, 1984). However, children who live in the far northern and southern latitudes, may be unable to synthesize enough vitamin D in their skin that can be stored for use in the winter. These children may need a vitamin D supplement (Oliveri et al., 1993).

AI Summary: Ages 9 through 13 and 14 through 18 Years

Vitamin D that is synthesized in the skin during the summer and fall months can be stored in the fat for use in the winter (Mawer et al., 1972), thereby minimizing the requirement for vitamin D. There is no reason to believe that the increased conversion of 25(OH)D to 1,25(OH)D seen in puberty results in a change in the borderline amount of circulating 25(OH)D that would be considered the minimum for adequacy. Thus, in the absence of additional data, 27.5 nmol/liter (11 ng/ml) is the appropriate cutoff for this age group. Most children aged 8 to 18 years who ingested 2.5 µg (100 IU)/day of vitamin D from margarine had no evidence of vitamin D deficiency and had a normal serum 25(OH)D level (Aksnes and Aarskog, 1982). To cover the needs of all children ages 9 through 18 years, regardless of exposure to sunlight, the above value is doubled for an AI of 5 µg (200 IU)/day.

AI for Boys	9 through 13 years	5.0 µg (200 IU)/day
	14 through 18 years	5.0 µg (200 IU)/day
AI for Girls	9 through 13 years	5.0 µg (200 IU)/day
	14 through 18 years	5.0 µg (200 IU)/day

Ages 19 through 30 and 31 through 50 Years

Indicator Used to Estimate the AI

Serum 25 (OH)D. There is little scientific information that relates vitamin D intake, bone health, and vitamin D status as determined by serum 25(OH)D and PTH concentrations in young adult and adult age groups. A descriptive longitudinal study of seven adult female patients in Great Britain (age range 20 to 46 years) who consumed a diet that contained from 0.4 to 1.7 µg (15 to 68 IU)/day of vitamin D revealed that the women developed clinical and biochemical features of osteomalacia after 1 to several years. No information about sunlight exposure was provided, and the patients achieved a positive calcium balance when consuming 2.5 µg (100 IU)/day of vitamin D (Smith and Dent, 1969).

Racial differences were not evident in measures of serum 25(OH)D and PTH in a cross-sectional study in 67 Caucasian (age

36.5 ± 6.4 years) and 70 African American (age 37 ± 6.7 years) premenopausal women living in the New York City area, who were active and exposed to sunlight. With an average daily intake of 3.5 ± 2.1 µg (139 ± 84 IU) and 3.6 ± 1.8 µg (145 ± 73 IU)/day, respectively, as measured by food frequency questionnaires and interviews, the Caucasian and African American women had similar normal serum 25(OH)D and PTH concentrations. However, BMD in both the lumbar spine and radius was significantly higher in the African American women (Meier et al., 1991). During the winter months (November through May) in Omaha, Nebraska, all except 6 percent of a group of young women aged 25 to 35 years (n = 52) maintained serum 25(OH)D levels greater than 30 nmol/liter (12 ng/ml) when daily vitamin D intake was estimated to be 3.3 to 3.4 µg (131 to 135 IU)/day (Kinyamu et al., 1997). Taken together, these studies suggest that adults younger than 50 years of age in the United States depend on sunlight for most of their vitamin D requirement. Physiological reliance on dietary vitamin D probably only occurs in the winter months in a small proportion who are not exposed to sunlight during the summer.

Indirect evidence of the importance of sunlight to vitamin D status was obtained from a recent study in 22 young male submariners (aged 18 to 32 years) who were not exposed to sunlight but who maintained their serum 25(OH)D at concentrations similar to those measured just before entering the submarine for 3 months with 15 µg (600 IU)/day of vitamin D (Holick, 1994). Those submariners who did not receive a vitamin D supplement had a 38 percent decline in serum 25(OH)D concentration after 1.5 and 3 months in the submarine. Lower supplement doses were not studied. The serum 25(OH)D levels of the nonsupplemented group increased by more than 80 percent when the submariners were exposed to sunlight for one month.

The importance of dietary sources of vitamin D was demonstrated by observations of significantly lower serum 25(OH)D (67.5 ± 47.5 nmol/liter [27 ± 19 ng/ml]) concentrations in males and females who were strictly vegetarian (mean age 42 ± 10 years) in the winter in Helsinki, Finland, compared with a control group of healthy omnivorous women with mean serum 25(OH)D concentration of 117.5 ± 37.5 nmol/liter (47 ± 15 ng/ml). Six of the 10 strict vegetarians had 25(OH)D levels below the lower reference limit of the group (62.5 nmol/liter [25 ng/ml]) indicating vitamin D deficiency (Lamberg-Allardt et al., 1993). Based on a 2-week food record, vitamin D intake in the strict vegetarians (0.3 µg or 10 IU/day) was markedly lower than in the control group (4.5 µg or 180 IU/day). Serum PTH concentrations were significantly higher in the vegetarians (57 ng/liter) compared with the control group (28 ng/liter), and 3 out of 10 subjects had concentrations that were higher than the upper reference limit (65 ng/liter), indicating secondary hyperparathyroidism.

AI Summary: Ages 19 through 30 and 31 through 50 Years

Based on the available literature, both sunlight and diet play an essential role in providing vitamin D to this age group. Because cutaneous vitamin D synthesis is markedly diminished or absent in the winter, young and middle-aged adults who live in northern (> 40°N) and southern latitudes (> 40°S) can become vitamin D deficient (Kinyamu et al., 1997). During the winter months in Omaha, Nebraska, most women with an average intake of 3.3 to 3.4 µg (131 to 135 IU)/day of vitamin D had serum 25(OH)D concentrations greater than 30 nmol/liter (12 ng/ml) (Kinyamu et al., 1997). Because there are no data for men only, other than those from submariners at a high supplement intake, it is assumed that the AI for men is similar to that for women. To cover the needs of adults ages 19 through 50 years, regardless of exposure to sunlight, the above value is rounded down to 2.5 µg (100 IU) and then doubled for an AI of 5.0 µg (200 IU)/day.

AI for Men	**19 through 50 years**	**5.0 µg (200 IU)/day**
AI for Women	**19 through 50 years**	**5.0 µg (200 IU)/day**

Ages 51 through 70 Years

Indicators Used to Estimate the AI

Serum 25(OH)D. Although this age group also depends on sunlight for most of its vitamin D requirement, this population may be more prone to developing vitamin D deficiency, owing to a variety of factors that reduce the cutaneous production of vitamin D_3. Increased use of clothing to cover the skin and prevent the damaging effects of sunlight (Matsuoka et al., 1992) and increased use of sunscreen can increase the risk of vitamin D deficiency (Holick, 1994). Aging also decreases the capacity of the skin to produce vitamin D (Holick et al., 1989; Need et al., 1993).

Bone Loss. Dietary supplementation of vitamin D in older women has been shown to influence bone loss. When vitamin D intake from food (2.5 to 5.0 µg or 100 to 200 IU/day) was supplemented with 2.5 or 17.5 µg (100 or 700 IU)/day in a double-blind, randomized 2-year trial in 247 postmenopausal women (mean age 64 ± 5 years) from Boston, loss of BMD of the femoral neck was less (–1.06 ± 0.34 percent) in the group supplemented with 17.5 µg (700 IU)/day than in the group supplemented with 2.5 µg (100 IU)/day (–2.54 ± 0.37 percent) (Dawson-Hughes et al., 1995).

Two further studies underline the importance of dietary intakes of vitamin D during the winter season in older adult populations. In 333 ambulatory Caucasian women (mean age 58 ± 6 years), serum PTH concentrations were elevated in winter (between March and May) in women consuming less than 5.5 µg (220 IU)/day of vitamin D, whereas no seasonal variation in serum PTH concentration occurred when vitamin D intakes were greater than 5.5 µg (220 IU)/day (Krall et al., 1989). In a study that measured bone loss between seasons in older women (62 ± 0.5 years) who had usual vitamin D intakes of 2.5 µg (100 IU)/day, dietary supplements of 10 µg (400 IU)/day appeared to reduce loss of spinal bone, at least during the 1 year of this randomized intervention trial (Dawson-Hughes et al., 1991). This finding is similar to that reported above regarding bone loss in the femoral neck, which was less in postmenopausal women who supplemented their diet containing 2.5 µg (100 IU)/day of vitamin D with 17.5 µg (700 IU)/day vitamin D compared with those who did not (Dawson-Hughes et al., 1995). Taken together, these studies provide evidence, at least in women, that dietary intakes of vitamin D higher than 2.5 µg (100 IU)/day are necessary at ages 51 through 70 years to prevent higher rates of bone loss during periods of low sun exposure.

AI Summary: Ages 51 through 70 Years

Using bone loss as an indicator of adequacy and data from studies of women, described above, a dietary vitamin D intake of 2.5 µg (100 IU)/day is inadequate. Although data do not exist for males in this age range, there is no reason to believe that their dietary vitamin D requirement should be different from that for females. At a vitamin D intake greater than 5.5 µg (220 IU)/day, there was no seasonal variation in serum PTH concentration (Krall et al., 1989). Given that there are few data from individuals with limited but uncertain sun exposure and stores to precisely determine a value between 2.5 µg (100 IU) and 17.5 µg (700 IU), 5 µg (200 IU) was chosen. To cover the needs of all adults ages 51 through 70 years, the above value was doubled for an AI of 10 µg (400 IU).

AI for Men	**51 through 70 years**	**10 µg (400 IU)/day**
AI for Women	**51 through 70 years**	**10 µg (400 IU)/day**

Ages > 70 Years

Indicator Used to Estimate the AI

Serum 25(OH)D. There is strong evidence for a decrease in circulating concentrations of 25(OH)D and increased risk of skeletal fractures with aging, and it is most apparent after the age of 70 years (Chevalley et al., 1994; Dawson-Hughes et al., 1991; Hordon and Peacock, 1987; Lamberg-Allardt et al., 1989; Lips et al., 1988; McGrath et al., 1993; Ng et al., 1994; Ooms et al., 1995; Villareal et al., 1991; Webb et al., 1990). Villareal et al. (1991) concluded that subclinical vitamin D deficiency with serum 25(OH)D concentrations of less than 37.5 nmol/liter (15 ng/ml) was associated with mild secondary hyperparathyroidism, lower serum calcium and phosphate levels, lower urinary calcium, and higher serum alkaline phosphatase.

Information from descriptive studies in the aging population suggests that both lack of sunlight and low intake of vitamin D influence serum 25(OH)D concentration in elderly subjects. During the winter months (November to May) in Omaha, Nebraska, all but 8 percent of 60 women living in nursing homes (mean age 84 years) and all but 1.6 percent of 64 free-living women (mean age 71 years) maintained serum 25(OH)D levels greater than 30 nmol/liter (12 ng/ml), when daily vitamin D intake was estimated to be 5.2 µg (207 IU) for the nursing home residents and 3.4 µg (135 IU) for the free-living women (Kinyamu et al., 1997). In another study during the winter months (January to May) in New York City with 109 male and female nursing home residents (mean age 82 years), serum 25(OH)D concentration was greater than 37.5 nmol/liter (15 ng/ml) in those taking a vitamin D supplement of 10 µg (400 IU)/ day (O'Dowd et al., 1993). In those residents with mean vitamin D intakes of 7.1 µg (283 IU)/day, 14 percent had serum 25(OH)D levels below 25 nmol/liter (10 ng/ml). Similarly, in 116 subjects (mean age 81) who were confined indoors for at least 6 months in Baltimore, serum 25(OH)D concentration was below 25 nmol/liter

(10 ng/ml) in 45 percent with vitamin D intakes ranging from 3.0 to 7.1 µg (121 to 282 IU)/day (Gloth et al., 1995).

Based on several randomized, double-blind clinical trials with elderly women or both men and women, a vitamin D intake of 10 µg (400 IU)/day is needed to maintain normal 25(OH)D and serum PTH status. This result was observed when the duration of the vitamin D intervention was for 1 year (Lips et al., 1988) or 3.5 years (Lips et al., 1996). In the latter study, there was no advantage to 10 µg (400 IU)/day versus placebo in the incidence of hip fractures or other peripheral fractures despite the better vitamin D status. However, a subset of the women who participated in the Lips et al. (1996) study and who were supplemented with 10 µg (400 IU)/day of vitamin D had a significant gain in change in BMD at the femoral neck after 2 years, in addition to increased 25(OH)D and decreased circulating PTH (Ooms et al., 1995). No significant BMD effects were found in the other bone sites measured: the femoral trochanter and the distal radius.

Studies in both women and men supplemented with 10 to 25 µg (400 to 1,000 IU)/day of vitamin D have shown reduced bone resorption by various urinary markers (Brazier et al., 1995; Chapuy et al., 1992; Egsmose et al., 1987; Fardellone et al., 1995; Kamel et al., 1996; Sebert et al., 1995; Sorva et al., 1991). In women supplemented for 18 months with both calcium and 20 µg (800 IU)/day of vitamin D, BMC increased significantly, and vertebral and nonvertebral fractures decreased significantly (Chapuy et al., 1992).

AI Summary: Ages > 70 Years

Evidence is strong that the elderly are at high risk for vitamin D deficiency, which causes secondary hyperparathyroidism and osteomalacia and exacerbates osteoporosis, resulting in increased risk of skeletal fractures (Chapuy et al., 1992; Egsmose et al., 1987; Honkanen et al., 1990; McKenna, 1992; Pietschmann et al., 1990). In a comparison of vitamin D status in the elderly in Europe and North America, Byrne et al. (1995) and McKenna (1992) concluded that the elderly are prone to hypovitaminosis D and associated abnormalities of bone chemistry and that a supplement of 10 to 20 µg (400 to 800 IU)/day would be of benefit. In support of this, 8, 14, and 45 percent of elderly subjects who had daily dietary vitamin D intakes of 9.6, 7.1, and 5.2 µg (384, 283, and 207 IU), respectively, were considered to be vitamin D deficient based on low serum 25(OH)D levels (Gloth et al., 1995; Kinyamu et al., 1997; O'Dowd et al., 1993). Therefore, based on the available literature, a value of 7.5 µg (300 IU)/day may be prudent for those individuals over 70 years of age with limited sun exposure and stores. In order to cover the needs of adults over age 70, regardless of exposure to sunlight and stores, the above value is doubled for an AI of 15 μg (600 IU)/day.

| AI for Men | > 70 years | 15 μg (600 IU)/day |
| AI for Women | > 70 years | 15 μg (600 IU)/day |

Special Consideration

Medications. Glucocorticoids are well known for their anti-inflammatory properties. One of the most undesirable side effects of glucocorticoid therapy is severe osteopenia. One of the mechanisms by which glucocorticoids induce osteopenia is by inhibiting vitamin D-dependent intestinal calcium absorption (Lukert and Raisz, 1990). Therefore, patients on glucocorticoid therapy may require additional vitamin D in order to maintain their serum 25(OH)D levels in the mid-normal range (25 to 45 ng/ml [62.5 to 112.5 nmol/liter]).

Medications to control seizures, such as phenobarbital and dilantin, can alter the metabolism and the circulating half-life of vitamin D (Favus and Christakos, 1996). Holick (1995) recommended that patients on at least two antiseizure medications who are institutionalized, and therefore not obtaining most of their vitamin D requirement from exposure to sunlight, increase their vitamin D intake to approximately 25 μg (1,000 IU)/day to maintain their serum 25(OH)D levels within the mid-normal range of 25 to 45 ng/ml (62.5 to 112.5 nmol/liter). This should prevent the osteomalacia and vitamin D deficiency associated with antiseizure medications.

Pregnancy

Indicators Used to Set the AI

Serum 25(OH)D. Paunier et al. (1978) evaluated the vitamin D intake from foods, supplements, and sunshine exposure of 40 healthy women at the time of delivery of their babies during the months of January and February. Women taking less than 3.8 μg (150 IU)/day had an average serum 25(OH)D concentration of 9.1 ± 1.5 ng/ml (22.75 ± 3.75 nmol/liter), while women taking more than 12.5 μg (500 IU)/day had a concentration of 11.1 ± 1.3 ng/ml (27.75 ± 3.25 nmol/liter). Although the authors noted no significant difference between these two values in the mothers, newborns of mothers who received the vitamin D supplement had a statistically higher serum calcium level on the fourth day of life than those from mothers with the lower vitamin D intake. Several studies have evaluated supplementation after the pregnant woman's first trimester with either 10 or 25 µg (400 or 1,000 IU)/day of vitamin D. It was concluded that vitamin D supplementation increased circulating concentrations of 25(OH)D in the mother (Anderson et al., 1988; Cockburn et al., 1980; Delvin et al., 1986; Mallet et al., 1986; Markested et al., 1986; Reddy et al., 1983) and may improve neonatal handling of calcium (Cockburn et al., 1980; Delvin et al., 1986).

During pregnancy, there is a gradual rise in a woman's serum $1,25(OH)_2D$ concentration that is paralleled by an increase in her blood concentration of vitamin D binding protein (Bikle et al., 1984; Bouillon et al., 1981). However, during the last trimester, the woman's serum $1,25(OH)_2D$ level continues to rise without any change in the vitamin D binding protein level, causing an increase in the free concentration of $1,25(OH)_2D$. Evidence is strong that the placenta metabolizes 25(OH)D to $1,25(OH)_2D$ and therefore contributes to the maternal and possibly fetal blood levels of $1,25(OH)_2D$ (Gray et al., 1979; Weisman et al., 1979).

AI Summary: Pregnancy

Although there is ample evidence for placental transfer of 25(OH)D from the mother to the fetus (Paunier et al., 1978), the quantities are relatively small and do not appear to affect the overall vitamin D status of pregnant women. Women, whether pregnant or not, who receive regular exposure to sunlight do not need vitamin D supplementation. However, at vitamin D intakes less than 3.8 µg (150 IU)/day, pregnant women during the winter months at high latitudes had a mean 25(OH)D concentration of 9.1 ng/ml (22.75 nmol/liter) at delivery (Paunier et al., 1978). Thus, there is no additional need to increase the vitamin D age-related AI during pregnancy above that required for nonpregnant women. However, an intake of 10 µg (400 IU)/day, which is supplied by prenatal vitamin supplements, would not be excessive.

AI for Pregnancy	14 through 18 years	5.0 µg (200 IU)/day
	19 through 30 years	5.0 µg (200 IU)/day
	31 through 50 years	5.0 µg (200 IU)/day

Lactation

Indicator Used to Set the AI

Serum 25(OH)D. During lactation, small and probably insignificant quantities of maternal circulating vitamin D and its metabolites are secreted into human milk (Nakao, 1988; Specker et al., 1985a). Although there is no reason to expect the mother's vitamin D requirement to be increased during lactation, some investigators have determined whether the infant can be supplemented via the mother's milk. Ala-Houhala (1985) and Ala-Houhala et al. (1986) evaluated the vitamin D status of mothers and their infants supplemented with vitamin D. Healthy mothers delivering in January received either 50 µg (2,000 IU)/day, 25 µg (1,000 IU)/day, or no vitamin D. Their infants were exclusively breast-fed and received 10 µg (400 IU)/day of vitamin D if their mothers received none. After 8 weeks of lactation, 25(OH)D concentrations of infants who were breast-fed from women receiving 50 µg (2,000 IU)/day of vitamin D were similar to those of infants supplemented with 10 µg (400 IU)/day. The serum 25(OH)D levels in the infants from mothers receiving 25 µg (1,000 IU)/day were significantly lower. None of the infants showed any clinical or biochemical signs of rickets, and all infants showed equal growth. Although it was concluded that postpartum maternal supplementation with 50 µg (2,000 IU)/day of vitamin D, but not 25 µg (1,000 IU)/day, seemed to normalize serum 25(OH)D concentration in infants fed human breast milk in the winter, the maternal 25(OH)D level increased in the two groups of mothers receiving 50 or 25 µg (2,000 or 1,000 IU)/day of vitamin D compared with mothers who received no vitamin D supplementation.

AI Summary: Lactation

There is no scientific literature that has determined a minimum vitamin D intake to sustain serum 25(OH)D concentration in the normal range during lactation, and there is no evidence that lactation increases a mother's AI for vitamin D. Therefore, it is reasonable to extrapolate from observations in nonlactating women that when sunlight exposure is inadequate, an AI of 5.0 µg (200 IU)/day is needed. However, an intake of 10 µg (400 IU)/day, which is supplied by postnatal vitamin supplements, would not be excessive.

AI for Lactation   14 through 18 years   **5.0 µg (200 IU)/day**
                       19 through 30 years   **5.0 µg (200 IU)/day**
                       31 through 50 years   **5.0 µg (200 IU)/day**

TOLERABLE UPPER INTAKE LEVELS

Hazard Identification

Hypervitaminosis D is characterized by a considerable increase in plasma 25(OH)D concentration to a level of approximately 400 to 1,250 nmol/liter (160 to 500 ng/ml) (Jacobus et al., 1992; Stamp et al., 1977). Because changes in circulating levels of 1,25(OH)$_2$D are generally small and unreliable, the elevated levels of 25(OH)D are considered the indicator of toxicity. However, increases in circulating levels of 1,25(OH)$_2$D in the range of 206.5 to 252.6 pmol/liter (85.9 to 105.1 pg/ml) have been reported (DeLuca, 1984; Holick, 1995; Reichel et al., 1989), which might contribute to the expression of toxic symptoms. As indicated earlier, serum 25(OH)D is a useful indicator of vitamin D status, both under normal conditions and in the context of hypervitaminosis D (Hollis, 1996; Jacobus et al., 1992).

The data in Table 7-1 suggest a direct relationship between vitamin D intake and 25(OH)D levels. Serum levels of 25(OH)D have diagnostic value, particularly in distinguishing the hypercalcemia due to hypervitaminosis D from that due to other causes, such as hyperparathyroidism, thyrotoxicosis, humoral hypercalcemia of malignancy, and lymphoma (Lafferty, 1991; Martin and Grill, 1995).

The adverse effects of hypervitaminosis D are probably largely mediated via hypercalcemia, but limited evidence suggests that direct effects of high concentrations of vitamin D may be expressed in various organ systems, including kidney, bone, central nervous system, and cardiovascular system (Holmes and Kummerow, 1983). Human case reports of pharmacologic doses of vitamin D over many years describe severe effects at intake levels of 250 to 1,250 µg/day (10,000 to 50,000 IU/day) (Allen and Shah, 1992). The available evidence concerning the adverse effects of hypervitaminosis D mediated by hypercalcemia and direct target tissue toxicity are briefly discussed below.

Hypercalcemia of Hypervitaminosis D

Hypercalcemia results primarily from the vitamin D-dependent increase in intestinal absorption of calcium (Barger-Lux et al., 1996) and the enhanced resorption of bone. Resorption of bone (hyperosteolysis) has been shown to be a major contributor to the hypercalcemia associated with hypervitaminosis D in studies that demonstrated rapid decreases in blood calcium levels following the

TABLE 7-1 Vitamin D Intake and Blood and Urinary Parameters in Adults Taking Vitamin D Supplements

Vitamin D Intake (IU/day)	Duration	Serum Calcium (mmol/L)	Serum 25(OH)D (nmol/L)	Serum Creatinine (μmol/liter)	Urinary Calcium (mmol/liter/GFR)	Study
800	4–6 months	NCa[a]	60–105 (5 studies; n = 188)	—	—	Byrne et al., 1995
1,800	3 months	NCa	65, 80 (2 studies; n = 55)	—	—	Byrne et al., 1995
1,800	3 months	NCa	57–86	82.4–83.8	—	Honkanen et al., 1990
2,000	6 months	NCa	—	—	—	Johnson et al., 1980
10,000	4 weeks	—	105[b]	—	—	Stamp et al., 1977
10,000	10 weeks	—	110[b]	—	—	Davies et al., 1982
20,000	4 weeks	—	150[b]	—	—	Stamp et al., 1977
50,000	6 weeks	3.75	320	388	—	Schwartzman and Franck, 1987
50,000	15 years	3.12	560	—	—	Davies and Adams, 1978
100,000	10 years	3.20	865	215	0.508	Selby et al., 1995
200,000	2 years	3.78	1202	207	—	Selby et al., 1995
300,000	6 years	3.30	1692	184	0.432	Rizzoli et al., 1994
300,000	3 weeks	2.82	800	339	0.065	Rizzoli et al., 1994
Vitamin D poisoning		4.0 (n = 11)	1162 (n = 11)	—	—	Pettifor et al., 1995
Overfortification of milk		3.28 (n = 35)	560 (n = 35)	—	—	Blank et al., 1995
Reference levels		2.15–2.65	20–100 (10) / 25–200 (9)	18–150	< 0.045	Blank et al., 1995 / Haddad, 1980

[a] NCa = normo-calcemic.
[b] Indicates extrapolation from graphic data.

administration of a bone resorption inhibitor, bisphosphonate (Rizzoli et al., 1994; Selby et al., 1995).

As Table 7-1 illustrates, hypercalcemias can result either from clinically prescribed intakes of vitamin D or from the inadvertent consumption of high amounts of the vitamin. The plasma (or serum) calcium levels reported range from 2.82 to 4.00 mmol/liter (normal levels are 2.15 to 2.62 mmol/liter) in those individuals with intakes of 1,250 μg (50,000 IU)/day or higher. There is no apparent trend relating "vitamin D intake-days" with plasma calcium levels.

The hypercalcemia associated with hypervitaminosis D gives rise to multiple debilitating effects (Chesney, 1990; Holmes and Kummerow, 1983; Parfitt et al., 1982). Specifically, hypercalcemia can result in a loss of the urinary concentrating mechanism of the kidney tubule (Galla et al., 1986), resulting in polyuria and polydipsia. A decrease in glomeruler filtration rate also occurs. Hypercalciuria results from the hypercalcemia and the disruption of normal reabsorption processes of the renal tubules. In addition, the prolonged ingestion of excessive amounts of vitamin D and the accompanying hypercalcemia can cause metastatic calcification of soft tissues, including the kidney, blood vessels, heart, and lungs (Allen and Shah, 1992; Moncrief and Chance, 1969; Taylor et al., 1972).

The central nervous system may also be involved: a severe depressive illness has been noted in hypervitaminosis D (Keddie, 1987). Anorexia, nausea, and vomiting have also been observed in hypercalcemic individuals treated with 1,250 to 5,000 μg (50,000 to 200,000 IU)/day of vitamin D (Freyberg, 1942). Schwartzman and Franck (1987) reviewed cases in which vitamin D was used to treat osteoporosis in middle-aged and elderly women. These women had health problems in addition to osteoporosis. Intake of vitamin D between 1,250 μg (50,000 IU)/week and 1,250 μg (50,000 IU)/day for 6 weeks to 5 years was found to be associated with reduced renal function and hypercalcemia.

Renal Disease

Some evidence supports calcification of renal and cardiac tissue following excess vitamin D intake that is not associated with hypercalcemia. In a study of 27 patients with hypoparathyroidism, Parfitt (1977) found that a mean intake of 2,100 μg (84,000 IU)/day of vitamin D for 5 years was associated with reduced renal function, nephrolithiasis, and nephrocalcinosis. Parfitt hypothesized that these results were a direct effect of vitamin D, since it was not associated with hypercalcemia in these patients. However, these results were judged inappropriate for use in deriving a tolerable upper intake level (UL) since the study subjects had hypoparathyroidism, which possibly increased their susceptibility to vitamin D toxicity. Irnell (1969) also reported a case of nephrocalcinosis and renal insufficiency in a thyroidectomized patient taking 1,125 µg (45,000 IU)/day of vitamin D for 6 years.

Cardiovascular Effects

Animal data in monkeys (Peng and Taylor, 1980; Peng et al., 1978), rabbits (Lehner et al., 1967), and pigs (Kummerow et al., 1976) suggest that calcification may also occur in nonrenal tissue. Human studies of cardiovascular effects are largely negative or equivocal. Although Linden (1974) observed that myocardial infarct patients in Tromso, Norway, were more likely to consume vitamin D in excess of 30 µg (1,200 IU)/day than were matched controls, two subsequent studies (Schmidt-Gayk et al., 1977; Vik et al., 1979) failed to confirm these results.

Although the data for nephrocalcinosis and arteriosclerosis are insufficient for determination of a UL, they point to the necessity for conservatism. There is a large uncertainty about progressive health effects, particularly on cardiovascular tissue and the kidney, with regular ingestion of even moderately high amounts of vitamin D over several decades.

Dose-Response Assessment

Adults: Ages > 18 Years

Data Selection. The most appropriate data available for the derivation of a UL for adults are provided by several studies evaluating the effect of vitamin D intake on serum calcium in humans (Honkanen et al., 1990; Johnson et al., 1980; Narang et al., 1984). The available animal data were not used to derive a UL for adults because the data were judged to have greater associated uncertainty than the human data.

Identification of a NOAEL (or LOAEL) and a Critical Endpoint. Narang et al. (1984) studied serum calcium levels in humans, with and without tuberculosis, where diet was supplemented with daily vitamin D doses of 10, 20, 30, 60, and 95 µg (400, 800, 1,200, 2,400, and 3,800 IU) for 3 months. Thirty healthy males and females ranging in age from 21 to 60 years and without tuberculosis were in one study group. Statistically significant increases in serum calcium were observed in these subjects at vitamin D doses of 60 and 95 µg (2,400 and 3,800 IU)/day. However, increases in serum calcium level in some subjects, while statistically significant, were not necessarily adverse, or indicative of hypercalcemia (for example, serum calcium levels above 2.75 mmol/liter). For example, the mean serum calcium level in normal controls following administration of 60 µg (2,400 IU)/day of vitamin D increased from 2.43 mmol/liter to 2.62 mmol/liter ($p < 0.01$). The mean serum calcium level in normal controls treated with 95 µg (3,800 IU)/day of vitamin D increased from 2.46 mmol/liter to 2.83 mmol/liter. At 30 µg (1,200 IU)/day, in normal controls, the increase was from 2.35 mmol/liter to 2.66 mmol/liter, but this was not a significant increase. The study thus demonstrates an effect of relatively low doses of supplementary vitamin D on serum calcium levels, although the degree of hypercalcemia was modest. It should also be noted that the effect developed over a relatively short time (3 months or less), so it is not known whether the effect would have progressed and worsened, or whether it would have disappeared, over a longer time period.

Hypercalcemia, defined as a serum calcium level above 2.75 mmol/liter (11 mg/dl), was observed at the highest dose of 95 µg (3,800 IU)/day, which is, therefore, the lowest-observed-adverse-effect level (LOAEL). Although a significant rise in serum calcium levels occurred at 60 µg (2,400 IU)/day, they were still within a normal range. Therefore, 60 µg (2400 IU)/day is designated as a no-observed-adverse-effect level (NOAEL).

Uncertainty and Uncertainty Factors. In using a NOAEL of 60 µg (2,400 IU)/day based only on the results of Narang et al. (1984) to derive a UL for adults, it appears to be uncertain whether any increase in serum calcium, even though still within normal limits, might be adverse for sensitive individuals and whether the short duration of this study and small sample size affected the results. The selected uncertainty factor (UF) of 1.2 was judged to be sufficiently conservative to account for the uncertainties in this data set. A larger UF was judged unnecessary due to the availability of human data and a reasonably well-defined NOAEL in a healthy population.

Derivation of a UL. Based on a NOAEL of 60 µg (2,400 IU)/day divided by a composite UF of 1.2, the estimated UL for adults is 50 µg (2,000 IU)/day. Supportive evidence for a UL of 50 µg (2,000 IU)/day is provided by Johnson et al. (1980) and Honkanen et al.

(1990). Johnson et al. (1980) conducted a double-blind clinical trial of men (all over 65 years) and women (all over 60 years) treated with 50 µg (2,000 IU)/day of vitamin D for approximately 6 months. Assuming a normally distributed population, these data as presented would appear to suggest that the risk of hypercalcemia in a population exposed to intakes of 50 µg (2,000 IU)/day ranges from 5/1,000 to less than 1/10,000. In addition, Honkanen et al. (1990) reported that 45 µg (1,800 IU)/day of supplementary vitamin D administered to Finnish women aged 65 to 72 years for 3 months produced no ill effects.

UL for Adults   > 18 years   50 µg (2,000 IU)/day

Infants: Ages 0 through 12 Months

Data Selection. Data from several studies in infants (Fomon et al., 1966; Jeans and Stearns, 1938; Stearns, 1968) were judged appropriate for use in deriving a UL for infants up to 1 year of age since the data document the duration and magnitude of intake, and as an aggregate, they define a dose-response relationship. Available data from animal studies were judged inappropriate due to their greater uncertainty.

Identification of a NOAEL (or LOAEL) and Critical Endpoint. Jeans and Stearns (1938) found retarded linear growth in 35 infants up to 1 year of age who received 45 to 112.5 µg (1,800 to 4,500 IU)/day of vitamin D as supplements (without regard to sunlight exposure, which was potentially considerable during the summer months) when compared with infants receiving supplemental doses of 8.5 µg (340 IU)/day or less for a minimum of 6 months. At 45 weeks of age, infants were found to have a linear growth rate 7 cm lower than the controls.

Fomon et al. (1966), in a similar study, explored the effects on linear growth in infants ($n = 13$) ingesting 34.5 to 54.3 µg (1,380 to 2,170 IU)/day of dietary vitamin D (mean = 44.4 µg or 1,775 IU/day) from fortified evaporated milk formulas as the only source of vitamin D compared with infants who were receiving 8.8 to 13.8 µg (350 to 550 IU)/day ($n = 11$) from another batch of formula. No effect was found in infants who were enrolled in the study during the first 9 days after birth up to 6 months of age. Given the small sample size used in this study, it was deemed appropriate to deviate from the model for the development of ULs (see Chapter 3 which defines a NOAEL as the highest intake at which no adverse effects have been observed) and identify the NOAEL for infants in this study based on the mean intake (for example, 44.4 µg or 1,775 IU/day) rather than the high end of the range. The NOAEL was rounded up to 45 µg (1,800 IU)/day. Stearns (1968) subsequently commented that Fomon et al. (1966) did not study the infants long enough since the greatest differences in the Jeans and Stearns (1938) study appeared after 6 months. However, taken together, these papers support a NOAEL of 45 µg (1,800 IU)/day.

In two different surveys at two different time periods, the British Paediatric Association (BPA) (BPA, 1956, 1964) reported a marked decline in hypercalcemia in infants, from 7.2 cases per month in a 1953–1955 survey, to 3.0 cases per month in a 1960–1961 survey. This change occurred at the same time as new guidelines were introduced for fortification of food products with vitamin D. Data from BPA (1956) and Bransby et al. (1964) also show the estimated total vitamin D intake in infants at the seventy fifth percentile of 100 µg (4,000 IU)/day declining to a range of 18.1 to 33.6 µg (724 to 1,343 IU)/day between the two surveys.

Graham (1959) studied 38 infants aged 3 weeks to 11 months with hypercalcemia in Glasgow from 1951 to 1957. The data as reported offer no definitive proof of a relationship between vitamin D intake and hypercalcemia. However, Graham does report that the highest serum calcium value obtained, 4.65 mmol/liter (18.6 mg/dl), occurred in an infant with an estimated daily intake of 33 µg (1,320 IU)/day of vitamin D and that the infant made a complete recovery when vitamin D was omitted from the diet.

Taken together, these data indicate that excessive vitamin D intake is probably a risk factor for hypercalcemia in a few sensitive infants. However, these data are inadequate for quantitative risk assessment because the daily dosage is so uncertain. This is because of the inaccuracies of survey data, but also and more importantly, because sunlight exposure was not reported, and the level of fortification of food was probably not accurately determined, and was most likely underestimated.

Uncertainty and Uncertainty Factors. Given the insensitivity of the endpoint, the fact that sample sizes were small, and that little data exist about sensitivity at the tails of the distributions, an adjustment in the NOAEL or use of a UF of 1.8 is warranted.

Derivation of the UL. Based on a NOAEL of 45 µg (1,800 IU)/day for infants and a UF of 1.8, the UL for infants up to 1 year of age is set at 25 µg (1,000 IU)/day.

UL for Infants   0 through 12 months   25 µg (1,000 IU)/day

Children: Ages 1 through 18 Years

No specific data are available for age groups other than adults and infants. Increased rates of bone formation in toddlers (1 year of age and older), children, and adolescents suggest that the adult UL is appropriate for these age groups. In addition, serum calcium levels must support the increased deposition occurring, and no data indicate impairment or insufficiency in renal handling mechanisms by 1 year of age. Therefore, the UL of 50 µg (2,000 IU)/day for adults is also specified for toddlers, children, and adolescents.

UL for Children   1 through 18 years   50 µg (2,000 IU)/day

Pregnancy and Lactation

The available data were judged inadequate to derive a UL for pregnant and lactating women that is different from other adults. Given the minor impact on either circulating vitamin D levels or serum calcium levels in utero or in infants seen with vitamin D supplements of 25 and 50 µg (1,000 and 2,000 IU)/day as previously discussed (Ala-Houhala et al., 1984, 1986), a concern about increased sensitivity during this physiologic period is not warranted.

UL for Pregnancy   14 through 50 years   50 µg (2,000 IU)/day
UL for Lactation   14 through 50 years   50 µg (2,000 IU)/day

Special Considerations

The UL for vitamin D, as with the ULs for other nutrients, only applies to healthy individuals. Granulomatous diseases (for example, sarcoidosis, tuberculosis, histoplasmosis) are characterized by hypercalcemia and/or hypercalciuria in individuals on normal or less-than-normal vitamin D intakes or with exposure to sunlight. This association is apparently due to the extrarenal conversion of 25(OH)D to $1,25(OH)_2D$ by activated macrophages (Adams, 1989; Sharma, 1996). Increased intestinal absorption of calcium and a proposed increase in bone resorption contributes to the hypercalcemia and hypercalciuria, and the use of glucocorticoids is a well-established treatment in these disorders (Grill and Martin, 1993).

Exposure Assessment

The vitamin D content of unsupplemented diets is, for the most part, low and averages about 2.5 µg (100 IU)/day for women (Krall et al., 1989; Murphy and Calloway, 1986). Diets high in fish, an exceptionally rich natural source of vitamin D (USDA, 1991) are considerably higher in vitamin D. Because milk is fortified to contain 10 µg (400 IU)/quart (9.6 µg [385 IU]/liter) of vitamin D, persons with high milk intakes also may have relatively high vitamin D intakes. A 1986 survey estimated that the ninety-fifth percentile of supplement intake by users of vitamin D supplements was 20 µg (800 IU)/day for men and 17.2 µg (686 IU)/day for women (Moss et al., 1989).

The endogenous formation of vitamin D_3 from sunlight irradiation of skin has never been implicated in vitamin intoxication. This is due to the destruction of the previtamin and vitamin D_3 remaining in skin with continued exposure to ultraviolet irradiation (Holick, 1996).

Risk Characterization

For most people, vitamin D intake from food and supplements is unlikely to exceed the UL. However, persons who are at the upper end of the ranges for both sources of intake, particularly persons who use many supplements and those with high intakes of fish or fortified milk, may be at risk for vitamin D toxicity.

RESEARCH RECOMMENDATIONS

• Research is needed to evaluate different intakes of vitamin D throughout the lifespan by geographical and racial variables that reflect the mix of the Canadian and American population and the influence of sunscreens.

• Regarding puberty and adolescence, research is needed to evaluate the effect of various intakes of vitamin D on circulating concentrations of 25 (OH)D and 1,25(OH)$_2$D during winter at a time when no vitamin D comes from sunlight exposure. During this time, the body adapts by increasing the renal metabolism of 25(OH)D to 1,25(OH)$_2$D and the efficiency of intestinal calcium absorption, thereby satisfying the increased calcium requirement by the rapidly growing skeleton.

• It is very difficult to determine the reference values for vitamin D in healthy young adults aged 18 through 30 and 31 through 50 years in the absence of sunlight exposure because of their typically high involvement in outdoor activity and the unexplored contribution of sunlight to vitamin D stores. More studies are needed that evaluate various doses of vitamin D in young and middle-aged adults in the absence of sunlight exposure.

• A major difficulty in determining how much vitamin D is adequate for the body's requirement is that a normal range for serum 25(OH)D is 25 to 137.5 nmol/liter (10 to 55 ng/ml) for all gender and life stage groups. However, there is evidence, especially in the elderly, that in order for the PTH to be at the optimum level, a 25(OH)D of 50 nmol/liter (20 ng/ml) or greater may be required. Therefore, more studies are needed to evaluate other parameters of calcium metabolism as they relate to vitamin D status including circulating concentrations of PTH.

• The development of methodologies to assess changes in body stores of vitamin D is needed to accurately assess requirements in the absence of exposure to sunlight. Such work would markedly assist in the estimation of reference values for all life stage groups.

8

Fluoride

BACKGROUND INFORMATION

Overview

Fluoride is the ionic form of fluorine, a halogen and the most electronegative of the elements of the periodic table. It is ubiquitous in nature. Fluoride combines reversibly with hydrogen to form the acid, hydrogen fluoride (HF). Much of the physiological behavior of fluoride (for example, its absorption from the stomach, distribution between extra- and intracellular fluid compartments and renal clearance) is due to the diffusion of HF (Whitford, 1996). Owing to its high affinity for calcium, fluoride is mainly associated with calcified tissues. Its ability to inhibit, and even reverse, the initiation and progression of dental caries is well known. It also has the unique ability to stimulate new bone formation, and as such, it has been used as an experimental drug for the treatment of osteoporosis (Kleerekoper and Mendlovic, 1993). Recent evidence has shown an especially positive clinical effect when fluoride (23 mg/day) is administered in a sustained release form (Pak et al., 1997) rather than in forms that are quickly absorbed from the GI tract.

The ingestion of fluoride during the pre-eruptive development of the teeth has a cariostatic effect (it reduces the risk of dental caries) due to the uptake of fluoride by enamel crystallites and formation of fluorhydroxyapatite, which is less acid soluble than hydroxyapatite (Brown et al., 1977; Chow, 1990). Fluoride in the oral fluids, including saliva and dental plaque, also contributes to the cariostat-

288

ic effect. This posteruptive effect is due mainly to reduced acid production by plaque bacteria and to an increased rate of enamel remineralization during an acidogenic challenge (Bowden, 1990; Hamilton, 1990; Marquis, 1995).

Physiology of Absorption, Metabolism, and Excretion

Fifty percent of orally ingested fluoride is absorbed from the gastrointestinal tract after approximately 30 minutes. In the absence of high dietary concentrations of calcium and certain other cations with which fluoride may form insoluble and poorly absorbed compounds, 80 percent or more is typically absorbed. Body fluid and tissue fluoride concentrations are proportional to the long-term level of intake; they are not homeostatically regulated (Guy, 1979). About 99 percent of the body's fluoride is found in calcified tissues—to which it is strongly but not irreversibly bound. Fluoride in bone appears to exist in both a rapidly exchangeable pool and a slowly exchangeable pool. The former is located in the hydration shells on bone crystallites, where fluoride may be exchanged isoionically or heteroionically with ions in the surrounding extracellular fluids. Mobilization from the slowly exchangeable pool results from the resorption associated with the process of bone remodeling.

The elimination of absorbed fluoride occurs almost exclusively via the kidneys. The renal handling of fluoride is characterized by unrestricted filtration through the glomeruli followed by a variable degree of tubular reabsorption. The extent of reabsorption is inversely related to tubular fluid pH. The renal clearance of fluoride in adults is about 30 to 40 ml/minute (Cowell and Taylor, 1981; Schiffl and Binswanger, 1982; Waterhouse et al., 1980). The rate of fluoride removal from plasma, which in healthy adults is approximately 75 ml/minute, is virtually equal to the sum of the renal and calcified tissues clearances.

The fractional retention or balance of fluoride at any age depends on the quantitative features of absorption and excretion. For healthy, young, or middle-aged adults, approximately 50 percent of absorbed fluoride is retained by uptake in calcified tissues, and 50 percent is excreted in the urine. For young children, as much as 80 percent can be retained owing to increased uptake by the developing skeleton and teeth (Ekstrand et al., 1994a, b). Such data are not available for persons in the later years of life, but based on bone mineral dynamics, it is likely that the fraction excreted is greater than the fraction retained.

Under most dietary conditions, fluoride balance is positive.

Whether it is positive or negative appears to be due to the blood-bone fluoride steady state. When chronic intake is insufficient to maintain or gradually increase plasma concentrations, fluoride excretion by infants (Ekstrand et al., 1984) and adults (Largent, 1952) can exceed the amounts ingested due to mobilization from calcified tissues.

Cariostatic Effect of Fluoride

The cariostatic action of fluoride on erupted teeth of children and adults is due to its effects on the metabolism of bacteria in dental plaque and on the dynamics of enamel de- and remineralization during an acidogenic challenge (Marquis, 1995; Tatevossian, 1990). Plaque fluoride concentrations are directly related to the fluoride concentrations in and frequencies of exposure to water, beverages, foods, and dental products. Fluoride can be deposited in plaque by direct uptake from these sources as well as from the saliva and gingival crevicular fluid after ingestion and absorption from the gastrointestinal tract. Its effects on plaque bacteria involve inhibition of several enzymes, which limits the uptake of glucose and thus reduces the amount of acid produced and secreted into the extracellular plaque fluid (Kanapka and Hamilton, 1971; Marquis, 1995). These effects attenuate the pH drop in plaque fluid that would otherwise occur and, hence, the severity of the acidic challenge to the enamel (Birkeland and Charlton, 1976).

The effects of fluoride on the processes of enamel de- and remineralization in erupted teeth include: (1) a reduction in the acid solubility of enamel; (2) promotion of remineralization of incipient enamel lesions, which are initiated at the ultrastructural level several times each day according to the frequency of eating or drinking foods containing carbohydrates metabolizable by plaque bacteria; (3) increasing the deposition of mineral phases in plaque, which, under acidic conditions produced during plaque metabolism, provide a source of mineral ions (calcium, phosphate, and fluoride) that retard demineralization and promote remineralization; and (4) a reduction in the net rate of transport of minerals out of the enamel surface by inducing the reprecipitation of fluoridated hydroxyapatite within the enamel (Margolis and Moreno, 1990; Ten Cate, 1990). These various mechanisms underlying the protective effects of fluoride on the erupted teeth of children and adults require frequent exposures to fluoride throughout life in order to achieve and maintain adequate concentrations of the ion in dental plaque and enamel.

Factors Affecting the Nutrient Requirement

Bioavailability

In general, the bioavailability of fluoride is high, but it can be influenced to some extent by the vehicle with which it is ingested. When a soluble compound such as sodium fluoride is ingested with water, absorption is nearly complete. If it is ingested with milk, baby formula, or foods, especially those with high concentrations of calcium or certain other divalent or trivalent ions that form insoluble compounds, absorption may be reduced by 10 to 25 percent (Ekstrand and Ehrnebo, 1979; Spak et al., 1982). The absorption of fluoride from ingested toothpaste, whether added as sodium fluoride or monofluorophosphate (MFP), is close to 100 percent (Ekstrand and Ehrnebo, 1980).

Fluoride-Food Component Interactions

The rate and extent of fluoride absorption from the gastrointestinal tract are reduced somewhat by ingestion with solid foods and some liquids, particularly those rich in calcium, such as milk or infant formulas (Spak et al., 1982). Results from studies with rats that had chronically elevated plasma fluoride concentrations showed that a diet high in calcium increases fecal fluoride excretion such that fluoride loss can equal or exceed fluoride intake (Whitford, 1994). It has been suggested that the co-ingestion of fluoride and caffeine or some other methylxanthines increases the bioavailability of fluoride (Chan et al., 1990), but other studies failed to confirm this effect (Chen and Whitford, 1994).

Intake of Fluoride

The *halo* or *diffusion* effect reduces the utility of the local water fluoride concentration for estimating daily fluoride intake. This effect results from the transport of foods and beverages prepared with fluoridated water to communities served with water having low fluoride concentrations, and vice versa. The consumption of beverages in the United States and Canada is displacing the consumption of tap or well water (Clovis and Hargreaves, 1988; Pang et al., 1992). In a study of fluoride intake by 225 children aged 2 to 10 years, Pang et al. (1992) reported that total fluid intake ranged from 970 to 1,240 ml/day. Consumption of soft drinks, juices, tea, and other beverages accounted for more than 50 percent of fluid intake and ranged from 585 to 756 ml/day. The fluoride concentrations ranged from nondetectable to 6.7 mg/liter. The estimated average (± standard deviation [SD]) fluoride intakes from beverages for children aged 2 to 3, 4 to 6 and 7 to 10 years were 0.36 ± 0.3, 0.54 ± 0.5, and 0.60 ± 0.5 mg/day. The maximum fluoride intakes for individual children within these age groups were 1.4, 2.4, and 2.0 mg/day.

The fluoride concentration in human milk ranges from 0.007 to 0.011 mg/liter (Ekstrand et al., 1984; Esala et al., 1982; Spak et al., 1982). Using the mean value of intake of human milk of 780 ml/day (Allen et al., 1991; Butte et al., 1984), this food provides about 0.005 to 0.009 mg/day of fluoride to the nursing infant. Intake by formula-fed infants spans a wide range depending on whether the product is ready to feed or requires the addition of water. The fluoride concentrations of ready-to-feed formulas currently made in the United States generally range from 0.1 to 0.2 mg/liter (Johnson and Bawden, 1987; McKnight-Hanes et al., 1988). Using a mean intake value of 860 ml/day of formula (Specker et al., 1997), bottle-fed infants receive about 0.09 to 0.17 mg/day of fluoride. Ready-to-feed formulas manufactured in Canada have concentrations ranging from 0.15 to 0.3 mg/liter (fluoride content of infant formulas as published by infant formula manufacturers, personal communication to Atkinson S, 1997).

The fluoride concentrations of powdered or liquid-concentrate infant formulas depend mainly on the fluoride concentration of the water used to reconstitute the products. They may be less than or several times higher than those of the ready-to-feed products. Thus, daily intakes by individual infants from these products are highly variable and can range from as little as 0.1 to over 1.0 mg/day of fluoride.

Table 8-1 summarizes the results of seven studies of dietary fluoride intake of children in the United States or Canada that were published from 1943 to 1988. The drinking water fluoride concentrations in fluoridated communities were between 0.7 and 1.1 mg/liter, whereas those in nonfluoridated communities were less than 0.4 mg/liter. The average daily dietary fluoride intakes (expressed on a body weight basis) in fluoridated areas have been relatively constant at about 0.05 mg/kg/day from infancy to early childhood since 1980. In communities without fluoridated water, average intakes have been about 50 percent lower than in fluoridated areas. As noted previously, as beverage consumption by children increases, particularly in communities without fluoridated water, fluoride intake may rise if the water source in the beverage is fluoridated (Pang et al., 1992).

TABLE 8-1 Dietary Fluoride (F) Intake by Children[a]

	mg F/day		mg F/kg body wt/day		
Age	Fluori-dated	Non-fluori-dated	Fluori-dated	Non-fluori-dated	Reference
1–3 years	0.42–0.83	—[b]	0.03–0.10	—	McClure, 1943
4–6 years	0.56–1.11	—	0.02–0.09	—	McClure, 1943
7–9 years	0.70–1.38	—	0.02–0.07	—	McClure, 1943
2 months	0.63	0.05	0.13	0.01	Singer and Ophaug, 1979
4 months	0.68	0.10	0.10	0.02	Singer and Ophaug, 1979
6 months	0.76	0.15	0.09	0.02	Singer and Ophaug, 1979
6 months	0.54	0.35	0.07	0.04	Ophaug et al., 1980a
2 years	0.61	0.32	0.05	0.03	Ophaug et al., 1980b
3–6 months	0.42	0.25	0.06	0.04	Dabeka et al., 1982
9–12 months	0.56	0.28	0.05	0.03	Dabeka et al., 1982
6 months	0.42	0.23	0.05	0.03	Ophaug et al., 1985
2 years	0.62	0.21	0.05	0.02	Ophaug et al., 1985
6 months	0.4	0.2	0.05	0.03	Featherstone and Shields, 1988

[a] Data presented as means or ranges.
[b] No data.

Ten independent U.S. and Canadian studies published from 1958 to 1987 have shown that dietary fluoride intakes by adults range from 1.4 to 3.4 mg/day in areas where the water fluoride concentration was 1.0 mg/liter. In areas where the water concentration was less than 0.3 mg/liter, the daily intakes ranged from 0.3 to 1.0 mg/day (Cholak, 1959; Dabeka et al., 1987; Filippo and Battistone, 1971; Kramer et al., 1974; McClure and Zipkin, 1958; Osis et al., 1974; Singer et al., 1980, 1985; Spenser et al., 1981; Taves, 1983). With the exception of the study by Taves (1983), each of these studies included fluoride intake from water. On a body weight basis, therefore, dietary fluoride intake by adults is generally lower than it was during the growth period. There was no evidence that dietary fluoride intake in the 1970s and 1980s had increased over that in the 1950s.

Intake from Food

Most foods have fluoride concentrations well below 0.05 mg/100 g (Taves, 1983). Exceptions to this include fluoridated water, beverages and some infant formulas that are made or reconstituted with

TABLE 8-2 Fluoride Concentrations of Foods

| Food | Fluoride Concentration (mg/liter or kg) | |
	Average	Range
Fruits	0.06	0.02–0.08
Meat, fish, poultry	0.22	0.04–0.51
Oils and fats	0.25	0.02–0.44
Dairy products	0.25	0.02–0.82
Leafy vegetables	0.27	0.08–0.70
Sugar and adjunct substances	0.28	0.02–0.78
Root vegetables	0.38	0.27–0.48
Grain and cereal products	0.42	0.08–2.01
Potatoes	0.49	0.21–0.84
Legume vegetables	0.53	0.49–0.57
Nonclassifiable	0.59	0.29–0.87
Beverages	0.76	0.02–2.74

SOURCE: Taves, 1983.

fluoridated water, teas, and some marine fish. Because of the ability of tea leaves to accumulate fluoride to concentrations exceeding 10 mg/100 g dry weight, brewed tea contains fluoride at concentrations ranging from 1 to 6 mg/liter depending on the amount of dry tea used, the water fluoride concentration, and brewing time (Cremer and Buttner, 1970; Wei et al., 1989). The concentrations in decaffeinated teas are approximately twice those of caffeinated teas (Chan and Koh, 1996). Muhler (1970) reported fluoride concentrations in marine fish ranging from 0.6 to 2.7 mg/100 g. The samples, however, may have contained bones. More recent studies reported average fluoride values for fish close to 0.05 mg/100 g and a range of 0.01 to 0.17 mg/100 g (Taves, 1983; Whitford, 1996).

Table 8-2 shows the fluoride concentrations of prepared foods that were served to adult hospital patients (Taves, 1983). When preparation required the use of water (for example, some juices, boiling vegetables), the local water, which contained 1.0 mg/liter fluoride, was used. Nonclassifiable foods included certain soups and puddings. The average daily fluoride intake was 1.8 mg, but intake from drinking water was not taken into account. Other investigators (Filippo and Battistone, 1971; Singer et al., 1980) reported an average intake of fluoride of 2.2 and 1.2 mg/day, respectively.

TABLE 8-3 Dietary Fluoride Supplement Dosage Schedule for U.S. and Canadian Children

Age of Child	Drinking Water Fluoride Concentration (mg/liter)		
	< 0.3	0.3–0.6	> 0.6
6 months to 3 years	0.25[a]	0	0
3 to 6 years	0.50	0.25	0
6 to 16 years	1.00	0.50	0

[a] Fluoride supplement values are given in mg of fluoride per day (2.2 mg sodium fluoride = 1.0 mg fluoride).
SOURCE: ADA, 1994; Canadian Paediatric Society, 1996.

Intake from Dietary Supplements

Table 8-3 shows the recently revised dietary fluoride supplement dosage schedule that was approved for U.S. and Canadian children by the American Dental Association and the American Academy of Pediatrics (ADA, 1994) and the Canadian Paediatric Society (1996). Supplements are available only by prescription and are intended for use by children living in areas with low water fluoride concentrations so that their intake is similar to that by children whose water fluoride concentrations are approximately 1.0 mg/liter. Based on the 1986 National Health Interview Survey (NHIS) data, it is estimated that 15 percent of children in the United States up to aged 5 years and 8 percent of those aged 5 to 17 years use dietary fluoride supplements (Wagener et al., 1995). Supplements are rarely prescribed for adults.

Intake from Dental Products

Intake from fluoridated dental products adds considerable fluoride (Burt, 1992; Whitford et al., 1987), often approaching or exceeding intake from the diet, particularly in young children who have poor control of the swallowing reflex. Although exposures to professionally applied products (for example, rinses and gels with high fluoride concentrations) occur less frequently, they also contribute to fluoride intake. The major contributors to nondietary fluoride intake are toothpastes (Osuji et al., 1988; Simard et al., 1989, 1991), mouth rinses (Bell et al., 1985), and dietary fluoride supplements (Ismail et al., 1990; Pendrys and Stamm, 1990).

Table 8-4 summarizes the findings from several studies of fluoride

TABLE 8-4 Fluoride Ingestion Resulting from the Use of Fluoride-Containing Toothpastes

Age (years)	Weight Used per Brushing (g) Mean	Range	Fluoride Ingested per Brushing (mg)[a] Mean	Range	% Ingested Mean	Range	Reference Study
3–6	—[b]	—	—	0–2.6[c]	—	—	Hargreaves et al., 1970
3–6	1.38	0.12–3.69	0.38	0–1.69	28	0–97	Hargreaves et al., 1972
2–4	0.86	0.19–2.41	0.30	—	35	—	Barnhart et al., 1974
5–7	0.94	0.15–2.08	0.13	—	14	—	Barnhart et al., 1974
11–13	1.10	0.31–2.00	0.07	—	6	—	Barnhart et al., 1974
20–25	1.39	0.42–3.29	0.04	—	3	—	Barnhart et al., 1974
8–10	1.04	0.23–2.57	0.12	0–0.41	12	0–32	Glass et al., 1975
2–5	0.66	—	0.33	—	45	—	Simard et al., 1989
3–10	1.00	1.00–1.00	0.36	0.08–0.82	36	8–82	Salama et al., 1989
3–5	0.49	—	0.14	—	29	—	Naccache et al., 1990
2	0.62	—	0.36	—	65	—	Naccache et al., 1992
3	0.53	—	0.28	—	49	—	Naccache et al, 1992
4	0.45	—	0.24	—	49	—	Naccache et al., 1992
5	0.52	—	0.23	—	42	—	Naccache et al, 1992
6	0.48	—	0.18	—	34	—	Naccache et al., 1992
7	0.50	—	0.18	—	34	—	Naccache et al., 1992

[a] Some studies measured the weight (g) of toothpaste ingested which, for a 1,000 ppm F product, would be proportional to the weight (mg) of fluoride ingested.
[b] No data.
[c] Toothpaste fluoride concentration = 2,400 ppm. Amounts of fluoride ingested were based on 24-hour urinary excretions and expressed as mg/day, not mg/brushing.

ingestion by children resulting from the use of toothpastes, the products of most interest because of their widespread and frequent use from an early age (Ronis et al., 1993). Dowell (1981) reported that brushing began for nearly 50 percent of his sample by the age of 12 months and that 75 percent had their teeth brushed at 18 months of age. As shown in Table 8-4, children 7 years of age or younger introduce approximately 0.8 mg of fluoride into the mouth with each brushing; the fraction that is swallowed and absorbed (Ekstrand and Ehrnebo, 1980) ranges from about 10 percent to nearly 100 percent. An average of about 0.30 mg of fluoride is ingested with each brushing by young children. Thus, brushing might contribute about 0.6 mg of fluoride daily, especially if a water rinse is not used after brushing. Similar findings were reported by Bruun and Thylstrup (1988), who studied Danish children.

Effects of Inadequate Fluoride Intake

Many studies conducted prior to the availability of fluoride-containing dental products demonstrated that dietary fluoride exposure is beneficial, owing to its ability to inhibit the development of dental caries in both children and adults (Russell and Elvove, 1951). The results of most of these studies showed that the prevalence of dental caries in communities with optimal water fluoride concentrations (range 0.7 to 1.2 mg/liter, depending on average regional temperature) was 40 to 60 percent lower than in areas with low water fluoride concentrations. The lower concentrations within the optimal range are recommended for warm climates where water intake tends to be greater than in cooler climates. Other studies have shown that the earlier children are exposed to fluoridated water or dietary fluoride supplements, the greater the reduction in dental caries in both the primary and permanent teeth (Hargreaves et al., 1988; Lewis, 1976; Stephen et al., 1987). The lack of exposure to fluoride or the ingestion of inadequate amounts of fluoride at any age places the individual at increased risk for dental caries.

Both the inter-community transport of foods and beverages and the use of fluoridated dental products have blurred the historical difference in the prevalence of dental caries between communities with and without water fluoridation. Brunelle and Carlos (1990) summarized the results of the 1986–1987 national survey conducted by the National Caries Program of the National Institute of Dental Research. The overall difference in caries prevalence between fluoridated and nonfluoridated regions in the United States was 18 percent whereas the majority of earlier studies reported differences of approximately 50 percent. After children with a reported history of exposure to dietary fluoride supplements or topical fluorides were excluded from the analysis, the difference increased to 25 percent. Further, the differences in the prevalence of caries in the seven geographic regions of the United States were inversely proportional to the percentages of water supplies that were fluoridated. In region VII (Pacific), where only 19 percent of the population is served with fluoridated water, the difference in caries scores between fluoridated and nonfluoridated areas was 61 percent. In region III (Midwest), where 74 percent of the population is served with fluoridated water, the difference was only 6 percent. These findings suggested an important role for the halo or diffusion effect. The results of this survey, like that of the 1979–1980 national survey conducted by the National Caries Program of the National Institute of Dental Research, indicate that water fluoridation continues to be of major importance in the control of dental caries.

ESTIMATING REQUIREMENTS FOR FLUORIDE

Selection of Indicators for Estimating the Fluoride Requirement

Dental Caries

The cariostatic effect of fluoride is a strong indicator for an Adequate Intake (AI) of the ion. Figure 8-1 summarizes the results of the pioneering epidemiological studies of the relationships between the concentration of fluoride in drinking water and dental caries and enamel fluorosis (mottling) (Dean, 1942). Enamel fluorosis is caused by excessive fluoride intake but only during the preeruptive development of the teeth. A fluorosis index value of 0.6 in a community was judged to represent the threshold for a problem of public health significance. As can be seen in Figure 8-1, this value occurred in communities having water fluoride concentrations in the 1.6 to 1.8 mg/liter range. The figure also shows that reduction in the average number of dental caries per child was nearly maximal in communities having water fluoride concentrations close to 1.0 mg/liter. This is how 1.0 mg/liter became the "optimal" concentration. That is, it was associated with a high degree of protection against caries and a low prevalence of the milder forms of enamel fluorosis. The average dietary fluoride intake by children living in optimally fluoridated communities was (and remains) close to 0.05 mg/kg/day (range 0.02 to 0.10 mg/kg/day; Table 8-1).

Both pre- and posteruptive exposures to fluoride have cariostatic effects (Dawes, 1989; Hargreaves, 1992; Horowitz, 1990). Based on data from their long-term study of the cariostatic effects of fluoridated water in the Netherlands, Groeneveld et al. (1990) concluded that: (1) the best effect on dental caries in the permanent teeth was achieved when fluoride was consumed from birth, (2) about 85 percent of the greatest reduction in caries was obtained when fluoride consumption started between ages 3 and 4, (3) about 66 percent of the protective effect for surfaces with high caries susceptibility (pits and fissures) derived from preeruptive fluoride exposure, and (4) about 25 percent of the protective effect for the lower risk, smooth surfaces was attributable to preeruptive fluoride exposure. Several other retrospective clinical studies have shown that the ear-

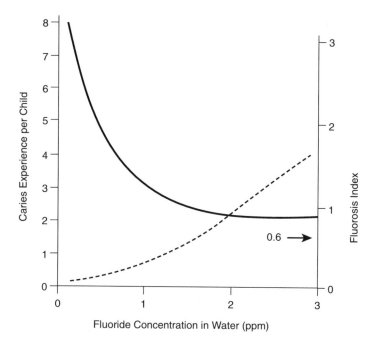

FIGURE 8-1 Relationships among caries experience (solid line), dental fluorosis index (dashed line), and the fluoride concentration of drinking water. A fluorosis index value of 0.6 was judged to represent the threshold for a problem of public health significance. The data are based on the examination of 7,257 12- to 14-year-old children (Dean, 1942).

lier children are exposed to fluoridated water or dietary fluoride supplements, the greater the reduction in dental caries in both the primary and permanent teeth (Hargreaves et al., 1988; Lewis, 1976; Stephen et al., 1987).

A large number of studies have shown that fluoridated drinking water increases resistance to dental caries at all ages. For example, Jackson et al. (1973) recorded caries experience among 3,902 residents of York and Hartlepool, England. The water fluoride concentrations in these cities were 0.2 mg/liter and 1.5 to 2.0 mg/liter, respectively. Caries experience in people in five different age groups (ranging from 15 to 19 to > 44 years) was significantly lower in Hartlepool (44 percent lower in the > 44-year-old group). In a study of Swedish subjects aged 30 to 40 years ($n = 496$), who were life-long residents of Uppsala (1.0 mg/liter fluoride in water) or Enköping (0.3 mg/liter fluoride in water), Wiktorsson et al. (1992) found that the percentage of decayed and filled surfaces was 21 percent lower in the fluoridated community. Multiple regression analysis indicated that this difference was due to the community of residence but not to differences in past dental treatment, frequency of toothbrushing with a fluoridated toothpaste, or the frequency of drinking tea.

Bone Mineral Content

Several reports published 30 to 40 years ago suggested that the long-term ingestion of fluoride at levels slightly above optimum for caries prevention improved the quality of the human skeleton and that the risk of osteoporosis might thereby be reduced (Bernstein et al., 1966; Leone et al., 1955, 1960). A recent Finnish study concluded that, compared with the low-fluoride control group, vertebral bone mineral density (BMD) was increased slightly while femoral neck BMD was not affected among perimenopausal women who had used fluoridated water (1.0 to 1.2 mg/liter) for 10 years or more (Kröger et al., 1994). There was no difference between the groups in the prevalence of self-reported bone fractures. Richards et al. (1994) reported that the normal, age-related increase in bone fluoride concentrations (range 463 to 4,000 mg/kg) had no effect on the compressive strength or ash density of vertebra in Danish men and women whose ages ranged from 20 to 91 years. Sowers et al. (1986, 1991), however, reported a marginal increase in bone fractures (self-reported) and lower bone densities among women whose drinking water contained 4 mg/liter of fluoride.

Some evidence exists that fluoride may inhibit the calcification of soft tissues (Taves and Neuman, 1964; Zipkin et al., 1970), including the aorta (Bernstein et al., 1966). Taves (1978) reported that the standardized mortality rate due to ischemic heart disease in cities with optimally fluoridated water was lower than in cities with low water fluoride concentrations. Data are insufficient to justify using these effects as the basis for estimating an AI for fluoride.

Fluoride Balance

As shown in studies with infants (Ekstrand et al., 1984, 1994a, b) and adults (Largent, 1952; Maheshwari et al., 1981), the balance of fluoride can be negative. This occurs when chronic intake is reduced sufficiently to allow plasma fluoride concentrations to fall, which promotes the mobilization of the ion from calcified tissues. However, no data document the effects of a long-term negative fluoride balance on enamel, on salivary or plaque concentrations, or on caries development. At this time, therefore, the use of balance data to estimate an adequate intake of fluoride is not warranted.

AI Definition

Because data are not available to determine an Estimated Average Requirement (EAR), the reference value that will be used for fluoride is the AI. The AI is based on estimated intakes that have been shown to reduce the occurrence of dental caries maximally in a population without causing unwanted side effects including moderate dental fluorosis.

FINDINGS BY LIFE STAGE AND GENDER GROUP

General Observations

The cariostatic effect associated with residence in communities served with optimally fluoridated water (ca. 1 mg/liter) has been confirmed by numerous epidemiological studies conducted in countries throughout the world (Horowitz, 1996). The average dietary intake by U.S. infants and children since 1980 in these areas has been close to 0.05 mg/kg/day (Table 8-1). The slightly higher average intakes by infants aged 2 to 6 months, reported by Singer and Ophaug (1979) were largely due to intake from formulas that had been manufactured with fluoridated water. Since then, most formula manufacturers in the United States have used low-fluoride water (Burt, 1992). Although the total amount of fluoride ingested daily by older children and adults is greater than by infants or young children, it is generally lower when expressed in terms of body weight. As noted earlier, average dietary fluoride intakes by adults living in fluoridated communities have ranged from 1.4 to 3.4 mg/day, or from 0.02 to 0.05 mg/kg/day for a 70 kg person.

Adequate Intake

Infants: Ages 0 through 6 Months

As noted earlier, fluoride intake among infants varies widely, especially during the first 6 months of life, depending on whether the infant is fed human milk or formula and whether the formula is ready-to-feed or requires reconstitution with water. Human milk-fed infants receive about 0.01 mg/day (0.001 to 0.003 mg/kg). Infants fed a formula reconstituted with fluoridated water may receive as much as 1.0 mg/day. Some evidence shows that the prevalence of mild enamel fluorosis in the primary teeth, but not the permanent teeth, is higher among formula-fed infants than infants fed cow's milk, which has a low fluoride concentration similar to that of human milk (Larsen et al., 1988). The current dosage schedule for dietary fluoride supplements in the United States (ADA, 1994) and Canada (Canadian Paediatric Society, 1996) recommends starting supplementation at 6 months of age. Since the intake of fluoride by human milk-fed infants during this period of life does not appear to significantly increase the risk of dental caries, fluoride from human milk is deemed adequate in early life.

AI for Infants   0 through 6 months   0.01 mg/day

Ages > 6 Months

Based on the extensively documented relationships between caries experience and both water fluoride concentrations and fluoride intake, the AI for fluoride from all sources is set at 0.05 mg/kg/day. This intake range is recommended for all ages greater than 6 months because it confers a high level of protection against dental caries and is associated with no known unwanted health effects. The cariostatic effect is due both to preeruptive fluoride incorporation into tooth enamel and to continuing, frequent posteruptive fluoride exposures of the teeth. Indicative of the benefit of continuing posteruptive exposures, several studies have shown that caries experience increases among persons who were raised in a fluoridated community but then moved to an area with a lower water fluoride concentration (Russell, 1949), or when a water system is defluoridated (Lemke et al., 1970).

AI Summary: Ages 7 through 12 Months

Based on an AI for fluoride from all sources of 0.05 mg/kg/day and a reference weight of children in this age range of 9 kg (Table 1-3), the AI is 0.5 mg/day.

AI for Children   7 through 12 months   0.5 mg/day

AI Summary: Ages 1 through 3 Years

Based on an AI for fluoride from all sources of 0.05 mg/kg/day and a reference weight of children 1 through 3 years of age of 13 kg (Table 1-3), the AI is 0.7 mg/day.

AI for Children   **1 through 3 years**   **0.7 mg/day**

AI Summary: Ages 4 through 8 Years

Based on an AI for fluoride from all sources of 0.05 mg/kg/day and a reference weight for children 4 through 8 years of age of 22 kg (Table 1-3), the AI is 1.1 mg/day.

AI for Children   **4 through 8 years**   **1 mg/day**

AI Summary: Ages 9 through 13 Years

Based on an AI for fluoride from all sources of 0.05 mg/kg/day and a reference weight for both boys and girls ages 9 through 13 years of 40 kg (Table 1-3), the AI is 2.0 mg/day.

AI for Boys   **9 through 13 years**   **2 mg/day**
AI for Girls   **9 through 13 years**   **2 mg/day**

AI Summary: Ages 14 through 18 Years

Based on an AI for fluoride from all sources of 0.05 mg/kg/day and a reference weight for boys ages 14 through 18 years of 64 kg (Table 1-3), the AI is 3.2 mg/day for boys. Based on a reference weight for girls ages 14 through 18 years of 57 kg, the AI is 2.9 mg/day for girls.

AI for Boys   **14 through 18 years**   **3 mg/day**
AI for Girls   **14 through 18 years**   **3 mg/day**

AI Summary: Ages 19 Years and Over

Based on an AI for fluoride from all sources of 0.05 mg/kg/day and a reference weight for males ages 19 and over of 76 kg (Table 1-3), the AI is 3.8 mg/day. Based on a reference weight for females ages 19 and above of 61 kg, the AI for females is 3.1 mg/day.

AI for Males   **19 years and over**   **4 mg/day**
AI for Females   **19 years and over**   **3 mg/day**

Pregnancy

It is known that fluoride crosses the placenta, enters the fetal circulation (Brambilla et al., 1994; Shen and Taves, 1974), and is incorporated into the developing primary teeth (Gedalia et al., 1964; Hargreaves, 1972; LeGeros et al., 1985). Studies conducted shortly after the beginning of water fluoridation indicated that the greatest reduction in caries was seen in children who had the longest exposure to fluoridated water (Arnold et al., 1956; Blayney and Hill, 1964). This raised the possibility of a beneficial effect of prenatal fluoride for the primary teeth. The results of several studies suggested that the ingestion of supplemental fluoride during pregnancy was beneficial to the primary teeth (Feltman and Kosel, 1961; Glenn, 1981; Glenn et al., 1984; Hoskova, 1968; Kailis et al., 1968; Prichard, 1969; Schutzmannsky, 1971). In contrast, other studies have reported no effects or statistically nonsignificant effects of prenatal fluoride administration on caries in the primary dentition (Carlos et al., 1962; Horowitz and Heifetz, 1967; Leverett et al., 1997). The Leverett et al. (1997) study was the first prospective, randomized, double blind study conducted in this area and the authors concluded that "the data do not support the hypothesis that the observed low carie levels are attributable to prenatal fluoride exposure." At this time, scientific evidence is insufficient to support a recommendation for prenatal fluoride supplementation. This is in line with the current recommendation of the American Dental Association. Further, when fluoride supplements are taken during pregnancy, the United States Food and Drug Administration prohibits making claims of benefit to the teeth of children.

The results from two studies indicated that fluoride balances in pregnant and nonpregnant women were not markedly different (Maheshwari et al., 1981, 1983). In the former study, 16 women aged 19 to 31 years were studied. Ten were in the second half of pregnancy, and six served as nonpregnant controls. The diets had a low fluoride content (less than 0.45 mg/day), which, as in some of the infant studies described above, resulted in negative fluoride balances. The average balances for the pregnant and nonpregnant groups were −0.32 and −0.15 mg/day, respectively. In the second study 18 women aged 19 to 33 years were supplemented with 1.0 mg/day so the average total intake was 1.35 mg/day. Seven of the women were not pregnant, six were in the second quarter of pregnancy, and five were in the fourth quarter of pregnancy. The higher fluoride intake in this study resulted in positive balances in each group. The differences among the groups were small and not statistically significant.

AI Summary: Pregnancy

There is no evidence at this time that the AI for women during pregnancy should be increased above the level recommended for women during the nonpregnant state.

AI for Pregnancy	**14 through 18 years**	**3 mg/day**
AI for Pregnancy	**19 through 50 years**	**3 mg/day**

Lactation

No data from human studies document the metabolism of fluoride during lactation. Because fluoride concentrations in human milk are very low and relatively insensitive to differences in the fluoride concentrations of the mother's drinking water, fluoride supplementation during lactation would not be expected to significantly affect fluoride intake by the nursing infant or the fluoride requirements of the mother. The AI for women during lactation is therefore not increased above that for women in the nonpregnant state.

AI for Lactation	**14 through 18 years**	**3 mg/day**
AI for Lactation	**19 through 50 years**	**3 mg/day**

Special Considerations

Fluoride Supplements in Areas without Water Fluoridation. Infants and children living in nonfluoridated water areas will not easily achieve the AI for fluoride. Thus, fluoride supplements have been recommended based on life stage and level of water fluoridation. Table 8-3 shows the recently revised dietary fluoride supplement dosage schedule that was approved for United States children by the American Dental Association and American Academy of Pediatrics (ADA, 1994) and for Canadian children by the Canadian Paediatric Society (1996). The daily fluoride dose is based on the age of the child and the fluoride concentration of the child's main drinking water source. Compared with the previous dosage schedule that was adopted in 1979, the current schedule represents a reduction of approximately 50 percent in the amount of fluoride to be prescribed for children up to the age of 6 years. Other changes from the previous schedule include starting supplementation at 6 months instead of at birth and reducing the water fluoride concentration to a level above which supplements should not be prescribed from 0.7 mg/liter to 0.6 mg/liter. The main reasons for these changes were the increased prevalence of enamel fluorosis in the United States and Canada and the identification of dietary supplements as one of the risk factors (see below). The decision to delay the start of supplementation until 6 months of age was based on the fact that approximately two-thirds of infants are formula-fed and that many human milk-fed infants receive nourishment from other sources that contain variable amounts of fluoride at an early age.

TOLERABLE UPPER INTAKE LEVELS

Hazard Identification

The primary adverse effects associated with chronic, excess fluoride intake are enamel and skeletal fluorosis.

Adverse Cosmetic Effect: Enamel Fluorosis

Enamel fluorosis is a dose-response effect caused by fluoride ingestion during the preeruptive development of the teeth. After the enamel has completed its preeruptive maturation, it is no longer susceptible. Inasmuch as enamel fluorosis is regarded as a cosmetic effect, it is the anterior teeth that are of most concern. The preeruptive maturation of the crowns of the anterior permanent teeth is finished and the risk of fluorosis is over by 8 years of age (Fejerskov et al., 1977). Therefore, fluoride intake up to the age of 8 years is of most interest. Several reports suggest that enamel in the transitional or early maturation stage of development is most susceptible to fluorosis, which for the anterior teeth, occurs during the second and third years of life (Evans, 1989; Evans and Darvell, 1995; Pendrys and Katz, 1989; Pendrys and Stamm, 1990). Some evidence indicates that the risk of mild enamel fluorosis in the primary teeth is somewhat increased as a result of the relatively high fluoride intake associated with feeding some infant formulas reconstituted with fluoridated water (Larsen et al., 1988).

Fluorosed enamel has a high protein content. This results in increased porosity which, in the moderate and severe forms, may eventually become stained and pitted (Fejerskov et al., 1977; Kaminsky et al., 1990). Clinically, the milder forms of enamel fluorosis are characterized by opaque striations that run horizontally across the surfaces of teeth. The striations may become confluent giving rise to white opaque patches, often most apparent on the incisal edges of anterior teeth or cusp tips of posterior teeth ("snow-capping"). Mild fluorosis has no effect on tooth function and may render the enamel more resistant to caries. It is not readily apparent to the affected individual or casual observer and often requires a trained specialist to detect. In contrast, the moderate and severe forms of enamel fluorosis are generally characterized by esthetically objectionable changes in tooth color and surface irregularities. Most investigators regard even the more advanced forms of enamel fluorosis as a cosmetic effect rather than a functional adverse effect (Clark et al., 1993; Kaminsky et al., 1990).

Adverse Functional Effect: Skeletal Fluorosis

Three recent reviews of the literature attempted to identify adverse functional effects of fluoride ingestion in adults (Kaminsky et al., 1990; NRC, 1993; USPHS, 1991). Fluoride exposures included those associated with drinking water containing as much as 8 mg/liter of fluoride and the use of dental products. These reviews indicate that the primary functional adverse effect associated with excess fluoride intake is skeletal fluorosis.

In the asymptomatic, preclinical stage of skeletal fluorosis, patients have slight increases in bone mass that are detectable radiographically, bone ash fluoride concentrations that range from 3,500 to 5,500 mg/kg, and bone concentrations that are 2 to 5 times higher than those of life-long residents of optimally fluoridated communities (Eble et al., 1992). Stage 1 skeletal fluorosis is characterized by occasional stiffness or pain in joints and some osteosclerosis of the pelvis and vertebra. Bone ash fluoride concentrations usually range from 6,000 to 7,000 mg/kg. In stages 2 and 3, bone ash concentrations exceed 7,500 to 8,000 mg/kg (Hodge and Smith, 1977). The clinical signs in stages 2 and 3, which may be crippling, may include dose-related calcification of ligaments, osteosclerosis, exostoses, possibly osteoporosis of long bones, muscle wasting, and neurological defects due to hypercalcification of vertebra (Krishnamachari, 1986).

The development of skeletal fluorosis and its severity is directly related to the level and duration of exposure. Most epidemiological research has indicated that an intake of at least 10 mg/day for 10 or more years is needed to produce clinical signs of the milder forms of the condition. Hodge (1979) reported that evidence of crippling fluorosis "was not seen in communities in the United States where water supplies contained up to 20 ppm." In such communities daily fluoride intakes of 20 mg would not be uncommon. In a recent case report, severe joint pain and stiffness in a 64-year-old man were attributed to a fluoride intake of approximately 50 mg/day for 6 years. The well water ingested had a fluoride concentration of 25 mg/liter and a low calcium concentration (Boyle and Chagnon,

1995). Stevenson and Watson (1957) surveyed 170,000 radiographs of patients from Texas and Oklahoma whose drinking water fluoride concentrations ranged from 4 to 8 mg/liter. They identified 23 cases of osteosclerosis but no evidence of skeletal fluorosis.

Crippling skeletal fluorosis continues to be extremely rare in the United States (only 5 cases have been confirmed during the last 35 years), even though for many generations there have been communities with drinking water fluoride concentrations in excess of those that have resulted in the condition in other countries (Singh and Jolly, 1970). This puzzling geographic distribution has usually been attributed to unidentified metabolic or dietary factors that rendered the skeleton more or less susceptible.

Dose-Response Assessment

Infants and Children Ages 0 through 8 Years

Data Selection. The most appropriate data available for identifying a no-observed-adverse-effect level (NOAEL) (or lowest-observed-adverse-effect level [LOAEL]) are provided by two studies evaluating the severity of enamel fluorosis in children (Dean, 1942; Dean and Elvove, 1937). In these early studies, fluoride intake was almost exclusively from the diet and not confounded by intake from dental products.

Identification of a NOAEL (or LOAEL) and Critical Endpoint. Dental fluorosis has a strong dose-response relationship with fluoride intake. Dean (1942) established that the milder forms of enamel fluorosis affected the permanent teeth of 10 to 12 percent of permanent residents in communities where the drinking water had a fluoride concentration close to 1.0 mg/liter. The fluoride intake of children with developing teeth in these communities averaged 0.05 mg/kg/day and ranged from 0.02 to 0.10 mg/kg/day. In areas where the water contained low concentrations of fluoride (0.3 mg/liter), fewer than 1 percent of the permanent residents had enamel fluorosis. Mild enamel fluorosis affected about 50 percent of residents where the water contained 2.0 mg/liter of fluoride. At this concentration, a few cases (< 5 percent) of moderate fluorosis were recorded (Dean, 1942). Fluoride intake by most children in these communities would have ranged from approximately 0.08 to 0.12 mg/kg/day. An average, chronic daily fluoride intake of 0.10 mg/kg appears to be the threshold beyond which moderate enamel fluorosis appears in some children. Where the water fluoride concentration was 4.0 mg/liter, nearly 90 percent of the residents had enamel fluorosis, and about one-half of the cases were classified as moderate or severe.

Because the cosmetic effects of the milder forms of enamel fluorosis are not readily apparent, moderate enamel fluorosis was selected as the *critical adverse effect* for susceptible age groups (infants, toddlers, and children through the age of 8 years). Thus, a fluoride intake of 0.10 mg/kg/day was identified as a LOAEL for moderate enamel fluorosis in children from birth through the age of 8 years, at which age the risk of developing fluorosis of the anterior teeth is over.

Uncertainty Assessment. The relationship between fluoride intake and enamel fluorosis is based on results from human studies and enamel fluorosis is considered a cosmetic effect rather than an adverse functional effect. Therefore, an uncertainty factor (UF) of 1 was selected.

Derivation of the UL. Based on a LOAEL of 0.10 mg/kg/day for moderate enamel fluorosis and a UF of 1, a Tolerable Upper Intake Level (UL) of 0.10 mg/kg/day was established for infants, toddlers, and children through 8 years of age. The extensive epidemiological research conducted in the United States during the 1930s and 1940s (Dean, 1942) established, with a high degree of certainty, that a chronic fluoride intake of less than 0.10 mg/kg/day by children at risk of enamel fluorosis was associated with a low prevalence (for example, approximately 10 percent) of the milder forms of the condition.

Based on a UL of 0.10 mg/kg/day of fluoride and a reference weight for infants ages 0 through 6 months of 7 kg (Table 1-3), the UL is 0.7 mg/day. For children ages 7 through 12 months with a reference weight of 9 kg, the UL is 0.9 mg/day.

| UL for Infants | 0 through 6 months | 0.7 mg/day |
| UL for Infants | 7 through 12 months | 0.9 mg/day |

Based on a UL of 0.10 mg/kg/day of fluoride and a reference weight for children ages 1 to 3 years of 13 kg (Table 1-3), the UL is 1.3 mg /day for children ages 1 through 3 years. For children ages 4 through 8 years with a reference weight of 22 kg, the UL is 2.2 mg/day.

| UL for Children | 1 through 3 years | 1.3 mg/day |
| UL for Children | 4 through 8 years | 2.2 mg/day |

Older Children and Adults: Ages > 8 Years

Data Selection. Although some recent recommendations have been made for additional research in the areas of intake, dental fluorosis, bone strength, and carcinogenicity, extensive reviews of the scientific literature revealed no adverse effects unless fluoride intakes were greater than 10 mg/day for 10 or more years (Kaminsky et al., 1990; NRC, 1993; USPHS, 1991). At these high, chronic intake levels, the risk of skeletal changes consistent with preclinical or stage 1 skeletal fluorosis increases. Therefore, the data deemed most appropriate for identifying a NOAEL (or LOAEL) for older children and adults are provided by studies on skeletal fluorosis.

Identification of a NOAEL (or LOAEL) and Critical Endpoint. Epidemiological studies reported no detectable radiographic changes in bone density in persons in the United States exposed to drinking water containing less than 4 mg/liter of fluoride (McCauley and McClure, 1954; Schlesinger et al., 1956; Sowers et al., 1986; Stevenson and Watson, 1957). Leone et al. (1955) compared bone x-rays of long-term residents of Bartlett and Cameron, Texas, which had water supplies with fluoride concentrations of 8.0 and 0.4 mg/liter, respectively. In this study, osteosclerosis was detected radiographically in 10 to 15 percent of individuals exposed to water containing 8.0 mg/liter of fluoride for an average of 37 years. However, no clinical symptoms of skeletal fluorosis were reported. Another report dealing with a variety of other medical conditions among residents of Bartlett and Cameron revealed no significant differences except for a slightly higher rate of cardiovascular abnormalities in Cameron residents (Leone et al., 1954). Therefore, based on the available data addressing the association between fluoride intake and skeletal fluorosis in North America, a NOAEL of 10 mg/day of fluoride was identified. This level of intake for some individuals would occur in areas where the drinking water has a fluoride concentration of 5 mg/liter and the diet is the main source of fluoride.

Uncertainty Assessment. Based on the fact that the NOAEL derives from human studies and the lack of evidence for symptomatic skeletal fluorosis observed at this level of fluoride intake, a UF of 1 was selected.

Derivation of the UL. The risk of developing early signs of skeletal fluorosis is associated with a fluoride intake greater than 10 mg/

day for 10 or more years. Therefore, a UL of 10 mg/day was established for children older than 8 years and for adults. Data from studies of fluoride exposure from dietary sources or work environments (Hodge and Smith, 1977) indicate that a UL of 10 mg/day for 10 or more years carries only a small risk for an individual to develop preclinical or stage 1 skeletal fluorosis.

UL for Children and Adults   > 8 years   10 mg/day

Pregnancy and Lactation

No data indicate an increased susceptibility to fluorosis during pregnancy. Therefore, the UL for adults of 10 mg/day was also established for pregnant women. A UL of 10 mg/day was established for lactation, because an extremely small proportion of fluoride in drinking water is transferred to the breast milk (Ekstrand et al., 1981, 1984; Esala et al., 1982; Spak et al., 1982).

UL for Pregnancy
and Lactation   14 through 50 years   10 mg/day

Special Considerations

Reports of relatively marked osteofluorotic signs and symptoms have been associated with concentrations of fluoride in drinking water of approximately 3 mg/liter in tropical climates. This adverse effect has been attributed to poor nutrition, hard manual labor, and high levels of water intake (Krishnamachari, 1986; Singh and Jolly, 1970; WHO, 1984). Therefore, an increased risk of skeletal fluorosis from excess fluoride intake may exist for malnourished individuals living in hot climates or tropical areas.

Exposure Assessment

Prior to the 1960s, the diet, including water, was the only significant source of fluoride. Since then, fluoride ingestion resulting from the use of dental products and fluoride supplements has increased the risk of enamel fluorosis in children. The results of several studies (Kumar et al., 1989; Leverett, 1986; Pendrys and Stamm, 1990; Williams and Zwemer, 1990) have indicated that mild enamel fluorosis in communities with optimally fluoridated water (1.0 mg/liter) is now more than twice as prevalent as in the 1930s and 1940s; that is, the prevalence has increased from an average of about 10 percent to an average approaching 25 percent. In communities where the water has a low fluoride concentration (0.3 mg/liter or less), the prevalence has increased from less than 1 percent to slightly more than 10 percent. These findings reflect levels of fluoride ingestion by some children with developing teeth that are higher than heretofore.

Moreover, a recent national survey (Wagener et al., 1995) found that dietary fluoride supplements were used by 15 percent of children under 2 years of age, 16 percent by those 2 through 4 years of age, and 8 percent by those 5 to 17 years of age. In their study of infants born in Iowa City, a university community with a high socioeconomic status, Levy et al. (1995) reported that from 19 to 25 percent of infants between the ages of 6 weeks and 9 months were given fluoride supplements. Pendrys and Morse (1990) and Levy and Muchow (1992) are among those who have found that supplements are often prescribed at the wrong dosage and in areas where they are not recommended because the water is already fluoridated at recommended levels. Recommendations have been made to reduce fluoride intake from nondietary sources (NRC, 1993; USPHS, 1991; Workshop Reports, 1992).

Risk Characterization

Although the prevalence of enamel fluorosis in both fluoridated and nonfluoridated communities in the United States and Canada is substantially higher than it was when the original epidemiological studies were done some 60 years ago, the severity remains largely limited to the very mild and mild categories. As recorded in the original studies, the prevalence of cases classified as moderate or severe increases with the concentration of fluoride in the drinking water. These relationships are illustrated in Table 8-5, which summarizes data from several U.S. studies done in the 1980s (USPHS, 1991).

These data suggest that the UL (0.1 mg/kg/day) is exceeded by approximately 1 in 100 children in areas where the water fluoride concentration is 1.0 mg/liter or slightly higher. In the 1930s and 1940s, no moderate or severe cases of enamel fluorosis were recorded in these areas, and because fluoride intake from water and the diet appears not to have increased since that time, the additional intake by children at risk of enamel fluorosis almost certainly derives from the use of fluoride-containing dental products.

The virtual absence of evidence of skeletal changes consistent with a diagnosis of skeletal fluorosis indicates that the UL for older children and adults is not being exceeded in the United States or Canada.

TABLE 8-5 Prevalence and Severity of Enamel Fluorosis as a Function of Drinking Water Fluoride Concentration

No. of Studies	No. of Subjects	Drinking Water Fluoride (mg/liter)	Prevalence of Enamel Fluorosis, %[a]	
			Very Mild/Mild	Moderate/Severe
4	1,885	ca. 1.0	21.5 (9.0–39.1)	1.0 (0–2.4)
3	526	1.3–1.4	25.1 (15.6–31.6)	0.7 (0–1.1)
6	1,080	2.0–3.0	64.5 (39.9–86.5)	12.6 (3.3–32.8)
4	631	3.0–4.3	53.1 (34.9–72.5)	21.7 (4.4–36.1)

[a] Range of the mean values of prevalence from the individual studies is shown in parentheses.
SOURCE: USPHS, 1991.

RESEARCH RECOMMENDATIONS

• Epidemiological studies (especially analytical studies) of the relationships among fluoride exposures from all major sources and the prevalence of dental caries and enamel fluorosis at specific life stages should continue for the purposes of detecting trends and determining the contribution of each source to the effects demonstrated.

• Epidemiological and basic laboratory studies should further refine our understanding of the effects of fluoride on the quality and biomechanical properties of bone and on the calcification of soft tissue.

• Studies are needed to define the effects of metabolic and environmental variables on the absorption, excretion, retention, and biological effects of fluoride. Such variables would include the composition of the diet (for example, calcium content), acid-base balance, and the altitude of residence.

9

Uses of Dietary
Reference Intakes

OVERVIEW

In the past, Recommended Dietary Allowances (RDAs) in the U.S. and Recommended Nutrient Intakes (RNIs) in Canada were the only values available to health professionals for planning and assessing diets of individuals and groups and for making judgments about excessive intake. However, the RDAs and RNIs were not ideally suited for many of these purposes (IOM, 1994). The Dietary Reference Intakes (DRIs) developed in this report—Estimated Average Requirements (EARs), RDAs, Adequate Intakes (AIs), and Tolerable Upper Intake Levels (ULs)—are a more complete set of reference values. Each type of DRI has specific uses. The most widespread uses of DRIs—diet assessment and planning—are described in this chapter. EARs, RDAs, AIs, and ULs refer to average *daily* intake over 1 or more weeks.

Three of the DRIs—the EAR, RDA, and AI—were set with reference to a specific criterion of adequacy. The criterion of adequacy may be the same for each gender and life stage group, but sometimes it is not. For example, the criterion of adequate calcium intake is *desirable calcium retention* for most age groups, but *calcium balance* is the criterion for men and women ages 31 through 50 years. Desirable calcium retention, in itself, would not be used to determine adequacy. Instead, it is the presumed relationship between desirable calcium retention and reduced risk of fracture in later life that provides a basis for selection of this indicator. Reduced fracture risk is the functional outcome chosen as the hall-

314

Dietary Reference Intakes (DRIs)*

EAR (Estimated Average Requirement): the intake that meets the estimated nutrient need of 50 percent of the individuals in that group.

RDA (Recommended Dietary Allowance): the intake that meets the nutrient need of almost all (97 to 98 percent) individuals in that group.

AI (Adequate Intake): observed or experimentally derived intake by a defined population or subgroup that, in the judgment of the DRI Committee, appears to sustain a defined nutritional state, such as normal circulating nutrient values, growth, or other functional indicators of health.

UL the highest level of daily nutrient intake that is likely to pose no risk of adverse health effects to almost all individuals in the general population. As intake increases above the UL, the risk of adverse effects increases.

---

*Refers to daily intakes, averaged over time.

---

mark of adequacy for calcium, and its indicator is desirable calcium retention to the extent that retention can be affected by dietary intake. Each nutrient chapter (Chapters 4 through 8) identifies the primary indicator or criterion that defines adequacy for the specific life stage and gender group. (See also Tables S-1 to S-5.)

USING RECOMMENDED DIETARY ALLOWANCES

Nutrient Recommendations for Individuals

The RDA is the value to be used in guiding individuals to achieve adequate nutrient intake. RDAs are given separately for specified life stage groups and by gender if applicable; they are intended to apply to healthy individuals. Due to the large variation in intakes, the RDAs are seldom appropriate for planning diets for or assessing the nutrient intakes of free-living groups (Beaton, 1994).

The RDA for each nutrient is set at a value that should be adequate for 97 to 98 percent of all individuals in a life stage group, given a specified definition of adequacy. The RDA is a target or recommended intake. Nutrient intake that is less than the RDA does not necessarily indicate that the criterion of adequacy has not been met by a given individual.

The RDA is expressed as a single absolute value and not in relation to weight or height. For example, from Chapter 5, the RDA and thus the recommended daily intake of phosphorus for women aged 19 through 30 years is 700 mg (22.6 mmol)/day. This would be the case for a woman in this age range weighing 50 kg (110 lb), 55 kg (121 lb), or 70 kg (154 lb).

One would expect larger individuals to have larger skeletal mass and therefore a greater requirement for calcium, phosphorus, magnesium, vitamin D, and fluoride. However, given the variety of research designs and subject variability used in the studies that provided the data for deriving the DRIs, it would be somewhat misleading to express them per kilogram of body weight or per centimeter of height. This would imply a greater precision in the estimate than is possible, given the available data. Reference weights are provided (Table 1-3) to allow a calculation, when necessary, of the amount per unit of body weight for individuals who are outside the typical range of body size. For some nutrients (for example magnesium), requirements may be closely related to lean tissue; for others, the relationship is weak.

Needs for energy are not necessarily useful for adjusting nutrient needs for this group of nutrients. For example, the RDA for phosphorus would be the same for an 18-year-old long-distance runner whose energy needs were 4,000 kcal/day and an 18-year-old sedentary individual with energy needs of 2,000 kcal/day.

From Chapter 6, the RDA for magnesium is 130 mg (5.4 mmol)/day for healthy boys and girls ages 4 through 8 years. This recommended intake, consumed on a daily basis, on average, would allow essentially all children to achieve the positive magnesium balance needed for normal growth. Because the RDA was based on studies of requirements in children or adolescents with a normal range of body weights for their age, a reference weight and height for the age group are given. It is thus possible to determine the amount of the nutrient per kilogram of body weight that is recommended and to use this value for adjusting the RDA for individuals in the age category whose weights and heights deviate substantially from the reference. This might be done, for example, for small 4-year-old children or for large 8-year-old children.

Assessing the Adequacy of Nutrient Intakes of an Individual

The RDA is of limited use in assessing the adequacy of an individual's nutrient intake. An individual's nutrient requirement is never known with certainty. If the individual's intake, on average, meets or exceeds the RDA, there is good assurance that the intake is adequate for the specified criterion, given current knowledge. When an individual's intake is less than the RDA, the risk of an inadequate intake is present. The risk increases as the intake falls further below the RDA. At 2 standard deviations (SD) below the EAR, it would be nearly certain that the individual's requirements would not be met (NRC, 1986). Neither reported dietary intake nor any other single criterion can be used, by itself, to evaluate the nutritional status of individuals. A usual intake that is well below the RDA may be an indication of the need for further assessment of nutritional status by biochemical tests or clinical examination.

USING ADEQUATE INTAKES

An AI is based on observed or experimentally determined approximations of the average nutrient intake, by a defined population or subgroup, that appears to be sufficient to sustain a defined nutritional state in the specified population. It is emphasized that, in contrast to the EAR, which is an estimate of the requirement that applies to individuals, the AI is usually derived from mean intakes of groups—the group rather than the individual is the unit of observation. The AI is therefore higher than the EAR would be, if it could be determined, since by definition, the EAR is the intake that meets the nutrient need of only 50 percent of the individuals in a group. Because of uncertainties about the relationship of the AI to the actual average requirement, the AI provides an imprecise basis for the assessment of nutrient intakes of population groups. Thus, the applications of the AI must be quite different from those of the EAR. However, healthy individuals with an intake at or above the AI are assumed to have a low risk of intake inadequate for a defined state of nutrition.

USING TOLERABLE UPPER INTAKE LEVELS

The UL is the highest level of daily nutrient intake that is likely to pose no risk of adverse health effects to almost all individuals in the general population. As intake increases above the UL, the risk of adverse effects increases. In most cases it applies to usual intakes from all sources, but in the case of magnesium, it does not apply to intake from food or local water supplies.

Similar to the situation for nutrient requirements, the intake at which a given individual will develop adverse effects as a result of taking high amounts of a nutrient from food and/or nonfood sources cannot be known with certainty. If the individual's intake is below the UL, there is good assurance that the intake will not cause adverse effects, given current knowledge. At intakes above the UL, the risk of adverse effects increases. Although there is no established benefit for healthy individuals associated with consumption of nutrients or food components above the RDA or AI, there is little concern of an increased risk of harmful effects of consumption up to the UL.

Ordinarily, the UL refers to intake from food, fortified food, water, and supplements. Nutrients are often available from a variety of food and nonfood sources. For fluoride, for example, intake from all sources must be considered, including water and dental products. Combined with other sources of fluoride, the over-use of fluoride-containing dental products may place many young children at risk of dental fluorosis.

To avoid exceeding the adult UL for calcium of 2.5 g (62.5 mmol)/day, intake from food, fortified food, and supplements must all be considered. The UL for calcium was determined based in part on studies in which hypercalciuria was related to both dietary and supplemental intakes of calcium. For phosphorus, intakes from both food and supplements are to be considered when comparing intakes with the UL of ~4.0 g (130 mmol)/day for adults. However, for individuals requiring very high energy intakes, phosphorus intake from diet alone may exceed the UL without adverse effects.

To avoid exceeding the UL for vitamin D of 50 µg (2,000 IU)/day, considering intake from all sources is important, but ordinarily only intake from food, fortified food, and nutrient supplements provides notable amounts. (Apart from fatty fish and liver, high concentrations of vitamin D do not occur naturally in commonly eaten foods in the United States and Canada.) Individuals who have high intakes of vitamin D-fortified foods (such as milk and margarine) and of vitamin D supplements (in multivitamin preparations, alone, or in fish oil) should keep the combined average daily intake below the UL of 50 µg (2,000 IU)/day to minimize the risk of developing hypercalcemia.

For many nutrients, such as magnesium, adverse effects associated with high levels of intake from food sources have not been reported. The UL of 350 mg (14.6 mmol)/day was set for magnesium from nonfood, over-the-counter pharmacologic products. This is the intake at which an individual might first experience an adverse effect (diarrhea) from ingestion of a nonfood source of magnesium for at least 1 week. Since the UL for magnesium applies only to nonfood sources, individuals should not be concerned with trying to avoid excessive amounts of magnesium from that occurring naturally in food or water.

USING ESTIMATED AVERAGE REQUIREMENTS

The EAR is particularly useful for evaluating the possible adequacy of nutrient intakes of population groups and for planning intakes of groups. In 1986, the National Research Council (NRC) proposed an approach to calculating the prevalence of inadequate nutrient intakes among a population group, using the mean (or EAR) and SD of the requirement (NRC, 1986). Beaton (1994) has noted that the prevalence of inadequate nutrient intakes can be estimated by the proportion of the population with intakes below the EAR, assuming that the variance of the intakes is greater than the variance of the EAR (which is generally the case). The EAR may also be used in setting a recommended mean intake for a population group, such that only 2 to 3 percent of the population falls below the EAR. These methods are described briefly below. A more detailed explanation of the methodology is given in Beaton (1994) and by the World Health Organization, Food and Agriculture Organization of the United Nations, and International Atomic Energy Agency (WHO/FAO/IAEA) Expert Consultation in *Trace Elements in Human Nutrition and Health* (WHO, 1996). It is anticipated that methods of using the EAR for these purposes will be addressed in a subsequent Food and Nutrition Board report.

Assessing the Adequacy of Nutrient Intake of Groups

An estimate of the prevalence of inadequate intakes of a nutrient by a specific gender or life stage group can be obtained by determining the percentage of the individuals in the group whose usual intakes are less than the EAR (Beaton, 1994) (see Figure 9-1). The estimate is most accurate if the requirements are symmetrically distributed and the SD of intakes is at least twice as large as the SD of requirements. It is also important that the intake data reflect usual intakes; methods have been developed to remove the day-to-day variance in the distributions of intake data (Nusser et al., 1996). This adjustment narrows the distribution and thus gives a better estimate of the proportion of the group with intakes below the EAR. This concept is illustrated in Figure 9-2. Estimates of the prevalence of inadequate intakes also can be affected by biases in the intake data (such as underreporting). (See Chapter 2 for a discussion of the many potential sources of error in self-reported dietary data.)

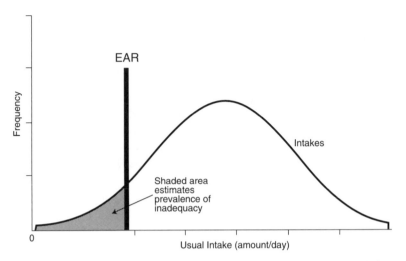

FIGURE 9-1 Prevalence of inadequate intakes in a population group. Adapted from Beaton (1994).

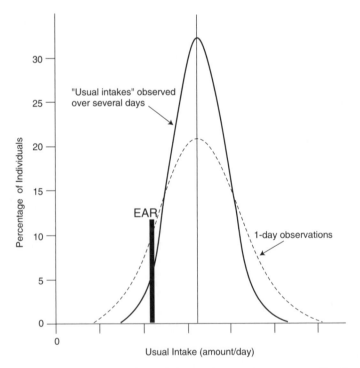

FIGURE 9-2 Effect of multiple days of observation on the apparent distribution of nutrient intake and how it changes the prevalence of inadequacy as estimated by comparison to EAR. Adapted from Hegsted (1972).

TABLE 9-1 Adjusted and Unadjusted Phosphorus Intakes (mg/day) of Young Women and Adolescent Boys in the United States

Category	Mean	SE[b]	Percentile						
			5th	10th	25th	50th	75th	90th	95th
Females 20–29[a]									
(n = 272)									
Unadjusted	1,098	54	342	465	694	1,041	1,376	1,722	2,066
Adjusted	1,097	61	703	780	917	1,080	1,259	1,436	1,551
Males 12–19									
(n = 286)									
Unadjusted	1,619	53	565	745	1,077	1,416	1,932	2,610	3,350
Adjusted	1,612	54	976	1,091	1,300	1,564	1,871	2,194	2,413

[a] Females include pregnant and lactating women.
[b] Standard error of the mean.

SOURCE: One-day unadjusted intake data from the 1994 CSFII, provided by USDA/ARS Food Survey Research Group, 1996. The data have been adjusted using the method developed by Nusser et al. (1996).

Table 9-1 illustrates the importance of adjusting distributions before calculating intake percentiles for groups. The means and seven percentiles of intakes of phosphorus from the 1994 CSFII are shown for teenage boys and for young women, with and without adjustment for usual intake using the Nusser et al. procedure (1996). If unadjusted 1-day intake data are used to estimate the prevalence of inadequate phosphorus intakes for young women, the actual prevalence of usual intakes below an EAR of 580 mg (18.7 mmol)/day will be overestimated. As shown in Table 9-1, between 10 and 25 percent of 1-day intakes fall below 580 mg (18.7 mmol)/day, while less than 5 percent of the adjusted intakes are below the EAR. For teenage boys, less than 10 percent would have inadequate intakes using the adjusted distribution and an EAR of 1,055 mg (34 mmol)/day, while almost 25 percent would have inadequate intakes if only the unadjusted distribution were examined.

The adjustment procedure is also crucial when examining the percentage of the population that is above the UL. Using an unadjusted distribution for adolescent boys, 5 percent of the population would have phosphorus intakes above 3,350 mg (108.1 mmol)/day, a level that is approaching the UL of 4,000 mg (129 mmol)/day. This might be considered unacceptably high unless the adjusted distribution were also examined: the ninety-fifth percentile of usual intakes is just 2,413 mg (77.8 mmol)/day implying that intakes seldom exceed the UL.

When assessing the intake of populations, a number of other questions need to be considered:

• To what extent does the nutrient requirement affect intake? Such a relationship, described by WHO/FAO/IAEA (WHO, 1996), would limit the validity of the probability approach.
• What kinds of adjustments can be made, if any, for biases in the food intake data?
• What factors should be considered in interpreting the findings in different populations?
• What is the allowable level of inadequate intake in a population before concern is raised?

Planning Nutrient Intakes of Groups

The EAR also may be used as a basis for planning or making recommendations for the nutrient intakes of free-living groups. If nutrient intakes are normally distributed, a target intake for a population group can be estimated based on the EAR and the variance of intake. The objective might be to set a value for the mean intake of the group that will ensure that most individuals (usually 97 to 98 percent) meet their nutrient requirement. In order that less than 2 to 3 percent of intakes fall below the EAR, a group's mean intake must be at least two SDs of intake above the EAR. Because the SD usually varies in relation to the magnitude of intake, the coefficient of variation (CV) of intake is used to calculate the target mean intake. The following formula has been derived for this calculation (see Beaton [1994] and WHO [1996] for more details):

Target mean intake for a group = EAR/(1 − [2 × CV of intake])
Where CV = SD of intake/mean intake.

For example, if a group of women in a nursing home had phosphorus intakes with a CV of 0.16, and intakes were normally distributed, achieving a group mean intake of 853 mg (27.5 mmol)/day would ensure that only 2 to 3 percent would have intakes below the EAR of 580 mg (18.7 mmol)/day (580/1-[2 × 0.16]) = 853). If intakes are not normally distributed, other mathematical approaches will be needed.

Another approach would be to implement programs that focus on increasing intakes at the lower end of the distribution, rather than trying to shift the entire distribution of intakes upward. For example, in a nursing home, persons with low phosphorus intakes could be given foods especially high in phosphorus, or meal planning could focus on increasing intakes of phosphorus from many sources. Although it is beyond the scope of this report, an evaluation of the various approaches that could be used to reduce the prevalence of inadequate intakes in population subgroups should be pursued. Such approaches include nutrition education, meal planning, nutrient fortification, and nutrient supplementation. The most efficient and effective strategy would vary from nutrient to nutrient and depend on the distribution of current intakes compared to the EAR.

The use of the EAR in planning intakes for groups is a process that involves a number of key decisions and analysis of questions such as the following:

• Should actual or ideal distributions of populations intakes be used to calculate recommendations for groups? (Actual distributions are seldom normally distributed.)
• What factors should influence the selection of the degree of risk that can be tolerated when planning for groups?
• Should other adjustments be made for factors that would reduce or increase actual intake of the nutrients?

OTHER USES OF DIETARY REFERENCE INTAKES

For many years, the U.S. Recommended Dietary Allowances and the Canadian Recommended Nutrient Intakes have been used by many national and federal agencies for a variety of purposes. For example, they have been considered in setting regulations for feeding programs, setting standards for feeding in group facilities (nursing homes, school cafeterias, correctional facilities), developing recommended intakes for the military, and setting reference values for food labels. They have been used for comparative purposes in many computer programs for nutrient analysis and by dietitians in modifying diets for patients. Guidance for using DRIs for these and many other purposes is beyond the scope of this report, but should be addressed in future reports.

ADDRESSING DISCREPANCIES BETWEEN USUAL INTAKE AND THE AI

Chapter 4 reveals major discrepancies between estimates of usual intakes of calcium and the AI for calcium for some of the life stage groups. For example, mean calcium intake from foods for U.S. females aged 9 years and older is about 650 mg (16.3 mmol)/day, but the AI for calcium ranges from 1,000 to 1,300 mg (25 to 32.5 mmol)/day, depending on the age group. However, this discrepancy does not necessarily mean that dietary intakes are generally inadequate because the relationship between the AI and the distribution of requirements for the nutrient is not known. Nevertheless, for individuals who wish to increase their calcium consumption, there are several possible strategies. These include increasing intake of foods high in calcium, such as low- or nonfat milk products, and increasing consumption of foods fortified with calcium, such as calcium-fortified orange juice or breakfast cereals. For those individuals at high risk, use of calcium supplements may be desirable in order to meet the AI. Identifying the most appropriate strategies to improve nutrient intake should be the focus of a research agenda.

SUMMARY

The correct reference value must be used for its intended purpose, which usually involves either planning for an adequate intake or the assessment of adequacy of intake. It is anticipated that future publications will address the interpretation and appropriate uses of DRIs in more detail in order to assist both the health professional and those interested in nutrition policy and analysis.

References

Abbott L, Nadler J, Rude RK. 1994. Magnesium deficiency in alcoholism: Possible contribution to osteoporosis and cardiovascular disease in alcoholics. *Alcohol Clin Exp Res* 18:1976–1082.

Abe E, Miyaura C, Sakagami H, Takeda M, Konno K, Yamazaki T, Yoshiki S, Suda T. 1981. Differentiation of mouse myeloid leukemia cells induced by 1α25-dihydroxyvitamin D$_3$. *Proc Natl Acad Sci USA* 78:4990–4994.

Abraham GE, Grewal H. 1990. A total dietary program emphasizing magnesium instead of calcium: Effect on the mineral density of calcaneous bone in post-menopausal women on hormonal therapy. *J Reprod Med* 35:503–507.

Abrams SA, Stuff JE. 1994. Calcium metabolism in girls: Current dietary intakes lead to low rates of calcium absorption and retention during puberty. *Am J Clin Nutr* 60:739–743.

Abrams SA, Sidbury JB, Muenzer J, Esteban NV, Vieira NE, Yergey AL. 1991. Stable isotopic measurement of endogenous fecal calcium excretion in children. *J Pediatr Gastroenterol Nutr* 12:469–473.

Abrams SA, Esteban NV, Vieira NE, Sidbury JB, Specker BL, Yergey AL. 1992. Developmental changes in calcium kinetics in children assessed using stable isotopes. *J Bone Miner Res* 7:287–293.

Abrams SA, Silber TJ, Esteban NV, Vieira NE, Stuff JE, Meyers R, Majd M, Yergey AL. 1993. Mineral balance and bone turnover in adolescents with anorexia nervosa. *J Pediatr* 123:326–331.

Abrams SA, O'Brien KO, Stuff JE. 1996a. Changes in calcium kinetics associated with menarche. *J Clin Endocrin Metab* 81:2017–2020.

Abrams SA, O'Brien KO, Wen J, Liang LK, Stuff JE. 1996b. Absorption by 1-year-old children of an iron supplement given with cow's milk or juice. *Pediatr Res* 39:171–175.

Abrams SA, Wen J, Stuff JE. 1997a. Absorption of calcium, zinc and iron from breast milk by 5- to 7-month-old infants. *Pediatr Res* 41:1–7.

Abrams SA, Grusak MA, Stuff J, O'Brien KO. 1997b. Calcium and magnesium balance in 9- to 14-year-old children. *Am J Clin Nutr* 66:1172-1177.

Abreo K, Adlakha A, Kilpatrick S, Flanagan R, Webb R, Shakamuri S. 1993. The Milk-Alkali Syndrome. A reversible form of acute renal failure. *Arch Intern Med* 153:1005–1010.

Ackerman PG, Toro G. 1953. Calcium and phosphorus balance in elderly men. *J Gerontol* 8:298–300.

ADA (American Dental Association Council on Dental Therapeutics). 1994. New fluoride guidelines proposed. *J Am Dent Assoc* 125:366.

Adams JS. 1989. Vitamin D metabolite-mediated hypercalcemia. *Endocrinol Metab Clin North Am* 18:765–778.

Adams JS, Beeker TG, Hongo T, Clemens TL. 1990. Constitutive expression of a vitamin D 1-hydroxylase in a myelomonocytic cell line: A model for studying 1,25-dihydroxyvitamin D production in vitro. *J Bone Miner Res* 5:1265–1269.

Affinito P, Tommaselli GA, DiCarlo C, Guida F, Nappi C. 1996. Changes in bone mineral density and calcium metabolism in breast-feeding women: A one year follow-up study. *J Clin Endocrinol Metab* 81:2314–2318.

Aksnes L, Aarskog D. 1982. Plasma concentrations of vitamin D metabolites in puberty: Effect of sexual maturation and implications for growth. *J Clin Endocrinol Metab* 55:94–101.

Ala-Houhala M. 1985. 25-Hydroxyvitamin D levels during breast-feeding with or without maternal or infantile supplementation of vitamin D. *J Pediatr Gastroenterol Nutr* 4:220–226.

Ala-Houhala M, Parvianinen MT, Pyykko K, Visakorpi JK. 1984. Serum 25-hydroxyvitamin D levels in Finnish children aged 2 to 17 years. *Acta Paediatr Scand* 73:232–236.

Ala-Houhala M, Koskinen T, Terho A, Koivula T, Visakorpi J. 1986. Maternal compared with infant vitamin D supplementation. *Arch Dis Child* 61:1159–1163.

Alaimo K, McDowell MA, Briefel RR, Bischof AM, Caughman CR, Loria CM, Johnson CL. 1994. *Dietary Intake of Vitamins, Minerals, and Fiber of Persons Ages 2 Months and Over in the United States: Third National Health and Nutrition Examination Survey, Phase I, 1988–91.* Advance data from vital and health statistics; no. 258. U.S. Department of Health and Human Services. Hyattsville, MD: National Center for Health Statistics.

Albert DG, Morita Y, Iseri LT. 1958. Serum magnesium and plasma sodium levels in essential vascular hypertension. *Circulation* 17:761–764.

Alderman BW, Weiss NS, Daling JR, Ure CL, Ballard JH. 1986. Reproductive history and postmenopausal risk of hip and forearm fracture. *Am J Epidemiol* 124:262–267.

Alfrey AC, Miller NL, Butkus D. 1974. Evaluation of body magnesium stores. *J Lab Clin Med* 84:153–162.

Allen JC, Keller RP, Archer P, Neville MC. 1991. Studies in human lactation: Milk composition and daily secretion rates of macronutrients in the first year of lactation. *Am J Clin Nutr* 54:69–80.

Allen SH, Shah JH. 1992. Calcinosis and metastatic calcification due to vitamin D intoxication. A case report and review. *Horm Res* 37:68–77.

Allender PS, Cutler JA, Follmann D, Cappuccio FP, Pryer J, Elliott P. 1996. Dietary calcium and blood pressure: A meta-analysis of randomized clinical trials. *Ann Intern Med* 124:825–831.

Aloia JF, Vaswani AN, Yeh JK, Ross P, Ellis K, Cohn SH. 1983. Determinants of bone mass in postmenopausal women. *Arch Intern Med* 143:1700–1704.

Aloia JF, Vaswani AN, Yeh JK, Ellis K, Cohn SH. 1984. Total body phosphorus in postmenospausal women. *Miner Electrolyte Metab* 10:73–76.

Aloia JF, Vaswani A, Yeh JK, Ross PL, Flaster E, Dilmanian FA. 1994. Calcium supplementation with and without hormone replacement therapy to prevent postmenopausal bone loss. *Ann Intern Med* 120:97–103.

Altura BT, Brust M, Bloom S, Barbour RL, Stempak JG, Altura BM. 1990. Magnesium dietary intake modulates blood lipid levels and atherogenesis. *Proc Natl Acad Sci USA* 87:1840–1844.

Altura BT, Shirey TL, Hiti J, Dell'Orfano K, Handwerker SM, Altura BM. 1992. A new method for the rapid determination of ionized Mg^{2+} in whole blood, serum and plasma. *Methods Find Exp Clin Pharmacol* 14:297–304.

Altura BT, Wilimizig C, Trnovec T, Nyulassy S, Altura BM. 1994. Comparative effects of a Mg-enriched diet and different orally administered magnesium oxide preparations on ionized Mg, Mg metabolism and electrolytes in serum of human volunteers. *J Am Coll Nutr* 13:447–454.

American Academy of Pediatrics. 1982. The promotion of breastfeeding: Policy statement based on task force report. *Pediatrics* 69:654–661.

Anderson DM, Hollis BW, LeVine BR, Pittard WB III. 1988. Dietary assessment of maternal vitamin D intake and correlation with maternal and neonatal serum vitamin D concentrations at delivery. *J Perinatol* 8:46–48.

Andon MB, Ilich JZ, Tzagournis MA, Matkovic V. 1996. Magnesium balance in adolescent females consuming a low- or high-calcium diet. *Am J Clin Nutr* 63:950–953.

Angus RM, Sambrook PN, Pockock NA, Eisman JA. 1988. Dietary intake and bone mineral density. *Bone Miner* 4:265–277.

Antman EM. 1996. Magnesium in acute myocardial infarction: Overview of available evidence. *Am Heart J* 132:487–495.

Appel LJ, Moore TJ, Obarzanek E, Vollmer WM, Svetkey LP, Sacks FM, Bray GA, Vogt TM, Cutler JA, Windhauser MM, Lin PH, Karanja N. 1997. A clinical trial of the effects of dietary patterns on blood pressure. *N Engl J Med* 336:1117–1124.

Arnold FA Jr, Dean HT, Jay P, Knutson JW. 1956. Effect of fluoridated public water supplies on dental caries prevalence. Tenth year of the Grand Rapids-Muskegon Study. *Pub Hlth Rep* 71:652–658.

Ascherio A, Rimm EB, Giovannucci EL, Colditz GA, Rosner B, Willett WC, Sacks F, Stampfer MJ. 1992. A prospective study of nutritional factors and hypertension among U.S. men. *Circulation* 86:1475–1484.

Ashe JR, Schofield FA, Gram MR. 1979. The retention of calcium, iron, phosphorus, and magnesium during pregnancy: The adequacy of prenatal diets with and without supplementation. *Am J Clin Nutr* 32:286–291.

Atkinson SA, Chappell JE, Clandinin MT. 1987. Calcium supplementation of mothers' milk for low birthweight infants: Problems related to absorption and excretion. *Nutr Res* 7:813–823.

Atkinson SA, Alston-Mills BP, Lonnerdal B, Neville MC, Thompson MP. 1995. Major minerals and ionic constituents of human and bovine milk. In: Jensen RJ, ed. *Handbook of Milk Composition*. California: Academic Press. Pp. 593–619.

Bainbridge RR, Mimouni FB, Landi T, Crossman M, Harris L, Tsang RC. 1996. Effect of rice cereal feedings on bone mineralization and calcium homeostatis in cow milk formula fed infants. *J Am Coll Nutr* 15:383–388.

Baran D, Sorensen A, Grimes J, Lew R, Karellas A, Johnson B, Roche J. 1990. Dietary modification with dairy products for preventing vertebral bone loss in premenopausal women: A three-year prospective study. *J Clin Endocrinol Metab* 70:264–270.

Bardicef M, Bardicef O, Sorokin Y, Altura BM, Altura BT, Cotton DB, Resnick LM. 1995. Extracellular and intracellular magnesium depletion in pregnancy and gestational diabetes. *Am J Obstet Gynecol* 172:1009–1013.

Barger-Lux MJ, Heaney RP. 1995. Caffeine and the calcium economy revisited. *Osteopor Int* 5:97–102.

Barger-Lux MJ, Heaney RP, Stegman MR. 1990. Effects of moderate caffeine intake on the calcium economy of premenopausal women. *Am J Clin Nutr* 52:722–725.

Barger-Lux MJ, Heaney RP, Lanspa SJ, Healy JC, DeLuca HF. 1995. An investigation of sources of variation in calcium absorption efficiency. *J Clin Endocrinol Metab* 80:406–411.

Barger-Lux MJ, Heaney RP, Dowell S, Bierman J, Holick MF, Chen TC. 1996. Relative molar potency of 25-hydroxyvitamin D indicates a major role in calcium absorption. *J Bone Miner Res* 11:S423.

Barnhart WE, Hiller LK, Leonard GJ, Michaels SE. 1974. Dentifrice usage and ingestion among four age groups. *J Dent Res* 53:1317–1322.

Barragry JM, France MW, Corless D, Gupta SP, Switala S, Boucher BJ, Cohen RD. 1978. Intestinal cholecalciferol absorption in the elderly and in younger adults. *Clin Sci Molec Med* 55:213–220.

Barrett-Connor E, Chang JC, Edelstein SL. 1994. Coffee-associated osteoporosis offset by daily milk consumption. The Rancho Bernardo Study. *J Am Med Assoc* 271:280–283.

Bashir Y, Sneddon JF, Staunton HA, Haywood GA, Simpson IA, McKenna WJ, Camm AJ. 1993. Effects of long-term oral magnesium chloride replacement in congestive heart failure secondary to coronary artery disease. *Am J Cardiol* 72:1156–1162.

Beall DP, Scofield RH. 1995. Milk-alkali syndrome associated with calcium carbonate consumption: Report of 7 patients with parathyroid hormone levels and an estimate of prevalence among patients hospitalized with hypercalcemia. *Medicine* 74:89–96.

Beaton GH. 1994. Criteria of an adequate diet. In: Shils RE, Olson JA, Shike M, eds. *Modern Nutrition in Health and Disease, 8th edition.* Philadelphia: Lea & Febiger. Pp. 1491–1505.

Beaton GH. 1996. Statistical approaches to establish mineral element recommendations. *J Nutr* 126:2302S–2328S.

Begum A, Pereira SM. 1969. Calcium balance studies on children accustomed to low calcium intakes. *Br J Nutr* 23:905–911.

Bell NH, Greene A, Epstein S, Oexmann MJ, Shaw S, Shary J. 1985. Evidence for alteration of the vitamin D-endocrine system in blacks. *J Clin Invest* 76:470–473.

Bell NH, Shary J, Stevens J, Garza M, Gordon L, Edwards J. 1991. Demonstration that bone mass is greater in black than in white children. *J Bone Miner Res* 6:719–723.

Bell NH, Yergey AL, Vieira NE, Oexmann MJ, Shary JR. 1993. Demonstration of a difference in urinary calcium, not calcium absorption, in black and white adolescents. *J Bone Miner Res* 8:1111–1115.

Bell RA, Whitford GM, Barenie JT, Myers DR. 1985. Fluoride retention in children using self-applied topical fluoride products. *Clin Prev Dent* 7:22–27.

Berkelhammer CH, Wood RJ, Sitrin MD. 1988. Acetate and hypercalciuria during total parenteral nutrition. *Am J Clin Nutr* 48:1482–1489.

Bernstein DS, Sadowsky N, Hegsted DM, Guri CD, Stare FJ. 1966. Prevalence of osteoporosis in high- and low-fluoride areas in North Dakota. *J Am Med Assoc* 198:499–504.

Bijvoet, OLM. 1969. Relation of plasma phosphate concentration to renal tubular reabsorption of phosphate. *Clin Sci* 37:23–26.

Bikle DD, Gee E, Halloran B, Haddad JG. 1984. Free 1,25-dihydroxyvitamin D levels in serum from normal subjects, pregnant subjects, and subjects with liver disease. *J Clin Invest* 74:1966–1971.

Birkeland JM, Charlton G. 1976. Effect of pH on the fluoride ion activity of plaque. *Caries Res* 10:72–80.

Bishop NJ, Dahlenburg SL, Fewtrell MS, Morley R, Lucas A. 1996. Early diet of pre-term infants and bone mineralization at age five years. *Acta Paediatr* 85:230–236.

Bizik BK, Ding W, Cerklewski FL. 1996. Evidence that bone resorption of young men is not increased by high dietary phosphorus obtained from milk and cheese. *Nutr Res* 16:1143–1146.

Black DM, Cummings SR, Genant HK, Nevitt MC, Palermo L, Browner W. 1992. Axial and appendicular bone density predict fractures in older women. *J Bone Miner Res* 7:633–638.

Blank S, Scanlon KS, Sinks TH, Lett S, Falk H. 1995. An outbreak of hypervitaminosis D associated with the overfortification of milk from a home-delivery dairy. *Am J Publ Health* 85:656–659.

Blayney JR, Hill IN. 1964. Evanston dental caries study XXIV. Prenatal fluorides—value of waterborne fluorides during pregnancy. *J Am Dent Assoc* 69:291–294.

Bodanszky H, Leleiko N. 1985. Metabolic alkalosis with hypertonic dehydration in a patient with diarrhoea and magnesium oxide ingestion. *Acta Paediatr Hung* 26:241–246.

Bogdonoff MD, Shock NW, Nichols MP. 1953. Calcium, phosphorus, nitrogen, and potassium balance studies in the aged male. *J Gerontol* 8:272–288.

Bostick RM, Potter JD, Fosdick L, Grambsch P, Lampe JW, Wood JR, Louis TA, Ganz R, Grandits G. 1993. Calcium and colorectal epithelial cell proliferation: A preliminary randomized, double-blinded, placebo-controlled clinical trial. *J Natl Cancer Inst* 85:132–141.

Boston JL, Beauchene RE, Cruikshank DP. 1989. Erythrocyte and plasma magnesium during teenage pregnancy: Relationship with blood pressure and pregnancy-induced hypertension. *Obstet Gynecol* 73:169–174.

Bouillon R, Van Assche FA, Van Baelen H, Heyns W, De Moor P. 1981. Influence of the vitamin D-binding protein on the serum concentration of 1,25-dihydroxyvitamin D_3. Significance of the free 1,25-dihydroxyvitamin D_3 concentration. *J Clin Invest* 67:589–596.

Bour NJS, Soullier BA, Zemel MB. 1984. Effect of level and form of phosphorus and level of calcium intake on zinc, iron and copper bioavailability in man. *Nutr Res* 4:371–379.

Bowden GH. 1990. Effects of fluoride on the microbial ecology of dental plaque. *J Dent Res* 69 (Spec Iss):653–659.

Boyle DR, Chagnon M. 1995. An incidence of skeletal fluorosis associated with groundwaters of the maritime carboniferous basin, Gaspe Region, Quebec, Canada. *Environ Geochem Health* 17:5–12.

BPA (British Paediatric Association). 1956. Hypercalcaemia in infants and Vitamin D. *Br Med J* 2:149.

BPA (British Paediatric Association). 1964. Infantile hypercalcaemia, nutritional rickets, and infantile scurvy in Great Britain. *Br Med J* 1:1659–1661.

Brambilla E, Belluomo G, Malerba A, Buscaglia M, Strohmenger L. 1994. Oral administration of fluoride in pregnant women, and the relation between concentration in maternal plasma and in amniotic fluid. *Arch Oral Biol* 39:991–994.

Brandwein SL, Sigman, KM. 1994. Case report: Milk-alkali syndrome and pancreatitis. *Am J Med Sci* 308:173–176.

Brannan PG, Vergne-Marini P, Pak CY, Hull AR, Fordtran JS. 1976. Magnesium absorption in the human small intestine. Results in normal subjects, patients with chronic renal disease, and patients with absorptive hypercalciuria. *J Clin Invest* 57:1412–1418.

Bransby ER, Berry WTC, Taylor DM. 1964. Study of the vitamin-D intakes of infants in 1960. *Br Med J* 1:1661–1663.

Brazier M, Kamel S, Maamer M, Agbomson F, Elesper I, Garabedian M, Desmet G, Sebert JL. 1995. Markers of bone remodeling in the elderly subject: Effects of vitamin D insufficiency and its correction. *J Bone Miner Res* 10:1753–1761.

Brickman AS, Coburn JW, Massry SG. 1974. 1,25 dihydroxy-vitamin D$_3$ in normal man and patients with renal failure. *Ann Intern Med* 80:161–168.

Brink EJ, Beynen AC. 1992. Nutrition and magnesium absorption: A review. *Prog Food Nutr Sci* 16:125–162.

Brodehl J, Gellissen K, Weber H-P. 1982. Postnatal development of tubular phosphate reabsorption. *Clin Nephrol* 17:163–171.

Brown WE, Gregory TM, Chow LC. 1977. Effects of fluoride on enamel solubility and cariostasis. *Caries Res* 11(Suppl 1):118–141.

Brunelle JA, Carlos JP. 1990. Recent trends in dental caries in U.S. children and the effect of water fluoridation. *J Dent Res* 69(Spec Iss):723–727.

Bruun C, Thylstrup A. 1988. Dentifrice usage among Danish children. *J Dent Res* 67:1114–1117.

Bucher HC, Cook RJ, Guyatt GH, Lang JD, Cook DJ, Hatala R, Hunt DL. 1996. Effects of dietary calcium supplementation on blood pressure: A meta-analysis of randomized controlled trials. *J Am Med Assoc* 275:1016–1022.

Bucuvalas JC, Heubi JE, Specker BL, Gregg DJ, Yergey AL, Vieira NE. 1990. Calcium absorption in bone disease associated with chronic cholestasis during childhood. *Hepatology* 12:1200–1205.

Bullamore JR, Wilkinson R, Gallagher JC, Nordin BEC, Marshall DH. 1970. Effects of age on calcium absorption. *Lancet* 2:535–537.

Bullimore DW, Miloszewski KJ. 1987. Raised parathyroid hormone levels in the milk-alkali syndrome: An appropriate response? *Postgrad Med J* 63:789–792.

Burt BA. 1992. The changing patterns of systemic fluoride intake. *J Dent Res* 71:1228–1237.

Burtis WJ, Gay L, Insogna KL, Ellison A, Broadus AE. 1994. Dietary hypercalciuria in patients with calcium oxalate kidney stones. *Am J Clin Nutr* 60:424–429.

Bushe CJ. 1986. Profound hypophosphataemia in patients collapsing after a "fun run." *Br Med J* 292:898–899.

Butte NF, Garza C, Smith EO, Nichols BL. 1984. Human milk intake and growth in exclusively breast-fed infants. *J Pediatr* 104:187–195.

Buzzard IM, Willett WC, eds. 1994. Dietary assessment methods. Proceedings of a conference held in St. Paul, MN. *Am J Clin Nutr* 59:143S–306S.

Byrne J, Thomas MR, Chan GM. 1987. Calcium intake and bone density of lactating women in their late childbearing years. *J Am Diet Assoc* 87:883–887.

Byrne PM, Freaney R, McKenna MJ. 1995. Vitamin D supplementation in the elderly: Review of safety and effectiveness of different regimes. *Calcif Tissue Int* 56:518–520.

Caddell JL, Ratananon N, Trangratapit P. 1973. Parenteral magnesium load tests in postpartum Thai women. *Am J Clin Nutr* 26:612–615.

Caddell JL, Saier FL, Thomason CA. 1975. Parenteral magnesium load tests in postpartum American women. *Am J Clin Nutr* 28:1099–1104.

Calvo MS. 1993. Dietary phosphorus, calcium metabolism and bone. *J Nutr* 123:1627–1633.

Calvo MS, Heath H III. 1988. Acute effects of oral phosphate-salt ingestion on serum phosphorus, serum ionized calcium, and parathyroid hormone in young adults. *Am J Clin Nutr* 47:1025–1029.

Calvo MS, Park YK. 1996. Changing phosphorus content of the U.S. diet: Potential for adverse effects on bone. *J Nutr* 126:1168S–1180S.

Calvo MS, Kumar R, Heath H III. 1988. Elevated secretion and action of serum parathyroid hormone in young adults consuming high phosphorus, low calcium diets assembled from common foods. *J Clin Endocrinol Metab* 66:823–829.

Calvo MS, Kumar R, Heath H. 1990. Persistently elevated parathyroid hormone secretion and action in young women after four weeks of ingesting high phosphorus, low calcium diets. *J Clin Endocrinol Metab* 70:1334–1340.

Campbell SB, MacFarlane DJ, Fleming SJ, Khafagi FA. 1994. Increased skeletal uptake of Tc-99m Methylene Disphosphonate in Milk-Alkali Syndrome. *Clin Nucl Med* 19:207–211.

Canadian Paediatric Society (Nutrition Committee). 1991. Meeting the iron needs of infants and young children: An update. *Can Med Assoc J* 144:1451–1454.

Canadian Paediatric Society. 1996. The use of fluoride in infants and children. *Paediatr Child Health* 1:131–134.

Cappuccio FP, Markandu ND, Beynon GW, Shore AC, Sampson B, MacGregor GA. 1985. Lack of effect of oral magnesium on high blood pressure: A double blind study. *Br Med J Clin Res Ed* 291:235–238.

Carlos JP, Gittelsohn AM, Haddon W Jr. 1962. Caries in deciduous teeth in relation to maternal ingestion of fluoride. *Pub Hlth Rep* 77:658–660.

Carroll MD, Abraham S, Dresser CM. 1983. Dietary intake source data: United States, 1976–1980. Data from the National Health Survey. Vital and Health Statistics series 11, no. 231. DHHS Publ. No. (PHS) 83-1681. Hyattsville, MD: National Center for Health Statistics, Public Health Service, U.S. Department of Health and Human Services.

Chan GM. 1991. Dietary calcium and bone mineral status of children and adolescents. *Am J Dis Child* 145:631–634.

Chan GM, Roberts CC, Folland D, Jackson R. 1982a. Growth and bone mineralization of normal breast-fed infants and the effects of lactation on maternal bone mineral status. *Am J Clin Nutr* 36:438–443.

Chan GM, Slater RN, Hollis J, Thomas MR. 1982b. Decreased bone mineral status in lactating adolescent mothers. *J Pediatr* 101:767–770.

Chan GM, Leeper L, Book LS. 1987. Effects of soy formulas on mineral metabolism in term infants. *Am J Dis Child* 141:527–530.

Chan GM, Hoffman K, McMurry M. 1995. Effects of dairy products on bone and body composition in pubertal girls. *J Pediatr* 126:551–556.

Chan JT, Koh SH. 1996. Fluoride content in caffeinated, decaffeinated and herbal teas. *Caries Res* 30:88–92.

Chan JT, Qui CC, Whitford GM, Weatherred JG. 1990. Influence of coffee on fluoride metabolism in rats. *Proc Soc Exp Biol Med* 194:43–47.

Chandra RK. 1984. Physical growth of exclusively breast-fed infants. *Nutr Res* 2:275–276.

Chapuy MC, Arlot ME, Duboeuf F, Brun J, Crouzet B, Arnaud S, Delmas PD, Meunier PJ. 1992. Vitamin D_3 and calcium to prevent hip fractures in elderly women. *N Engl J Med* 327:1637–1642.

Charles P, Jensen FT, Mosekilde L, Hansen HH. 1983. Calcium metabolism evaluated by ^{47}Ca kinetics: Estimation of dermal calcium loss. *Clin Sci* 65:415–422.

Chen TC, Castillo L, Korycka-Dahl M, DeLuca HF. 1974. Role of vitamin D metabolites in phosphate transport of rat intestine. *J Nutr* 104:1056–1060.

Chen TC, Shao A, Heath H III, Holick MF. 1993. An update on the vitamin D content of fortified milk from the United States and Canada. *N Engl J Med* 329:1507.

Chen X, Whitford GM. 1994. Lack of significant effect of coffee and caffeine on fluoride metabolism in rats. *J Dent Res* 73:1173–1179.

Chesney RW. 1990. Requirements and upper limits of vitamin D intake in the term neonate, infant, and older child. *J Pediatr* 116:159–166.

Chevalley T, Rizzoli R, Nydegger V, Slosman D, Rapin CH, Michel JP, Vasey H, Bonjour JP. 1994. Effects of calcium supplements on femoral bone mineral density and vertebral fracture rate in vitamin D-replete elderly patients. *Osteopor Int* 4:245–252.

Chinn HI. 1981. Effects of dietary factors on skeletal integrity in adults: Calcium, phosphorus, vitamin D, and protein. Prepared for Bureau of Foods, Food and Drug Administration, U.S. Department of Health and Human Services, Washington, D.C.

Cholak J. 1959. Fluorides: A critical review. I. The occurrence of fluoride in air, food and water. *J Occup Med* 1:501–511.

Chow LC. 1990. Tooth-bound fluoride and dental caries. *J Dent Res* 69(Spec Iss):595–600.

Clark DC, Hann HJ, Williamson MF, Berkowitz J. 1993. Aesthetic concerns of children and parents in relation to different classifications of the Tooth Surface Index of Fluorosis. *Community Dent Oral Epidemiol* 21:360–364.

Clarkson EM, Warren RL, McDonald SJ, de Wardener HE. 1967. The effect of a high intake of calcium on magnesium metabolism in normal subjects and patients with chronic renal failure. *Clin Sci* 32:11–18.

Clarkson PM, Haymes EM. 1995. Exercise and mineral status of athletes: Calcium, magnesium, phosphorus, and iron. *Med Sci Sports Exerc* 27:831–843.

Clemens TL, Adams JS. 1996. Vitamin D metabolites. In: Favus MJ, Christakos S, eds. *Primer on the Metabolic Bone Diseases and Disorders of Mineral Metabolism, 3rd edition*. Philadelphia, PA: Lippincott-Raven. Pp. 109–114.

Clemens TL, Adams JS, Henderson SL, Holick MF. 1982. Increased skin pigment reduces the capacity of skin to synthesise vitamin D_3. *Lancet* 1:74–76.

Clemens TL, Zhou X, Myles M, Endres D, Lindsay R. 1986. Serum vitamin D_2 and vitamin D_3 metabolite concentrations and absorption of vitamin D_2 in elderly subjects. *J Clin Endocrinol Metab* 63:656–660.

Cleveland LE, Goldman JD, Borrud LG. 1996. *Data Tables: Results from USDA's 1994 Continuing Survey of Food Intakes by Individuals and 1994 Diet and Health Knowledge Survey*. Beltsville, MD: Agricultural Research Service, U.S. Department of Agriculture.

Clovis J, Hargreaves JA. 1988. Fluoride intake from beverage consumption. *Community Dent Oral Epidemiol* 16:11–15.

CNPP, USDA (Center for Nutrition Policy and Promotion, U.S. Department of Agriculture). 1996. Nutrient Content of the U.S. Food Supply, 1990–1994. Preliminary Data. Washington, DC: U.S. Department of Agriculture.

Cockburn F, Belton NR, Purvis RJ, Giles MM, Brown JK, Turner TL, Wilkinson EM, Forfar JO, Barrie WJM, McKay GS, Pocock SJ. 1980. Maternal vitamin D intake and mineral metabolism in mothers and their newborn infants. *Br Med J* 281:11–14.

Coffin B, Azpiroz F, Guarner F, Malagelada JR. 1994. Selective gastric hypersensitivity and reflex hyporeactivity in functional dyspepsia. *Gastroenterology* 107:1345–1351.

Cohen L. 1988. Recent data on magnesium and osteoporosis. *Magnes Res* 1:85–87.

Cohen L, Laor A. 1990. Correlation between bone magnesium concentration and magnesium retention in the intravenous magnesium load test. *Magnes Res* 3:271–274.

Cohn SH, Abesamis C, Yasumura S, Aloia JF, Zanzi I, Ellis KJ. 1977. Comparative skeletal mass and radial bone mineral content in black and white women. *Metabolism* 26:171–178.

Colston K, Colston MJ, Feldman D. 1981. 1,25-dihydroxyvitamin D_3 and malignant melanoma: The presence of receptors and inhibition of cell growth in culture. *Endocrinol* 108:1083–1086.

COMA (Committee on Medical Aspects of Food Policy). 1991. *Dietary Reference Values for Food Energy and Nutrients for the United Kingdom. Report on Health and Social Subjects, No. 41.* London: HMSO.

Comstock GW. 1979. Water hardness and cardiovascular diseases. *Am J Epidemiol* 110:375–400.

Conradt A, Weidinger H, Algayer H. 1984. On the role of magnesium in fetal hypotrophy, pregnancy induced hypertension and pre-eclampsia. *Magnes Bull* 2:68–76.

Cooper C, Melton LJ III. 1992. Epidemiology of osteoporosis. *Trends Endocrinol Metab* 3:224–229.

Cooper C, Campion G, Melton LJ III. 1992. Hip fractures in the elderly: A worldwide projection. *Osteopor Int* 2:285–289.

Costello RB, Moser-Veillon PB, DiBianco R. 1997. Magnesium supplementation in patients with congestive heart failure. *J Am Coll Nutr* 16:22–31.

Cowell DC, Taylor WH. 1981. Ionic fluoride: A study of its physiological variation in man. *Ann Clin Biochem* 18:76–83.

Craig JM. 1959. Observations on the kidney after phosphate loading in the rat. *Arch Pathol* 68:306–315.

Cramer CF. 1961. Progress and rate of absorption of radiophosphorus through the intestinal tract of rats. *Can J Biochem Physiol* 39:499–503.

Cremer HD, Buttner W. 1970. *Absorption of Fluorides. Fluoride and Human Health.* Geneva, Switzerland: World Health Organization.

Cross NA, Hillman LS, Allen SH, Krause GF, Vieira NE. 1995a. Calcium homeostasis and bone metabolism during pregnancy, lactation, and postweaning: A longitudinal study. *Am J Clin Nutr* 61:514–523.

Cross NA, Hillman LS, Allen SH, Krasue GF. 1995b. Changes in bone mineral density and markers of bone remodeling during lactation and postweaning in women consuming high amounts of calcium. *J Bone Miner Res* 10:1312–1320.

Cumming RG, Cummings SR, Nevitt MC, Scott J, Ensrud KE, Vogt TM, Fox K. 1997. Calcium intake and fracture risk: Results from the study of osteoporotic fractures. *Am J Epidemiol* 145:926–934.

Cummings SR, Black DM, Nevitt MC, Browner W, Cauley J, Ensrud K, Genant HK, Palermo L, Scott J, Vogt TM. 1993. Bone density at various sites for prediction of hip fractures. The Study of Osteoporotic Fractures Research Group. *Lancet* 341:72–75.

Cummings SR, Nevitt MC, Browner WS, Stone K, Fox KM, Ensrud KE, Cauley J, Black D, Vogt TM. 1995. Risk factors for hip fracture in white women: Study of Osteoporotic Fractures Research Group. *N Engl J Med* 332:767–773.

Cunningham AS, Mazess RB. 1983. Bone mineral loss in lactating adolescents. *J Pediatr* 101:338–339.

Curhan GC, Willett WC, Rimm EB, Stampfer MJ. 1993. A prospective study of dietary calcium and other nutrients and the risk of symptomatic kidney stones. *N Engl J Med* 328:833–838.

334   DIETARY REFERENCE INTAKES

Curhan GC, Willett WC, Speizer FE, Spiegelman D, Stampfer MJ. 1997. Comparison of dietary calcium with supplemental calcium and other nutrients as factors affecting the risk for kidney stones in women. *Ann Intern Med* 126:497–504.

Dabeka RW, McKenzie AD, Conacher HBS, Kirkpatrick DC. 1982. Determination of fluoride in Canadian infant foods and calculation of fluoride intakes by infants. *Can J Pub Hlth* 73:188–191.

Dabeka RW, McKenzie AD, Lecroix GM. 1987. Dietary intakes of lead, cadmium, arsenic and fluoride by Canadian adults: A 24-hour duplicate diet study. *Food Addit Contam* 4:89–101.

Dale G, Fleetwood JA, Inkster JS, Sainsbury JR. 1986. Profound hypophosphataemia in patients collapsing after a "fun run." *Br Med J (Clin Res)* 292:447–448.

Dalton MA, Sargent JD, O'Connor GT, Olmstead EM, Klein RZ. 1997. Calcium and phosphorus supplementation of iron-fortified infant formula: No effect on iron status of healthy full-term infants. *Am J Clin Nutr* 65:921–926.

Davies M, Adams PH. 1978. The continuing risk of vitamin D intoxication. *Lancet* 2(8090):621–623.

Davies M, Lawson DEM, Emberson C, Barnes JLC, Roberts GE, Barnes ND. 1982. Vitamin D from skin: Contribution to vitamin D status compared with oral vitamin D in normal and anti-convulsant-treated subjects. *Clin Sci* 63:461–472.

Davies M, Hayes ME, Yin JA, Berry JL, Mawer EB. 1994. Abnormal synthesis of 1,25-dihydroxyvitamin D in patients with malignant lymphoma. *J Clin Endocrinol Metab* 78:1202–1207.

Davis RH, Morgan DB, Rivlin RS. 1970. The excretion of calcium in the urine and its relation to calcium intake, sex and age. *Clin Sci* 39:1–12.

Dawes C. 1989. Fluorides: Mechanisms of action and recommendations for use. *J Can Dent Assoc* 55:721–723.

Dawson-Hughes B. 1996. Calcium. In: Marcus R, Feldman D, Kelsey J, eds. *Osteoporosis*. Orlando, FL: Academic Press, Inc. Pp. 1103, 1105.

Dawson-Hughes B, Stern DT, Shipp CC, Rasmussen HM. 1988. Effect of lowering dietary calcium intake on fractional whole body calcium retention. *J Clin Endocrinol Metab* 67:62–68.

Dawson-Hughes B, Dallal GE, Krall EA, Sadowski L, Sahyoun N, Tannenbaum S. 1990. A controlled trial of the effect of calcium supplementation on bone density in postmenopausal women. *N Engl J Med* 323:878–883.

Dawson-Hughes B, Dallal GE, Krall EA, Harris S, Sokoll LJ, Falconer G. 1991. Effect of vitamin D supplementation on wintertime and overall bone loss in healthy postmenopausal women. *Ann Intern Med* 115:505–512.

Dawson-Hughes B, Harris S, Kramich C, Dallal G, Rasmussen HM. 1993. Calcium retention and hormone levels in black and white women on high- and low-calcium diets. *J Bone Miner Res* 8:779–787.

Dawson-Hughes B, Harris SS, Krall EA, Dallal GE, Falconer G, Green CL. 1995. Rates of bone loss in postmenopausal women randomly assigned to one of two dosages of vitamin D. *Am J Clin Nutr* 61:1140–1145.

Dawson-Hughes B, Fowler SE, Dalsky G, Gallagher C. 1996. Sodium excretion influences calcium homeostasis in elderly men and women. *J Nutr* 126:2107–2112.

Dawson-Hughes B, Harris SS, Krall EA, Dallal GE. 1997. Calcium and vitamin D supplementation on bone density in men and women 65 years of age or older. *N Engl J Med* 337:670–676.

Dean HT. 1942. The investigation of physiological effects by the epidemiological method. In: Moulton FR, ed. *Fluorine and Dental Health*. Washington, DC: American Association for the Advancement of Science. Pp. 23–31.

Dean HT, Elvove E. 1937. Further studies on the minimal threshold of chronic endemic dental fluorosis. *Pub Hlth Rep* 52:1249–1264.

Delmas PD. 1992. Clinical use of biochemical markers of bone remodeling in osteoporosis. *Bone* 13:S17–S21.

Delmi M, Rapin CH, Bengoa JM, Delmas PD, Vasey H, Bonjour JP. 1990. Dietary supplementation in elderly patients with fractured neck of the femur. *Lancet* 335:1013–1016.

DeLuca HF. 1984. The metabolism, physiology, and function of vitamin D. In: Kumar R, ed. *Vitamin D: Basic and Clinical Aspects.* Boston: M. Nijhoff Publishers.

DeLuca HF. 1988. The vitamin D story: A collaborative effort of basic science and clinical medicine. *FASEB J* 2:224–236.

Delvin EE, Salle BL, Glorieux FH, Adeleine P, David LS. 1986. Vitamin D supplementation during pregnancy: Effect on neonatal calcium homeostasis. *J Pediatr* 109:328–334.

Demay MB. 1995. Hereditary defects in vitamin D metabolism and vitamin D receptor defects. In: DeGroot LJ, Besser M, Burger HG, Jameson JL, Loriaux DL, Marshall JC, O'Dell WD, Potts JT, Rubenstein AH, eds. *Endocrinology, Vol 2, Third edition.* Philadelphia, PA: WB Saunders. Pp. 1173–1178.

Demirjian A. 1980. *Anthropometry Report. Height, Weight, and Body Dimensions: A Report from Nutrition Canada.* Ottawa: Minister of National Health and Welfare, Health and Promotion Directorate, Health Services and Promotion Branch.

Dengel JL, Mangels AR, Moser-Veillon PB. 1994. Magnesium homeostasis: Conservation mechanism in lactating women consuming a controlled-magnesium diet. *Am J Clin Nutr* 59:990–994.

Deurenberg P, Pieters JJ, Hautvast JG. 1990. The assessment of the body fat percentage by skinfold thickness measurements in childhood and young adolescence. *Br J Nutr* 63:293–303.

Deuster PA, Singh A. 1993. Responses of plasma magnesium and other cations to fluid replacement during exercise. *J Am Coll Nutr* 12:286–293.

Devine A, Criddle RA, Dick IM, Kerr DA, Prince RL. 1995. A longitudinal study of the effect of sodium and calcium intakes on regional bone density in postmenopausal women. *Am J Clin Nutr* 62:740–745.

DeVizia B, Mansi A. 1992. Calcium and phosphorus metabolism in full-term infants. *Monatsschr Kinderheilkd* 140:S8–S12.

DeVizia B, Fomon SJ, Nelson SE, Edwards BE, Zeigler EE. 1985. Effect of dietary calcium on metabolic balance of normal infants. *Pediatr Res* 19:800–806.

Dewey KG, Finley DA, Lonnerdal B. 1984. Breast milk volume and composition during late lactation (7–20 months). *J Pediatr Gastroenterol Nutr* 3:713–720.

DHHS (Department of Health and Human Services). 1988. *The Surgeon General's Report on Nutrition and Health.* Washington, DC: US Department of Health and Human Services, Public Health Service.

DHHS (Department of Health and Human Services). 1990. *Healthy People 2000: National Health Promotion and Disease Prevention Objectives.* DHHS Publ. No. (PHS) 91-50212. Washington, DC: US Government Printing Office. Pp. 466–467.

Diem K. 1970. *Documenta Geigy.* Ardsley, NY: Geigy Pharmaceuticals.

Dobnig H, Kainer F, Stepan V, Winter R, Lipp R, Schaffer M, Kahr A, Nocnik S, Patterer G, Leb G. 1995. Elevated parathyroid hormone-related peptide levels after human gestation: Relationship to changes in bone and mineral metabolism. *J Clin Endocrinol Metab* 80:3699–3707.

Dorsch TR. 1986. The milk-alkali syndrome, vitamin D, and parathyroid hormone. *Ann Intern Med* 105:800–801.

Dorup I, Clausen T. 1993. Correlation between magnesium and potassium contents in muscle: Role of Na(+)-K+ pump. *Am J Physiol* 264:C457–C463.

Dourson ML, Stara JF. 1983. Regulatory history and experimental support of uncertainty (safety) factors. *Regul Toxicol Pharmacol* 3:224–238.

Dowell TB. 1981. The use of toothpaste in infancy. *Br Dent J* 150:247–249.

Drinkwater BL, Chesnut CH III. 1991. Bone density changes during pregnancy and lactation in active women: A longitudinal study. *Bone Miner* 14:153–160.

Drinkwater B, Bruemner B, Chesnut C. 1990. Menstrual history as a determinant of current bone density in young athletes. *J Am Med Assoc* 263:545–548.

Dwyer JT, Dietz WH, Hass G, Suskind R. 1979. Risk of nutritional rickets among vegetarian children. *Am J Dis Child* 133:134–140.

Dyckner T, Wester PO. 1983. Effect of magnesium on blood pressure. *Br Med J (Clin Res)* 286:1847–1849.

Dyckner T, Wester PO. 1985. Skeletal muscle magnesium and potassium determinations: Correlation with lymphocyte contents of magnesium and potassium. *J Am Coll Nutr* 4:619–625.

Ebeling PR, Yergey AL, Vieira NE, Burritt MF, O'Fallon WM, Kumar R, Riggs BL. 1994. Influence of age on effects on endogenous 1,25-dihydroxy-vitamin D on calcium absorption in normal women. *Calcif Tissue Int* 55:330–334.

Eble DM, Deaton TG, Wilson FC, Bawden JW. 1992. Fluoride concentrations in human and rat bone. *J Pub Hlth Dent* 52:288–291.

Egsmose C, Lund B, McNair P, Lund B, Storm T, Sorensen OH. 1987. Low serum levels of 25-hydroxyvitamin D and 1,25-dihydroxyvitamin D in institutionalized old people: Influence of solar exposure and vitamin D supplementation. *Age Ageing* 16:35–40.

Eisman JA, Suva LJ, Sher E, Pearce PJ, Funder JW, Martin TJ. 1981. Frequency of 1,25-dihydroxyvitamin D_3 receptor in human breast cancer. *Cancer Res* 41:5121–5124.

Ekstrand J, Ehrnebo M. 1979. Influence of milk products on fluoride bioavailability in man. *Eur J Clin Pharmacol* 16:211–215.

Ekstrand J, Ehrnebo M. 1980. Absorption of fluoride from fluoride dentifrices. *Caries Res* 14:96–102.

Ekstrand J, Boreus LO, de Chateau P. 1981. No evidence of transfer of fluoride from plasma to breast milk. *Br Med J* 283:761–762.

Ekstrand J, Spak CJ, Falch J, Afseth J, Ulvestad H. 1984. Distribution of fluoride to human breast milk following intake of high doses of fluoride. *Caries Res* 18:93–95.

Ekstrand J, Fomon SJ, Ziegler EE, Nelson SE. 1994a. Fluoride pharmacokinetics in infancy. *Pediatr Res* 35:157–163.

Ekstrand J, Ziegler EE, Nelson SE, Fomon SJ. 1994b. Absorption and retention of dietary and supplemental fluoride by infants. *Adv Dent Res* 8:175–180.

Elders PJ, Netelenbos JC, Lips P, van Ginkel FC, Khoe E, Leeuwenkamp OR, Hackeng WH, van der Stelt PF. 1991. Calcium supplementation reduces vertebral bone loss in perimenopausal women: A controlled trial in 248 women between 46 and 55 years of age. *J Clin Endocrinol Metab* 73:533–540.

Elders PJ, Lips P, Netelenbos JC, van Ginkel FC, Khoe E, van der Vijgh WJ, van der Stelt PF. 1994. Long-term effect of calcium supplementation on bone loss in perimenopausal women. *J Bone Miner Res* 9:963–970.

Elia M. 1992. Energy expenditure and the whole body. In: Kinney JM, Tucker HN, eds. *Energy Metabolism: Tissue Determinants and Cellular Corollaries.* New York: Raven Press Ltd. Pp. 19–59.

Elin RJ. 1987. Assessment of magnesium status. *Clin Chem* 33:1965–1970.

Elin RJ, Hosseini JM. 1985. Magnesium content of mononuclear blood cells. *Clin Chem* 31:377–380.

Ellis KJ, Shypailo RJ, Hergenroeder A, Perez M, Abrams S. 1996. Total body calcium and bone mineral content: Comparison of dual-energy X-ray absorptiometry (DXA) with neutron activation analysis (NAA). *J Bone Miner Res* 11:843–848.

Ellis KJ, Abrams SA, Wong WW. 1997. Body composition of a young, multiethnic female population. *Am J Clin Nutr* 65:724–731.

EPA (U. S. Environmental Protection Agency). 1986. Guidelines for Carcinogen Risk Assessment. *Federal Register* 51(185):33992–34003.

EPA (U. S. Environmental Protection Agency). 1996. Proposed Guidelines for Carcinogen Risk Assessment; Notice. *Federal Register* 61(79):17960–18011.

Esala S, Vuori E, Helle A. 1982. Effect of maternal fluorine intake on breast milk fluorine content. *Br J Nutr* 48:201–204.

Esvelt RP, DeLuca HF. 1981. Calcitroic acid: Biological activity and tissue distribution studies. *Arch Biochem Biophys* 206:403–413.

European Community. 1993. *Nutrient and Energy Intakes for the European Community.* Reports of the Scientific Committee for Food, Thirty-first Series.

Evans RW. 1989. Changes in dental fluorosis following an adjustment to the fluoride concentration of Hong Kong's water supplies. *Adv Dent Res* 3:154–160.

Evans RW, Darvell BW. 1995. Refining the estimate of the critical period for susceptibility to enamel fluorosis in human maxillary central incisors. *J Pub Hlth Dent* 55:238–249.

Fairweather-Tait S, Prentice A, Heumann KG, Landing MAJ, Stirling DM, Wharf SG, Turnlund JR. 1995. Effect of calcium supplements and stage of lactation on the calcium absorption efficiency of lactating women accustomed to low calcium intakes. *Am J Clin Nutr* 62:1188–1192.

FAO/WHO (Food and Agriculture Organization of the United Nations/World Health Organization). 1982. *Evaluation of Certain Food Additives and Contaminants.* Twenty-sixth report of the Joint FAO/WHO Expert Committee on Food Additives (WHO Technical Report Series No. 683).

FAO/WHO (Food and Agriculture Organization of the United Nations/World Health Organization, Expert Consultation). 1995. *The Application of Risk Analysis to Food Standard Issues.* Recommendations to the Codex Alimentarius Commission (ALINORM 95/9, Appendix 5).

FAO/WHO/UNA (Food and Agriculture Organization of the United Nations/ World Health Organization/United Nations). 1985. *Energy and Protein Requirements.* Report of a joint FAO/WHO/UNA Consultation Technical Report Series. No. 724. Geneva, Switzerland: World Health Organization.

Fardellone P, Sebert JL, Garabedian M, Bellony R, Maamer M, Agbomson F, Brazier M. 1995. Prevalence and biological consequences of vitamin D deficiency in elderly institutionalized subjects. *Rev Rhum* 62:576–581.

Farmer ME, White LR, Brody JA, Bailey KR. 1984. Race and sex differences in hip fracture incidence. *Am J Publ Health* 74:1374–1380.

Fatemi S, Ryzen E, Flores J, Endres DB, Rude RK. 1991. Effect of experimental human magnesium depletion on parathyroid hormone secretion and 1,25-dihydroxyvitamin D metabolism. *J Clin Endocrinol Metab* 73:1067–1072.

Faulkner KG, Cummings SR, Black D, Palermo L, Gluer CC, Genant HK. 1993. Simple measurement of femoral geometry predicts hip fracture: The study of osteoporotic fractures. *J Bone Miner Res* 8:1211–1217.

Favus MJ, Christakos S. 1996. *Primer on the Metabolic Bone Diseases and Disorders of Mineral Metabolism, 3rd Edition.* Philadelphia, PA: Lippincott-Raven.

Featherstone JDB, Shields CP. 1988. *A Study of Fluoride in New York State Residents.* Final report to New York State Department of Health.

Fehily AM, Coles RJ, Evans WD, Elwood PC. 1992. Factors affecting bone density in young adults. *Am J Clin Nutr* 56:579–586.

Fejerskov O, Thylstrup A, Larsen MJ. 1977. Clinical and structural features and possible pathogenic mechanisms of dental fluorosis. *Scand J Dent Res* 85:510–534.

Feldblum PJ, Zhang J, Rich LE, Fortney JA, Talmage RV. 1992. Lactation history and bone mineral density among perimenopausal women. *Epidemiology* 3:527–531.

Feliciano ES, Ho ML, Specker BL, Falciglia G, Shui QM, Yin TA, Chen XC. 1994. Seasonal and geographical variations in the growth rate of infants in China receiving increasing dosages of vitamin D supplements. *J Trop Pediatr* 40:162–165.

Feltman R, Kosel G. 1961. Prenatal and postnatal ingestion of fluorides—fourteen years of investigation. Final report. *J Dent Med* 16:190–198.

Fieser LF, Fieser M. 1959. Vitamin D. In: *Steroids.* New York: Reinhold. Pp. 90–168.

Filippo FA, Battistone GC. 1971. The fluoride content of a representative diet of the young adult male. *Clin Chim Acta* 31:453–457.

Fine KD, Santa Ana CA, Porter JL, Fordtran JS. 1991a. Intestinal absorption of magnesium from food and supplements. *J Clin Invest* 88:396–402.

Fine KD, Santa Ana CA, Fordtran JS. 1991b. Diagnosis of magnesium-induced diarrhea. *N Engl J Med* 324:1012–1017.

Fink RI, Kolterman OG, Griffin J, Olefsky JM. 1983. Mechanisms of insulin resistance in aging. *J Clin Invest* 71:1523–1535.

Fitzgerald MG, Fourman P. 1956. An experimental study of magnesium deficiency in man. *Clin Sci* 15:635.

Fomon SJ, Nelson SE. 1993. Calcium, phosphorus, magnesium, and sulfur. In: Fomon SJ, ed. *Nutrition of Normal Infants.* St. Louis: Mosby-Year Book, Inc. Pp. 192–216.

Fomon SJ, Younoszai MK, Thomas LN. 1966. Influence of vitamin D on linear growth of normal full-term infants. *J Nutr* 88:345–50.

Fomon SJ, Haschke F, Ziegler EE, Nelson SE. 1982. Body composition of reference children from birth to age 10 years. *Am J Clin Nutr* 35:1169–1175.

Franz KB. 1987. Magnesium intake during pregnancy. *Magnesium* 6:18–27.

Franz KB. 1989. Influence of phosphorus on intestinal absorption of calcium and magnesium. In: Itokawa Y, Durlach J, eds. *Magnesium in Health and Disease.* London: John Libbey & Co. Pp. 71–78.

Fraser DR. 1980. Regulation of the metabolism of vitamin D. *Physiol Rev* 60:551–613.

Fraser DR. 1983. The physiological economy of vitamin D. *Lancet* 1:969–972.

Freiman I, Pettifor JM, Moodley GM. 1982. Serum phosphorus in protein energy malnutrition. *J Pediatr Gastroenterol Nutr* 1:547–550.

French JK, Koldaway IM, Williams LC. 1986. Milk-alkali syndrome following over-the-counter antacid self-medication. *N Zeal Med J* 99:322–323.

Freudenheim JL, Johnson NE, Smith EL. 1986. Relationships between usual nutrient intake and bone-mineral content of women 35–65 years of age: Longitudinal and cross-sectional analysis. *Am J Clin Nutr* 44:863–876.

Freyberg RH. 1942. Treatment of arthritis with vitamin and endocrine preparations. *J Am Med Assoc* 119:1165–1171.

Frithz G, Wictorin B, Ronquist G. 1991. Calcium-induced constipation in a prepubescent boy. *Acta Paediatr Scand* 80:964–965.

Frost HM. 1973. The origin and nature of transients in human bone remodeling dynamics. In: Frame B, Parfitt AM, Duncan H, eds. *Clinical Aspects of Metabolic Bone Disease.* Amsterdam: Excerpta Medica Series. Pp. 124–137.

Frost HM. 1987. The mechanostat: A proposed pathogenic mechanism of osteoporosis and the bone mass effects of mechanical and nonmechanical agents. *Bone Miner* 2:73–85.

Frost HM. 1997. Why do marathon runners have less bone than weight lifters? A vital-biomechanical view and explanation. *Bone* 20:183–189.

Gadallah M, Massry SG, Bigazzi R, Horst RL, Eggena P, Campese VM. 1991. Intestinal absorption of calcium and calcium metabolism in patients with essential hypertension and normal renal function. *Am J Hypertens* 4:404–409.

Galla JH, Booker BB, Luke RG. 1986. Role of the loop segment in the urinary concentrating defect of hypercalcemia. *Kidney Int* 29:977–982.

Gallagher JC, Riggs BL, DeLuca HF. 1980. Effect of estrogen on calcium absorption and serum vitamin D metabolites in postmenopausal osteoporosis. *J Clin Endocrinol Metab* 51:1359–1364.

Gallagher JC, Goldgar D, Moy A. 1987. Total bone calcium in women: Effect of age and menopause status. *J Bone Miner Res* 2:491–496.

Garby L, Lammert O. 1984. Within-subjects between-days-and-weeks variation in energy expenditure at rest. *Human Nutr Clin Nutr* 38:395–397.

Garfinkel L, Garfinkel D. 1985. Magnesium regulation of the glycolytic pathway and the enzymes involved. *Magnesium* 4:60–72.

Garland C, Shekelle RB, Barrett-Connor E, Criqui MH, Rossof AH, Paul O. 1985. Dietary vitamin D and calcium and risk of colorectal cancer: A 19-year prospective study in men. *Lancet* 1:307–309.

Garland FC, Garland CF, Gorham ED, Young JF. 1990. Geographic variation in breast cancer mortality in the United States: A hypothesis involving exposure to solar radiation. *Prev Med* 19:614–622.

Garn SM. 1972. The course of bone gain and the phases of bone loss. *Orthop Clin North Am* 3:503–520.

Gartside PS, Glueck CJ. 1995. The important role of modifiable dietary and behavioral characteristics in the causation and prevention of coronary heart disease hospitalization and mortality: The prospective NHANES I follow-up study. *J Am Coll Nutr* 14:71–79.

Gedalia I, Brzezinski A, Portuguese N, Bercovici B. 1964. The fluoride content of teeth and bones of human foetuses. *Arch Oral Biol* 9:331–340.

Geleijnse JM, Witteman JC, Bak AA, den Breeijen JH, Grobbee DE. 1994. Reduction in blood pressure with a low sodium, high potassium, high magnesium salt in older subjects with mild to moderate hypertension. *Br Med J* 309:436–440.

German Society of Nutrition. 1991. *Recommendations on Nutrient Intake.* Abstract and Tables of the 157 Pages Booklet, 5th revised edition. Frankfurt: Druckerei Henrich.

Gershoff SN, Legg MA, Hegsted DM. 1958. Adaptation to different calcium intakes in dogs. *J Nutr* 64:303–312.

Gertner JM, Coustan DR, Kliger AS, Mallette LE, Ravin N, Broadus AE. 1986. Pregnancy as state of physiologic absorptive hypercalciuria. *Am J Med* 81:451–456.

Gillman MW, Hood MY, Moore LL, Nguyen US, Singer MR, Andon MB. 1995. Effect of calcium supplementation on blood pressure in children. *J Pediatr* 127:186–192.

Gilsanz V, Roe TF, Mora S, Costin G, Goodman WG. 1991. Changes in vertebral bone density in black girls and white girls during childhood and puberty. *N Engl J Med* 325:1597–1600.

Glaser K, Parmelee AH, Hoffman WS. 1949. Comparative efficacy of vitamin D preparations in prophylactic treatment of premature infants. *Am J Dis Child* 77:1–14.

Glass RL, Peterson JK, Zuckerberg DA, Naylor MN. 1975. Fluoride ingestion resulting from the use of a monofluorophosphate dentifrice by children. *Br Dent J* 138:423–426.

Glenn FB. 1981. The rationale for the administration of a NaF tablet supplement during pregnancy and postnatally in a private practice setting. *J Dent Child* 48:118–122.

Glenn FB, Glenn WD III, Duncan RC. 1984. Prenatal fluoride tablet supplementation and the fluoride content of teeth: Part VII. *J Dent Child* 51:344–351.

Gloth FM III, Gundberg CM, Hollis BW, Haddad JG Jr, Tobin JD. 1995. Vitamin D deficiency in homebound elderly persons. *J Am Med Assoc* 274:1683–1686.

Goeree R, O'Brien B, Pettitt D, Cuddy L, Ferraz M, Adachi J. 1996. An assessment of the burden of illness due to osteoporosis in Canada. *J SOGC*:15S–24S.

Golden BE, Golden MH. 1981. Plasma zinc, rate of weight gain, and the energy cost of tissue deposition in children recovering from severe malnutrition on a cow's milk or soya protein-based diet. *Am J Clin Nutr* 34:892–899.

Goldfarb S. 1994. Diet and nephrolithiasis. *Ann Rev Med* 45:235–243.

Goldring SR, Krane SM, Avioli LV. 1995. Disorders of calcification: Osteomalacia and rickets. In: DeGroot LJ, ed. *Endocrinology, Vol 2, Third Edition*. Philadelphia: WB Saunders. Pp. 1204–1227.

Golzarian J, Scott HW Jr, Richards WO. 1994. Hypermagnesemia-induced paralytic ileus. *Dig Dis Sci* 39:1138–1142.

Gora ML, Seth SK, Bay WH, Visconti JA. 1989. Milk-alkali syndrome associated with use of chlorothiazide and calcium carbonate. *Clin Pharm* 8:227–229.

Goren S, Silverstein LJ, Gonzales N. 1993. A survey of food service managers of Washington State boarding homes for the elderly. *J Nutr Elderly* 12:27–42.

Graham S. 1959. Idiopathic hypercalcemia. *Postgraduate Med* 25:67–72.

Gray TK, Lester GE, Lorenc RS. 1979. Evidence for extra-renal 1-hydroxylation of 25-hydroxyvitamin D_3 in pregnancy. *Science* 204:1311–1313.

Greer FR. 1989. Calcium, phosphorus, and magnesium: How much is too much for infant formulas? *J Nutr* 119:1846–1851.

Greer FR, Garn SM. 1982. Loss of bone mineral content in lactating adolescents. *J Pediatr* 101:718–719.

Greer FR, Searcy JE, Levin RS, Steichen JJ, Steichen-Asche PS, Tsang RC. 1982a. Bone mineral content and serum 25-hydroxyvitamin D concentrations in breast-fed infants with and without supplemental vitamin D: One-year follow-up. *J Pediatr* 100:919–922.

Greer FR, Tsang RC, Levin RS, Searcy JE, Wu R, Steichen JJ. 1982b. Increasing serum calcium and magnesium concentrations in breast-fed infants: Longitudinal studies of minerals in human milk and in sera of nursing mothers and their infants. *J Pediatr* 100:59–64.

Greer FR, Steichen JJ, Tsang RC. 1982c. Effects of increased calcium, phosphorus, and vitamin D intake on bone mineralization in very low-birth-weight infants fed formulas with polycose and medium-chain triglycerides. *J Pediatr* 100:951–955.

Greer FR, Lane J, Ho M. 1984. Elevated serum parathyroid hormone, calcitonin, and 1,25-dihydroxyvitamin D in lactating women nursing twins. *Am J Clin Nutr* 40:562–568.

Greger JL, Baier MJ. 1983. Effect of dietary aluminum on mineral metabolism of adult males. *Am J Clin Nutr* 38:411–419.

Greger JL, Baligar P, Abernathy RP, Bennett OA, Peterson T. 1978. Calcium, magnesium, phosphorus, copper, and manganese balance in adolescent females. *Am J Clin Nutr* 31:117–121.

Greger JL, Huffman J, Abernathy RP, Bennett OA, Resnick SE. 1979. Phosphorus and magnesium balance of adolescent females fed two levels of zinc. *J Food Sci* 44:1765–1767.

Greger JL, Smith SA, Snedeker SM. 1981. Effect of dietary calcium and phosphorus levels on the utilization of calcium, phosphorus, magnesium, manganese, and selenium by adult males. *Nutr Res* 1:315–325.

Grill V, Martin TJ. 1993. Non-parathyroid hypercalcaemias. In: Nordin BEC, Need AG, Morris HA, eds. *Metabolic Bone and Stone Disease.* Edinburgh: Churchill Livingstone. Pp. 133–145.

Grimston SK, Morrison K, Harder JA, Hanley DA. 1992. Bone mineral density during puberty in Western Canadian children. *Bone Miner* 19:85–96.

Groeneveld A, Van Eck AA, Backer-Dirks O. 1990. Fluoride in caries prevention: Is the effect pre- or post-eruptive? *J Dent Res* 69(Spec Iss):751–755.

Gullestad L, Dolva LO, Waage A, Falch D, Fagerthun H, Kjekshus J. 1992. Magnesium deficiency diagnosed by an intravenous loading test. *Scan J Clin Lab Invest* 52:245–253.

Gullestad L, Nes M, Ronneberg R, Midtvedt K, Falch D, Kjekshsu J. 1994. Magnesium status in healthy free-living elderly Norwegians. *J Am Coll Nutr* 13:45–50.

Gultekin A, Ozalp I, Hasanoglu A, Unal A. 1987. Serum-25-hydroxycholecalciferol levels in children and adolescents. *Turk J Pediatr* 29:155–162.

Gunther T. 1993. Mechanisms and regulation of Mg2+ efflux and Mg2+ influx. *Miner Electrolyte Metab* 19:259–265.

Guy WS. 1979. Inorganic and organic fluorine in human blood. In: Johansen E, Taves DR, Olsen TO, eds. *Continuing Evaluation of the Use of Fluorides.* AAAS Selected Symposium. Boulder, CO: Westview Press.

Haddad JG, Jr. 1980. Competitive protein-binding radioassays for 25-OH-D; clinical applications. In: Norman, ed. *Vitamin D, vol. 2.* New York: Marcel Dekker, Inc., P. 587.

Haddad JG, Hahn TJ. 1973. Natural and synthetic sources of circulating 25-hydroxyvitamin D in man. *Nature* 244:515–517.

Hakim R, Tolis G, Goltzman D, Meltzer S, Friedman R. 1979. Severe hypercalcemia associated with hydrochlorothiazide and calcium carbonate therapy. *Can Med Assoc J* 21:591–594.

Halioua L, Anderson JJ. 1989. Lifetime calcium intake and physical activity habits: Independent and combined effects on the radial bone of healthy premenopausal Caucasian women. *Am J Clin Nutr* 49:534–541.

Hallberg L, Rossander-Hulten L, Brune M, Gleerup A. 1992. Calcium and iron absorption: Mechanism of action and nutritional importance. *Eur J Clin Nutr* 46:317–327.

Hallfrisch J, Muller DC. 1993. Does diet provide adequate amounts of calcium, iron, magnesium, and zinc in a well-educated adult population? *Exper Gerontol* 28:473–483.

Hamilton IR. 1990. Biochemical effects of fluoride on oral bacteria. *J Dent Res* 69(Spec Iss):660–667.

Hammer DI, Heyden S. 1980. Water hardness and cardiovascular mortality. *J Am Med Assoc* 243:2399–2400.

Hamuro Y, Shino A, Suzuoki Z. 1970. Acute induction of soft tissue calcification with transient hyperphosphatemia in the KK mouse by modification in dietary contents of calcium, phosphorus, and magnesium. *J Nutr* 100:404–412.

Handwerker SM, Altura BT, Altura BM. 1996. Serum ionized magnesium and other electrolytes in the antenatal period of human pregnancy. *J Am Coll Nutr* 15:36–43.

Hardwick LL, Jones MR, Brautbar N, Lee DB. 1991. Magnesium absorption: Mechanisms and the influence of vitamin D, calcium and phosphate. *J Nutr* 121:13–23.

Hargreaves JA. 1972. Fluoride content of deciduous tooth enamel from three different regions (Abstract). *J Dent Res* 51:274.

Hargreaves JA. 1992. The level and timing of systemic exposure to fluoride with respect to caries resistance. *J Dent Res* 71:1244–1248.

Hargreaves JA, Ingram GS, Wagg BJ. 1970. An extended excretion study on the ingestion of a monofluorophosphate toothpaste by children. *Acta Med Sci Hung* 27:413–419.

Hargreaves JA, Ingram FF, Wagg BJ. 1972. A gravimetric based study of the ingestion of toothpaste by children. *Caries Res* 6:237–243.

Hargreaves JA, Thompson GW, Pimlott JFL, Norbert LD. 1988. Commencement date of fluoride supplementation related to dental caries. *J Dent Res* 67:230.

Harris SS, Dawson-Hughes B. 1994. Caffeine and bone loss in healthy postmenopausal women. *Am J Clin Nutr* 60:573–578.

Hart M, Windle J, McHale M, Grissom R. 1982. Milk-alkali syndrome and hypercalcemia: A case report. *Nebr Med J* 67:128–130.

Hasling C, Charles P, Jensen FT, Mosekilde L. 1990. Calcium metabolism in postmenopausal osteoporosis: The influence of dietary calcium and net absorbed calcium. *J Bone Miner Res* 5:939–946.

Hayslip CC, Klein TA, Wray HL, Duncan WE. 1989. The effects of lactation on bone mineral content in healthy postpartum women. *Obstet Gynecol* 73:588–592.

Health Canada. 1990. *Nutrition Recommendations. The Report of the Scientific Review Committee 1990*. Ottawa: Canadian Government Publishing Centre.

Health Canada. 1993. *Health Risk Determination—The Challenge of Health Protection*. Health Canada, Health Protection Branch. Ottawa: Health Canada.

Heaney RP. 1993. Protein intake and the calcium economy. *J Am Diet Assoc* 93:1259–1260.

Heaney RP. 1997. Vitamin D: Role in the calcium economy. In: Feldman D, Glorieux FH, Pike JW, eds. *Vitamin D*. San Diego, CA: Academic Press. Pp. 485–497.

Heaney RP, Recker RR. 1982. Effects of nitrogen, phosphorus, and caffeine on calcium balance in women. *J Lab Clin Med* 99:46–55.

Heaney RP, Recker RR. 1987. Calcium supplements: Anion effects. *Bone Miner* 2:433–439.

Heaney RP, Recker RR. 1994. Determinants of endogenous fecal calcium in healthy women. *J Bone Miner Res* 9:1621–1627.

Heaney RP, Skillman TG. 1964. Secretion and excretion of calcium by the human gastrointestinal tract. *J Lab Clin Med* 64:29–41.

Heaney RP, Skillman TG. 1971. Calcium metabolism in normal human pregnancy. *J Clin Endocrinol* 33:661–670.

Heaney RP, Saville PD, Recker RR. 1975. Calcium absorption as a function of calcium intake. *J Lab Clin Med* 85:881–890.

Heaney RP, Recker RR, Saville PD. 1977. Calcium balance and calcium requirements in middle-aged women. *Am J Clin Nutr* 30:1603–1611.

Heaney RP, Recker RR, Saville PD. 1978. Menopausal changes in calcium balance performance. *J Lab Clin Med* 92:953–963.

Heaney RP, Recker RR, Hinders SM. 1988. Variability of calcium absorption. *Am J Clin Nutr* 47:262–264.

Heaney RP, Recker RR, Stegman MR, Moy AJ. 1989. Calcium absorption in women: Relationships to calcium intake, estrogen status, and age. *J Bone Miner Res* 4:469–475.

Heaney RP, Recker RR, Weaver CM. 1990a. Absorbability of calcium sources: The limited role of solubility. *Calcif Tissue Int* 46:300–304.

Heaney RP, Weaver CM, Fitzsimmons ML. 1990b. Influence of calcium load on absorption fraction. *J Bone Miner Res* 5:1135–1138.

Heaney RP, Weaver CM, Fitzsimmons ML. 1991. Soybean phytate content: Effect on calcium absorption. *Am J Clin Nutr* 53:745–747.

Heaton FW. 1969. The kidney and magnesium homeostasis. *Ann NY Acad Sci* 162:775–785.

Hegsted DM. 1972. Problems in the use and interpretation of the Recommended Dietary Allowances. *Ecol Food Nutr* 1:255–265.

Heinig MJ, Nommsen LA, Peerson JM, Lonnderal B, Dewey KG. 1993. Energy and protein intakes of breast-fed and formula-fed infants during the first year of life and their association with growth velocity: The DARLING study. *Am J Clin Nutr* 58:152–161.

Hemmingsen C, Staun M, Olgaard K. 1994. Effects of magnesium on renal and intestinal calbindin-D. *Miner Electrolyte Metab* 20:265–273.

Herman-Giddens ME, Slora EJ, Wasserman RC, Bourdony CJ, Bhapkar MV, Koch GG, Hasemeier CM. 1997. Secondary sexual characteristics and menses in young girls seen in office practice: A study from the Pediatric Research in Office Settings Network. *Pediatrics* 99:505–512.

Hill AB. 1971. *Principles of Medical Statistics, 9th Ed.* New York: Oxford University Press.

Hillman LS. 1990. Mineral and vitamin D adequacy in infants fed human milk or formula between 6 and 12 months of age. *J Pediatr* 117:S134–S142.

Hillman L, Sateesha S, Haussler M, Wiest W, Slatopolsky E, Haddad J. 1981. Control of mineral homeostasis during lactation: Interrelationships of 25-hydroxyvitamin D, 24,25-dihydroxyvitamin D, 1,25-dihydroxyvitamin D, parathyroid hormone, calcitonin, prolactin, and estradiol. *Am J Obstet Gynecol* 139:471–476.

Hillman LS, Chow W, Salmons SJ, Weaver E, Erickson M, Hansen J. 1988. Vitamin D metabolism, mineral homeostasis and bone mineralization in term infants fed human milk, cow milk-based formula or soy-based formula. *J Pediatr* 112:864–874.

Hodge HC, Smith FA. 1977. Occupational fluoride exposure. *J Occup Med* 19:12–39.

Hodge HC. 1979. The safety of fluoride tablets or drops. In: Johansen E, Taves DR, Olson, TO, eds. *Continuing Evaluation of the Use of Fluorides, AAAS Selected Symposium 1.* Boulder, CO: Westview Press. Pp. 253–274.

Hodgson E, Mailman RB, Chamber JE. 1988. *Dictionary of Toxicology.* New York: Van Nostrand Reinhold, Inc.

Hoffman S, Grisso JA, Kelsey JL, Gammon MD, O'Brien LA. 1993. Parity, lactation and hip fracture. *Osteopor Int* 3:171–176.

Hofvander Y, Hagman U, Hillervik C, Sjolin S. 1982. The amount of milk consumed by 1–3 months old breast- or bottle-fed infants. *Acta Pediatr Scand* 71:953–958.

Holbrook TL, Barrett-Connor E, Wingard DL. 1988. Dietary calcium and risk of hip fracture: 14-year prospective population study. *Lancet* 2:1046–1049.

Holick MF. 1986. Vitamin D requirements for the elderly. *Clin Nutr* 5:121–129.

Holick MF. 1994. McCollum Award Lecture, 1994: Vitamin D: New horizons for the 21st century. *Am J Clin Nutr* 60:619–630.

Holick MF. 1995. Vitamin D: Photobiology, metabolism, and clinical applications. In: DeGroot LJ, Besser M, Burger HG, Jameson JL, Loriaux DL, Marshall JC, O'Dell WD, Potts JL, Rubenstein AH, eds. *Endocrinology, 3rd Edition*. Philadelphia, PA: WB Saunders.

Holick MF. 1996. Vitamin D: Photobiology, metabolism, mechanism of action, and clinical application. In: Favus MJ, ed. *Primer on the Metabolic Bone Diseases and Disorders of Mineral Metabolism, 3rd Edition*. Philadelphia, PA: Lippincott-Raven. Pp. 74–81.

Holick MF, Clark MB. 1978. The photobiogenesis and metabolism of vitamin D. *Fed Proc* 37:2567–2574.

Holick MF, Schnoes HK, DeLuca HF. 1971. Identification of 1,25-dihydroxychole-calciferol, a form of vitamin D_3 metabolically active in the intestine. *Proc Natl Acad Sci USA* 68:803–804.

Holick MF, Uskokovic M, Henley JW, MacLaughlin J, Holick SA, Potts JT Jr. 1980. The photoproduction of 1α, 25-dihydroxyvitamin D_3 in skin: An approach to the therapy of vitamin-D-resistant syndromes. *N Engl J Med* 303:349–354.

Holick MF, MacLaughlin JA, Doppelt SH. 1981. Regulation of cutaneous previta-min D_3 photosynthesis in man: Skin pigment is not an essential regulator. *Science* 211:590–593.

Holick MF, Matsuoka LY, Wortsman J. 1989. Age, vitamin D, and solar ultraviolet. *Lancet* 2:1104–1105.

Holick MF, Shao Q, Liu WW, Chen TC. 1992. The vitamin D content of fortified milk and infant formula. *N Engl J Med* 326:1178–1181.

Hollifield JW. 1987. Magnesium depletion, diuretics, and arrythmias. *Am J Med* 82(Suppl 3A):30–37.

Hollis BW. 1996. Assessment of vitamin D nutritional and hormonal status: What to measure and how to do it. *Calcif Tissue Int* 58:4–5.

Holmes RP, Kummerow FA. 1983. The relationship of adequate and excessive intake of vitamin D to health and disease. *J Am Coll Nutr* 2:173–199.

Honkanen R, Alhava E, Parviainen M, Talasniemi S, Monkkonen R. 1990. The necessity and safety of calcium and vitamin D in the elderly. *J Am Geriatr Soc* 38:862–866.

Hordon LD, Peacock M. 1987. Vitamin D metabolism in women with femoral neck fracture. *Bone Miner* 2:413–426.

Horowitz HS. 1990. The future of water fluoridation and other systemic fluorides. *J Dent Res* 69(Spec Iss):760–764.

Horowitz HS. 1996. The effectiveness of community water fluoridation in the United States. *J Pub Hlth Dent* 56:253–258.

Horowitz HS, Heifetz SB. 1967. Effects of prenatal exposure to fluoridation on dental caries. *Pub Hlth Rep* 82:297–304.

Horowitz M, Wishart J, Mundy L, Nordin BEC. 1987. Lactose and calcium absorp-tion in postmenopausal osteoporosis. *Arch Intern Med* 147:534–536.

Hoskova M. 1968. Fluoride tablets in the prevention of tooth decay. *Cesk Pediatr* 23:438–441.

Howard JE, Hopkins TR, Connor TB. 1953. On certain physiologic responses to intravenous injection of calcium salts into normal, hyperparathyroid and hy-poparathyroid persons. *J Clin Endocrinol Metab* 13:1–19.

Hreshchyshyn MM, Hopkins A, Zylstra S, Anbar M. 1988. Associations of parity, breast-feeding, and birth control pills with lumbar spine and femoral neck bone densities. *Am J Obstet Gynecol* 159:318–322.

Hua H, Gonzales J, Rude RK. 1995. Magnesium transport induced ex vivo by a pharmacological dose of insulin is impaired in non-insulin-dependent diabetes mellitus. *Magnes Res* 8:359–366.

Huang Z, Himes JH, McGovern PG. 1996. Nutrition and subsequent hip fracture risk among a national cohort of white women. *Am J Epidemiol* 144:124–134.

Hunt CD, Nielsen FH. 1981. Interaction between boron and cholecalciferol in the chick. In: McC Howell J, Gawthorne JM, White CL, eds. *Trace Element Metabolism in Man and Animals, TEMA-4*. Canberra: Australian Academy of Science. Pp. 597–600.

Hunt MS, Schofield FA. 1969. Magnesium balance and protein intake level in adult human female. *Am J Clin Nutr* 22:367–373.

Hwang DL, Yen CF, Nadler JL. 1993. Insulin increases intracellular magnesium transport in human platelets. *J Clin Endocrinol Metab* 76:549–553.

IOM (Institute of Medicine). 1990. *Nutrition During Pregnancy*. Report of the Subcommittee on Nutritional Status and Weight Gain During Pregnancy, Subcommittee on Dietary Intake and Nutrient Supplements During Pregnancy, Committee on Nutritional Status During Pregnancy and Lactation, Food and Nutrition Board. Washington, DC: National Academy Press.

IOM (Institute of Medicine). 1991. *Nutrition During Lactation*. Report of the Subcommittee on Nutrition During Lactation, Committee on Nutritional Status During Pregnancy and Lactation, Food and Nutrition Board. Washington, DC: National Academy Press.

IOM (Institute of Medicine). 1994. *How Should the Recommended Dietary Allowances Be Revised?* Food and Nutrition Board. Washington, DC: National Academy Press.

Ireland P, Fordtran JS. 1973. Effect of dietary calcium and age on jejunal calcium absorption in humans studied by intestinal perfusion. *J Clin Invest* 52:2672–2681.

Irnell L. 1969. Metastatic calcification of soft tissue on overdose of vitamin D. *Acta Med Scand* 185:147–152.

Iseri LT, French JH. 1984. Magnesium: Nature's physiologic calcium blocker. *Am Heart J* 108:188–193.

ISIS-4 (Fourth International Study of Infarct Survival) Collaborative Group. 1995. ISIS-4: A randomised factorial trial assessing early oral captopril, oral mononitrate, and intravenous magnesium sulphate in 58,050 patients with suspected acute myocardial infarction. *Lancet* 345:669–685.

Ismail AI, Brodeur JM, Kavanagh M, Boisclair G, Tessier C, Picotte L. 1990. Prevalence of dental caries and dental fluorosis in students, 11–17 years of age, in fluoridated and non-fluoridated cities in Quebec. *Caries Res* 24:290–297.

Jackman LA, Millane SS, Martin BR, Wood OB, McCabe GP, Peacock M, Weaver CM. 1997. Calcium retention in relation to calcium intake and postmenarcheal age in adolescent females. *Am J Clin Nutr* 66:327–333.

Jackson D, Murray JJ, Fairpo CG. 1973. Life-long benefits of fluoride in drinking water. *Br Dent J* 134:419–422.

Jacobus CH, Holick MF, Shao Q, Chen TC, Holm IA, Kolodny JM, Fuleihan GE, Seely EW. 1992. Hypervitaminosis D associated with drinking milk. *N Engl J Med* 326:1173–1177.

Janas LM, Picone TA, Benson JD, MacLean WC. 1988. Influence of dietary calcium to phosphorus and parathormone during the first two weeks of life. *Pediatr Res* 23:485A.

Janelle KC, Barr SI. 1995. Nutrient intakes and eating behavior scores of vegetarian and nonvegetarian women. *J Am Diet Assoc* 95:180–186.

Jeans PC. 1950. Vitamin D. *J Am Med Assoc* 143:177–181.

Jeans PC, Stearns G. 1938. The effect of vitamin D on linear growth in infancy. II. The effect of intakes above 1,800 USP units daily. *J Pediatr* 13:730–740.

Joffres MR, Reed DM, Yano K. 1987. Relationship of magnesium intake and other dietary factors to blood pressure: The Honolulu heart study. *Am J Clin Nutr* 45:469–475.

Johansson C, Mellström D, Milsom I. 1993. Reproductive factors as predictors of bone density and fractures in women at the age of 70. *Maturitas* 17:39–50.

Johnson AO, Semenya JG, Buchowski MS, Enwonwu CO, Scrimshaw NS. 1993a. Correlation of lactose maldigestion, lactose intolerance, and milk intolerance. *Am J Clin Nutr* 57:399–401.

Johnson AO, Semenya JG, Buchowski MS, Enwonwu CO, Scrimshaw NS. 1993b. Adaptation of lactose maldigesters to continued milk intakes. *Am J Clin Nutr* 58:879–881.

Johnson CM, Wilson DM, O'Fallon WM, Malek RS, Kurland LT. 1979. Renal stone epidemiology: A 25-year study in Rochester, Minn. *Kidney Int* 16:624–631.

Johnson J Jr, Bawden JW. 1987. The fluoride content of infant formulas available in 1985. *Pediatr Dent* 9:33–37.

Johnson KR, Jobber J, Stonawski BJ. 1980. Prophylactic vitamin D in the elderly. *Age Ageing* 9:121–127.

Johnston CC, Miller JZ, Slemenda CW, Reister TK, Hui S, Christian JC, Peacock M. 1992. Calcium supplementation and increases in bone mineral density in children. *N Engl J Med* 327:82–87.

Jones JE, Manalo R, Flink EB. 1967. Magnesium requirements in adults. *Am J Clin Nutr* 20:632–635.

Jowsey J, Balasubramaniam P. 1972. Effect of phosphate supplements on soft tissue calcification and bone turnover. *Clin Sci* 42:289–299.

Junor JR, Catto GRD. 1976. Renal biopsy in the milk-alkali syndrome. *J Clin Path* 29:1074–1076.

Kailis DG, Taylor SR, Davis GB, Bartlett LG, Fitzgerald DJ, Grose IJ, Newton PD. 1968. Fluoride and caries: Observations of the effects of prenatal and postnatal fluoride on some Perth pre-school children. *Med J Austral* 2:1037–1040.

Kalkwarf HJ, Specker BL. 1995. Bone mineral loss during lactation and recovery after weaning. *Obstet Gynecol* 86:26–32.

Kalkwarf HJ, Specker BL, Heubi JE, Vieira NE, Yergey AL. 1996. Intestinal calcium absorption of women during lactation and after weaning. *Am J Clin Nutr* 63:526–531.

Kalkwarf HJ, Specker BL, Bianchi DC, Ranz J, Ho M. 1997. The effect of calcium supplementation on bone density during lactation and after weaning. *N Engl J Med* 337:523–528.

Kallmeyer JC, Funston MR. 1983. The milk-alkali syndrome: A case report. *S Afr Med J* 64:287–288.

Kamel S, Brazier M, Picard C, Boitte F, Samson L, Desmet G, Sebert JL. 1994. Urinary excretion of pyridinolines crosslinks measured by immunoassay and HPLC techniques in normal subjects and in elderly patients with vitamin D deficiency. *Bone Miner* 26:197–208.

Kamel S, Brazier M, Rogez JC, Vincent O, Maamer M, Desmet G, Sebert JL. 1996. Different responses of free and peptide-bound cross-links to vitamin D and calcium supplementation in elderly women with vitamin D insufficiency. *J Clin Endocrinol Metab* 81:3717–3721.

Kaminsky LS, Mahoney MC, Leach J, Melius J, Miller MJ. 1990. Fluoride: Benefits and risks of exposure. *Crit Rev Oral Biol Med* 1:261–281.

Kanapka JA, Hamilton IR. 1971. Fluoride inhibition of enolase activity in vivo and its relationship to the inhibition of glucose-6-P formation in *Streptococcus salivarius*. *Arch Biochem Biophys* 146:167–174.

Kanemitsu T, Koike A, Yamamoto S. 1985. Study of the cell proliferation kinetics in ulcerative colitis, adenomatous polyps, and cancer. *Cancer* 56:1094–1098.

Kanis JA, Melton LJ III, Christiansen C, Johnston CC, Khaltaev N. 1994. The diagnosis of osteoporosis. *J Bone Miner Res* 9:1137–1141.

Kapsner P, Langsdorf L, Marcus R, Kraemer FB, Hoffman AR. 1986. Milk-alkali syndrome in patients treated with calcium carbonate after cardiac transplantation. *Arch Intern Med* 146:1965–1968.

Katzman DK, Bachrach LK, Carter DR, Marcus R. 1991. Clinical and anthropometric correlates of bone mineral acquisition in healthy adolescent girls. *J Clin Endocrinol Metab* 73:1332–1339.

Kayne LH, Lee DB. 1993. Intestinal magnesium absorption. *Miner Electrolyte Metab* 19:210–217.

Keddie KMG. 1987. Case report: Severe depressive illness in the context of hypervitaminosis D. *Br J Psych* 150:394–396.

Kellie SE, Brody JA. 1990. Sex-specific and race-specific hip fracture rates. *Am J Pub Hlth* 80:326–328.

Kelsay JL, Prather ES. 1983. Mineral balances of human subjects consuming spinach in a low-fiber diet and in a diet containing fruits and vegetables. *Am J Clin Nutr* 38:12–19.

Kelsay JL, Behall KM, Prather ES. 1979. Effect of fiber from fruits and vegetables on metabolic responses of human subjects. II. Calcium, magnesium, iron, and silicon balances. *Am J Clin Nutr* 32:1876–1880.

Kent GN, Price RI, Gutteridge DH, Smith M, Allen JR, Bhagat CI, Barnes MP, Hickling CJ, Retallack RW, Wilson SG, Devlin RD, Davies C, St. John A. 1990. Human lactation: Forearm trabecular bone loss, increased bone turnover, and renal conservation of calcium and inorganic phosphate with recovery of bone mass following weaning. *J Bone Miner Res* 5:361–369.

Kent GN, Price RI, Gutteridge DH, Rosman KJ, Smith M, Allen JR, Hickling CJ, Blakeman SL. 1991. The efficiency of intestinal calcium absorption is increased in late pregnancy but not in established lactation. *Calcif Tissue Int* 48:293–295.

Kesteloot H, Joossens JV. 1990. The relationship between dietary intake and urinary excretion of sodium, potassium, calcium and magnesium: Belgian Interuniversity Research on Nutrition and Health. *J Hum Hypertension* 4:527–533.

Kiel DP, Felson DT, Hannan MT, Anderson JJ, Wilson PW. 1990. Caffeine and the risk of hip fracture: The Framingham Study. *Am J Epidemiol* 132:675–684.

Kinyamu HK, Gallagher JC, Balhorn KE, Petranick KM, Rafferty KA. 1997. Serum vitamin D metabolites and calcium absorption in normal young and elderly free-living women and in women living in nursing homes. *Am J Clin Nutr* 65:790–797.

Klaassen CD, Amdur MO, Doull J. 1986. *Casarett and Doull's Toxicology: The Basic Science of Poisons, Third Edition.* New York: Macmillan Publishing Company.

Kleerekoper M, Mendlovic DB. 1993. Sodium fluoride therapy of postmenopausal osteoporosis. *Endocrinol Rev* 14:312–323.

Kleibeuker JH, Welberg JW, Mulder NH, van der Meer R, Cats A, Limburg AJ, Kreumer WM, Hardonk MJ, de Vries EG. 1993. Epithelial cell proliferation in the sigmoid colon of patients with adenomatous polyps increases during oral calcium supplementation. *Br J Cancer* 67:500–503.

Klein CJ, Moser-Veillon PB, Douglass LW, Ruben KA, Trocki O. 1995. A longitudinal study of urinary calcium, magnesium, and zinc excretion in lactating and nonlactating postpartum women. *Am J Clin Nutr* 61:779–786.

Kleiner SM, Bazzarre TL, Ainsworth BE. 1994. Nutritional status of nationally ranked elite bodybuilders. *Int J Sport Nutr* 4:54–69.

Kleinman GE, Rodriquez H, Good MC, Caudle MR. 1991. Hypercalcemic crisis in pregnancy associated with excessive ingestion of calcium carbonate antacid (milk-alkali syndrome): Successful treatment with hemodialysis. *Obstet Gynecol* 73:496–499.

Knochel JP. 1977. The pathophysiology and clinical characteristics of severe hypophosphatemia. *Arch Intern Med* 137:203–220.

Knochel JP. 1985. The clinical status of hypophosphatemia: An update. *N Engl J Med* 313:447–449.

Kobayashi A, Kawai S, Ohbe Y, Nagashima Y. 1975. Effects of dietary lactose and a lactase preparation on the intestinal absorption of calcium and magnesium in normal infants. *Am J Clin Nutr* 28:681–683.

Kochersberger G, Westlund R, Lyles KW. 1991. The metabolic effects of calcium supplementation in the elderly. *J Am Geriatr Soc* 39:192–196.

Koetting CA, Wardlaw GM. 1988. Wrist, spine, and hip bone density in women with variable histories of lactation. *Am J Clin Nutr* 48:1479–1481.

Kohlmeier L, Mendez M, McDuffie J, Miller M. 1997. Computer-assisted self-interviewing: A multimedia approach to dietary assessment. *Am J Clin Nutr* 65:1275S–1281S.

Koo W, Tsang R. 1997. Calcium, magnesium, phosphorus and vitamin D. In: *Nutrition During Infancy, 2nd Edition*. Cincinnati: Digital Education. Pp. 175–189.

Koo W, Krug-Wispe S, Neylen M, Succop P, Oestreich AE, Tsang RC. 1995. Effect of three levels of vitamin D intake in preterm infants receiving high mineral-containing milk. *J Pediatr Gastroenterol Nutr* 21:182–189.

Krall EA, Sahyoun N, Tannenbaum S, Dallal GE, Dawson-Hughes B. 1989. Effect of vitamin D intake on seasonal variations in parathyroid hormone secretion in postmenopausal women. *N Engl J Med* 321:1777–1783.

Kramer L, Osis D, Wiatrowski E, Spenser H. 1974. Dietary fluoride in different areas of the United States. *Am J Clin Nutr* 27:590–594.

Kreiger N, Kelsey JL, Holford TR, O'Connor T. 1982. An epidemiologic study of hip fracture in postmenopausal women. *Am J Epidemiol* 116:141–148.

Krejs GJ, Nicar MJ, Zerwekh HE, Normal DA, Kane MG, Pak CY. 1983. Effect of 1,25-dihydroxyvitamin D_3 on calcium and magnesium absorption in the healthy human jejunum and ileum. *Am J Med* 75:973–976.

Krishnamachari KA. 1986. Skeletal fluorosis in humans: A review of recent progress in the understanding of the disease. *Prog Food Nutr Sci* 10:279–314.

Krook L, Whalen JP, Lesser GV, Berens DL. 1975. Experimental studies on osteoporosis. *Methods Achiev Exp Pathol* 7:72–108.

Kröger H, Kotaniemi A, Vainio P, Alhava E. 1992. Bone densitometry of the spine and femur in children by dual-energy x-ray absorptiometry. *Bone Miner* 17:75–85.

Kröger H, Kotaniemi A, Kröger L, Alhava E. 1993. Development of bone mass and bone density of the spine and femoral neck—a prospective study of 65 children and adolescents. *Bone Miner* 23:171–182.

Kröger H, Alhava E, Honkanen R, Tuppurainen M, Saarikoski S. 1994. The effect of fluoridated drinking water on axial bone mineral density: A population-based study. *Bone Miner* 27:33–41.

Kruse K, Bartels H, Kracht U. 1984. Parathyroid function in different stages of vitamin D deficiency rickets. *Eur J Pediatr* 141:158–162.

Kumar JV, Green EL, Wallace W, Carnahan T. 1989. Trends in dental fluorosis and dental caries prevalences in Newburgh and Kingston, NY. *Am J Pub Hlth* 79:565–569.

Kumar R. 1986. The metabolism and mechanism of action of 1,25-dihydroxyvitamin D_3. *Kidney Int* 30:793–803.

Kumar R, Cohen WR, Silva P, Epstein FH. 1979. Elevated 1,25-dihydroxyvitamin D plasma levels in normal human pregnancy and lactation. *J Clin Invest* 63:342–344.

Kummerow FA, Simon Cho BH, Huang Y-T, Imai H, Kamio A, Deutsch MJ, Hooper WM. 1976. Additive risk factors in atherosclerosis. *Am J Clin Nutr* 29:579–584.

Kurtz TW, Al-Bander HA, Morris RC. 1987. "Salt sensitive" essential hypertension in men. *N Engl J Med* 317:1043–1048.

Kurzel RB. 1991. Serum magnesium levels in pregnancy and preterm labor. *Am J Perinatol* 8:119–127.

Kuti V, Balazs M, Morvay F, Varenka Z, Szekely A, Szucs M. 1981. Effect of maternal magnesium supply on spontaneous abortion and premature birth and on intrauterine fetal development: Experimental epidemiological study. *Magnes Bull* 3:73–79.

Ladizesky M, Lu Z, Oliveri B, San Roman N, Diaz S, Holick MF, Mautalen C. 1995. Solar ultraviolet B radiation and photoproduction of vitamin D_3 in central and southern areas of Argentina. *J Bone Miner Res* 10:545–549.

Lafferty FW. 1991. Differential diagnosis of hypercalcemia. *J Bone Miner Res* 6:S51–S59.

Lakshmanan LF, Rao RB, Kim WW, Kelsay JL. 1984. Magnesium intakes, balances, and blood levels of adults consuming self-selected diets. *Am J Clin Nutr* 40:1380–1389.

Lamberg-Allardt C, vonKnorring J, Slatis P, Holmstrom T. 1989. Vitamin D status and concentrations of serum vitamin D metabolites and osteocalcin in elderly patients with femoral neck fracture: A follow-up study. *Eur J Clin Nutr* 43:355–361.

Lamberg-Allardt C, Karkkainen M, Seppanen R, Bistrom H. 1993. Low serum 25-hydroxyvitamin D concentrations and secondary hyperparathyroidism in middle-aged white strict vegetarians. *Am J Clin Nutr* 58:684–689.

Largent EJ. 1952. Rates of elimination of fluoride stored in the tissues of man. *Arch Ind Hyg* 6:37–42.

Larsen MJ, Senderovitz F, Kirkegaard E, Poulsen S, Fejerskov O. 1988. Dental fluorosis in the primary and permanent dentition in fluoridated areas with consumption of either powdered milk or natural cow's milk. *J Dent Res* 67:822–825.

Lawson DE, Fraser DR, Kodicek E, Morris HR, Williams DH. 1971. Identification of 1,25-dihydroxycholecalciferol, a new kidney hormone controlling calcium metabolism. *Nature* 230:228–230.

Lealman GT, Logan RW, Hutchison JH, Kerr MM, Fulton AM, Brown CA. 1976. Calcium, phosphorus, and magnesium concentrations in plasma during first week of life and their relation to type of milk feed. *Arch Dis Child* 51:377–384.

LeBlanc A, Schneider V, Spector E, Evans H, Rowe R, Lane H, Demers L, Lipton A. 1995. Calcium absorption, endogenous excretion, and endocrine changes during and after long-term bed rest. *Bone* 16:301S–304S.

Lebrun JB, Moffatt ME, Mundy RJ, Sangster RK, Postl BD, Dooley JP, Dilling LA, Godel JC, Haworth JC. 1993. Vitamin D deficiency in a Manitoba community. *Can J Pub Hlth* 84:394–396.

Lee WT, Leung SS, Wang SH, Xu YC, Zeng WP, Lau J, Oppenheimer SJ, Cheng JC. 1994. Double-blind, controlled calcium supplementation and bone mineral accretion in children accustomed to a low-calcium diet. *Am J Clin Nutr* 60:744–750.

Lee WT, Leung SS, Leung DM, Tsang HS, Lau J, Cheng JC. 1995. A randomized double-blind controlled calcium supplementation trial, and bone and height acquisition in children. *Br J Nutr* 74:125–139.

Lee WT, Leung SS, Leung DM, Cheng JC. 1996. A follow-up study on the effects of calcium-supplement withdrawal and puberty on bone acquisition of children. *Am J Clin Nutr* 64:71–77.

LeGeros RZ, Glenn FB, Lee DD, Glenn WD. 1985. Some physico-chemical properties of deciduous enamel with and without pre-natal fluoride supplementation (PNF). *J Dent Res* 64:465–469.

Lehner NDM, Bullock BC, Clarkson TB, Lofland HB. 1967. Biologic activities of vitamin D_2 and D_3 for growing squirrel monkeys. *Lab Anim Care* 17:483.

Leitch I, Aitken FC. 1959. The estimation of calcium requirement: A re-examination. *Nutr Abs Rev* 29:393–409.

Lemann J Jr. 1996. Calcium and phosphate metabolism: An overview in health and in calcium stone formers. In: Coe FL, Favus MJ, Pak CY, Parks JH, Preminger GM, eds. *Kidney Stones: Medical and Surgical Management.* Philadelphia, PA: Lippincott-Raven. Pp. 259–288.

Lemann J Jr, Worcester EM, Gray RW. 1991. Hypercalciuria and stones. *Am J Kidney Dis* 17:386–391.

Lemke CW, Doherty JM, Arra MC. 1970. Controlled fluoridation: The dental effects of discontinuation in Antigo, Wisconsin. *J Am Dent Assoc* 80:782–786.

Leone NC, Shimkin MB, Arnold FA, Stevenson CA, Zimmerman ER, Geiser PB, Lieberman JE. 1954. Medical aspects of excessive fluoride in a water supply. *Pub Hlth Rep* 69:925–936.

Leone NC, Stevenson CA, Hilbish TF, Sosman MC. 1955. A roentgenologic study of a human population exposed to high-fluoride domestic water: A ten-year study. *Am J Roentg* 74:874–885.

Leone NC, Stevenson CA, Besse B, Hawes, LE, Dawber TA. 1960. The effects of the absorption of fluoride. II. A radiological investigation of 546 human residents of an area in which the drinking water contained only a minute trace of fluoride. *Archs Ind Hlth* 21:326–327.

Leoni V, Fabiani L, Ticchiarelli L. 1985. Water hardness and cardiovascular mortality rate in Abruzzo, Italy. *Arch Environ Health* 40:274–278.

Leung SSF, Lui S, Swaminathan R. 1989. Vitamin D status of Hong Kong Chinese infants. *Acta Paediatr Scand* 78:303–306.

Leverett DH. 1986. Prevalence of dental fluorosis in fluoridated and nonfluoridated communities—a preliminary investigation. *J Pub Hlth Dent* 46:184–187.

Leverett DH, Adair SM, Vaughan BW, Proskin HM, Moss ME. 1997. Randomized clinical trial of the effect of prenatal fluoride supplements in preventing dental caries. *Caries Res* 31:174–179.

Levine RJ, Hauth JC, Curet LB, Sibai BM, Catalano PM, Morris CD, DerSimonian R, Esterlitz JR, Raymond EG, Bild DE, Clemens JD, Cutler JA. 1997. Trial of calcium to prevent preeclampsia. *N Engl J Med* 337:69–76.

Levy SM, Muchow G. 1992. Provider compliance with recommended dietary fluoride supplement protocol. *Am J Pub Hlth* 82:281–283.

Levy SM, Kohout FJ, Kiritsy MC, Heilman JR, Wefel JS. 1995. Infants' fluoride ingestion from water, supplements and dentifrice. *J Am Dent Assoc* 126:1625–1632.

Lewis DW. 1976. *An Evaluation of the Effects of Water Fluoridation, City of Toronto, 1963–1975.* Toronto, Canada: The Corporation of the City of Toronto.

Lewis NM, Marcus MSK, Behling AR, Greger JL. 1989. Calcium supplements and milk: Effects on acid-base balance and on retention of calcium, magnesium, and phosphorus. *Am J Clin Nutr* 49:527–533.

Liel Y, Edwards J, Shary J, Spicer KM, Gordon L, Bell NH. 1988. The effects of race and body habitus on bone mineral density of the radius, hip, and spine in premenopausal women. *J Clin Endocrinol Metab* 66:1247–1250.

Lin S-H, Lin Y-F, Shieh S-D. 1996. Milk-alkali syndrome in an aged patient with osteoporosis and fractures. *Nephron* 73:496–497.

Linden V. 1974. Vitamin D and myocardial infarction. *Br Med J* 3:647–650.

Linkswiler HM, Zemel MB, Hegsted M, Schuette S. 1981. Protein-induced hypercalciuria. *Fed Proc* 40:2429–2433.

Lips P, Wiersinga A, vanGinkel FC, Jongen MJ, Netelenbos JC, Hackeng WH, Delmas PD, vanderVijgh WJ. 1988. The effect of vitamin D supplementation on vitamin D status and parathyroid function in elderly subjects. *J Clin Endocrinol Metab* 67:644–650.

Lips P, Graafmans WC, Ooms ME, Bezemer D, Bouter LM. 1996. Vitamin D supplementation and fracture incidence in elderly persons: A randomized, placebo-controlled clinical trial. *Ann Intern Med* 124:400–406.

Lipski PS, Torrance A, Kelly PJ, James OF. 1993. A study of nutritional deficits of long-stay geriatric patients. *Age Aging* 22:244–255.

Lissner L, Bengtsson C, Hansson T. 1991. Bone mineral content in relation to lactation history in pre- and postmenopausal women. *Calcif Tissue Int* 48:319–325.

Livingstone MB, Prentice AM, Coward WA, Strain JJ, Black AE, Davies PS, Stewart CM, McKenna PG, Whitehead RG. 1992. Validation estimates of energy intake by weighted dietary record and diet history in children and adolescents. *Am J Clin Nutr* 56:29–35.

Lloyd T, Schaeffer JM, Walker MA, Demers LM. 1991. Urinary hormonal concentrations and spinal bone densities of premenopausal vegetarian and nonvegetarian women. *Am J Clin Nutr* 54:1005–1010.

Lloyd T, Andon MB, Rollings N, Martel JK, Landis R, Demers LM, Eggli DF, Kieselhorst K, Kulin HE. 1993. Calcium supplementation and bone mineral density in adolescent girls. *J Am Med Assoc* 270:841–844.

Lo CW, Paris PW, Clemens TL, Nolan J, Holick MF. 1985. Vitamin D absorption in healthy subjects and in patients with intestinal malabsorption syndromes. *Am J Clin Nutr* 42:644–649.

Lonnerdal B. 1997. Effects of milk and milk components on calcium, magnesium, and trace element absorption during infancy. *Physiol Rev* 77:643–669.

Looker AC, Harris TB, Madans JH, Sempos CT. 1993. Dietary calcium and hip fracture risk: The NHANES I Epidemiology Follow-Up Study. *Osteopor Int* 3:177–184.

Looker AC, Johnston CC Jr, Wahner HW, Dunn WL, Calvo MS, Harris TB, Heyse SP, Lindsay RL. 1995. Prevalence of low femoral bone density in older US women from NHANES III. *J Bone Miner Res* 10:796–802.

Lopez JM, Gonzalez G, Reyes V, Campino C, Diaz S. 1996. Bone turnover and density in healthy women during breastfeeding and after weaning. *Osteopor Int* 6:153–159.

Lotz M, Zisman E, Bartter FC. 1968. Evidence for a phosphorus-depletion syndrome in man. *N Engl J Med* 278:409–415.

Lowenstein FW, Stanton MF. 1986. Serum magnesium levels in the United States, 1971–1974. *J Am Coll Nutr* 5:399–414.

Lowik MR, van Dokkum W, Kistemaker C, Schaafsma G, Ockhuizen T. 1993. Body composition, health status and urinary magnesium excretion among elderly people (Dutch Nutrition Surveillance System). *Magnes Res* 6:223–232.

LSRO/FASEB (Life Sciences Research Office/Federation of American Societies for Experimental Biology). 1986. *Guidelines for Use of Dietary Intake Data.* Anderson SA, ed. Bethesda, MD: LSRO/FASEB.

Lu PW, Briody JN, Ogle GD, Morley K, Humphries IR, Allen J, Howman-Giles R, Sillence D, Cowell CT. 1994. Bone mineral density of total body, spine, and femoral neck in children and young adults: A cross-sectional and longtitudinal study. *J Bone Miner Res* 9:1451–1458.

Luckey MM, Meier DE, Mandeli JP, DaCosta MC, Hubbard ML, Goldsmith SJ. 1989. Radial and vertebral bone density in white and black women: Evidence for racial differences in premenopausal bone homeostasis. *J Clin Endocrinol Metab* 69:762–770.

Lukert BP, Raisz LG. 1990. Glucocorticoid-induced osteoporosis: Pathogenesis and management. *Ann Intern Med* 112:352–364.

Lund B, Sorensen OH. 1979. Measurement of 25-hydroxyvitamin D in serum and its relation to sunshine, age and vitamin D intake in the Danish population. *Scand J Clin Lab Invest* 39:23–30.

Luoma H, Aromaa A, Helminen S, Murtomaa H, Kiviluoto L, Punsar S, Knekt P. 1983. Risk of myocardial infarction in Finnish men in relation to fluoride, magnesium and calcium concentration in drinking water. *Acta Med Scand* 213:171–176.

Lutwak L, Laster L, Gitelman HJ, Fox M, Whedon GD. 1964. Effects of high dietary calcium and phosphorus on calcium, phosphorus, nitrogen and fat metabolism in children. *Am J Clin Nutr* 14:76–82.

Ma J, Folsom AR, Melnick SL, Eckfeldt JH, Sharrett AR, Nabulsi AA, Hutchinson RG, Metcalf PA. 1995. Associations of serum and dietary magnesium with cardiovascular disease, hypertension, diabetes, insulin, and carotid arterial wall thickness: The ARIC study. Atherosclerosis Risk in Community Study. *J Clin Epidemiol* 48:927–940.

MacLaughlin J, Holick MF. 1985. Aging decreases the capacity of human skin to produce vitamin D_3. *J Clin Invest* 76:1536–1538.

MacLaughlin JA, Anderson RR, Holick MF. 1982. Spectral character of sunlight modulates photosynthesis of previtamin D_3 and its photoisomers in human skin. *Science* 216:1001–1003.

Maguire ME. 1984. Hormone-sensitive magnesium transport and magnesium regulation of adenylate cyclase. *Trends Pharmacol Sci* 5:73–77.

Mahalko JR, Sandstead HH, Johnson LK, Milne DB. 1983. Effect of a moderate increase in dietary protein on the retention and excretion of Ca, Cu, Fe, Mg, P, and Zn by adult males. *Am J Clin Nutr* 37:8–14.

Maheshwari UR, McDonald JT, Schneider VS, Brunetti AJ, Leybin L, Newbrun E, Hodge HC. 1981. Fluoride balance studies in ambulatory healthy men with and without fluoride supplements. *Am J Clin Nutr* 34:2679–2684.

Maheshwari UR, King JC, Leybin L, Newbrun E, Hodge HC. 1983. Fluoride balances during early and late pregnancy. *J Occup Med* 25:587–590.

Mallet E, Gugi B, Brunelle P, Henocq A, Basuyau JP, Lemeur H. 1986. Vitamin D supplementation in pregnancy: A controlled trial of two methods. *Obstet Gynecol* 68:300–304.

Malm OJ. 1958. Calcium requirement and adaptation in adult men. *Scand J Clin Lab Invest* 10(Suppl 36):1–280.

Malone DNS, Horn DB. 1971. Acute hypercalcemia and renal failure after antacid therapy. *Br Med J* 1:709–710.

Manz F. 1992. Why is the phosphorus content of human milk exceptionally low? *Monatsschr Kinderheilkd* 140:S35–S39.

Marcus R, Cann C, Madvig P, Minkoff J, Goddard M, Bayer M, Martin M, Gaudiani L, Haskell W, Genant H. 1985. Menstrual function and bone mass in elite women distance runners. Endocrine and metabolic features. *Ann Intern Med* 102:158–163.

Margen S, Chu JY, Kaufmann NA, Calloway DH. 1974. Studies in calcium metabolism I. The calciuretic effect of dietary protein. *Am J Clin Nutr* 27:584–589.

Margolis HC, Moreno EC. 1990. Physicochemical perspectives on the cariostatic mechanisms of systemic and topical fluorides. *J Dent Res* 69(Spec Iss):606–613.

Marier JR. 1986. Magnesium content of the food supply in the modern-day world. *Magnesium* 5:1–8.

Marken PA, Weart CW, Carson DS, Gums JG, Lopes-Virella MF. 1989. Effects of magnesium oxide on the lipid profile of healthy volunteers. *Atherosclerosis* 77:37–42.

Markestad T, Elzouki AY. 1991. Vitamin-D deficiency rickets in northern Europe and Libya. In: Glorieux FH, ed. *Rickets: Nestle Nutrition Workshop Series, Vol 21*. New York, NY: Raven Press.

Markestad T, Ulstein M, Bassoe HH, Aksnes L, Aarskog D. 1983. Vitamin D metabolism in normal and hypoparathyroid pregnancy and lactation. Case report. *Br J Obstet Gynaecol* 90:971–976.

Markestad T, Ulstein M, Aksnes L, Aarskog D. 1986. Serum concentrations of vitamin D metabolites in vitamin D supplemented pregnant women. A longitudinal study. *Acta Obstet Gynecol Scand* 65:63–67.

Marquis RE. 1995. Antimicrobial actions of fluoride for oral bacteria. *Can J Microbiol* 41:955–964.

Marsh AG, Sanchez TV, Midkelsen O, Keiser J, Mayor G. 1980. Cortical bone density of adult lacto-ovo-vegetarian and omnivorous women. *J Am Diet Assoc* 76:148–151.

Marshall DH, Nordin BEC, Speed R. 1976. Calcium, phosphorus and magnesium requirement. *Proc Nutr Soc* 35:163–173.

Martin AD, Bailey DA, McKay HA. 1997. Bone mineral and calcium accretion during puberty. *Am J Clin Nutr* 66:611–615.

Martin BJ. 1990. The magnesium load test: Experience in elderly subjects. *Aging (Milano)* 2:291–296.

Martin TJ, Grill V. 1995. Hypercalcemia. *Clin Endocrinol* 42:535–538.

Martinez ME, Salinas M, Miguel JL, Herrero E, Gomez P, Garcia J, Sanchez-Sicilia L, Montero A. 1985. Magnesium excretion in idiopathic hypercalciuria. *Nephron* 40: 446–450.

Massey LK, Wise KJ. 1984. The effect of dietary caffeine on urinary excretion of calcium, magnesium, sodium and potassium in healthy young females. *Nutr Res* 4:43–50.

Massey LK, Roman-Smith H, Sutton RA. 1993. Effect of dietary oxalate and calcium on urinary oxalate and risk of formation of calcium oxalate kidney stones. *J Am Diet Assoc* 93:901–906.

Matkovic V. 1991. Calcium metabolism and calcium requirements during skeletal modeling and consolidation of bone mass. *Am J Clin Nutr* 54:245S–260S.

Matkovic V, Heaney RP. 1992. Calcium balance during human growth: Evidence for threshold behavior. *Am J Clin Nutr* 55:992–996.

Matkovic V, Fontana D, Tominac C, Goel P, Chesnut CH III. 1990. Factors that influence peak bone mass formation: A study of calcium balance and the inheritance of bone mass in adolescent females. *Am J Clin Nutr* 52:878–888.

Matkovic V, Jelic T, Wardlaw GM, Illich JZ, Goel PK, Wright JK, Andon MB, Smith KT, Heaney RP. 1994. Timing of peak bone mass in Caucasian females and its implication for the prevention of osteoporosis. *J Clin Invest* 93:799–808.

Matkovic V, Ilich JZ, Andon MB, Hsieh LC, Tzagournis MA, Lagger BJ, Goel PK. 1995. Urinary calcium, sodium, and bone mass of young females. *Am J Clin Nutr* 62:417–425.

Matsuda H. 1991. Magnesium gating of the inwardly rectifying K+ channel. *Ann Rev Physiol* 53:289–298.

Matsuoka LY, Ide L, Wortsman J, MacLaughlin JA, Holick MF. 1987. Sunscreens suppress cutaneous vitamin D₃ synthesis. *J Clin Endocrinol Metab* 64:1165–1168.

Matsuoka LY, Wortsman J, Dannenberg MJ, Hollis BW, Lu Z, Holick MF. 1992. Clothing prevents ultraviolet-B radiation-dependent photosynthesis of vitamin D₃. *J Clin Endocrinol Metab* 75:1099–1103.

Mawer EB, Schaefer K, Lumb GA, Stanbury SW. 1971. The metabolism of isotopically labelled vitamin D₃ in man: The influence of the state of vitamin D nutrition. *Clin Sci* 40:39–53.

Mawer EB, Backhouse J, Holman CA, Lumb GA, Stanbury DW. 1972. The distribution and storage of vitamin D and its metabolites in human tissues. *Clin Sci* 43:413–431.

Mazariegos-Ramos E, Guerrero-Romero F, Rodriguez-Moran M, Lazcano-Burciaga G, Paniagua R, Amato D. 1995. Consumption of soft drinks with phosphoric acid as a risk factor for the development of hypocalcemia in children: A case-control study. *J Pediatr* 126:940–942.

McCarron DA. 1983. Calcium and magnesium nutrition in human hypertension. *Ann Int Med* 98:800–805.

McCarron DA, Morris CD. 1985. Blood pressure response to oral calcium in persons with mild to moderate hypertension: A randomized, double-blind, placebo-controlled, crossover trial. *Ann Intern Med* 103:825–831.

McCarron DA, Morris CD, Young E, Roullet C, Drüeke T. 1991. Dietary calcium and blood pressure: Modifying factors in specific populations. *Am J Clin Nutr* 54:215S–219S.

McCauley HB, McClure FJ. 1954. Effect of fluoride in drinking water on the osseous development of the hand and wrist in children. *Pub Hlth Rep* 69:671–683.

McClure FJ. 1943. Ingestion of fluoride and dental caries. Quantitative relations based on food and water requirements of children one to twelve years old. *Am J Dis Child* 66:362–369.

McClure FJ, Zipkin I. 1958. Physiologic effects of fluoride as related to water fluoridation. *Dent Clin North Am* 2:441–458.

McCrory WW, Forman CW, McNamara H, Barnett HL. 1950. Renal excretion of phosphate in newborn infants: Observations in normal infants and in infants with hypocalcemic tetany. *Am J Dis Child* 80:512–513.

McFarlane D. 1941. Experimental phosphate nephritis in the rat. *J Pathol* 52:17–24.

McGrath N, Singh V, Cundy T. 1993. Severe vitamin D deficiency in Auckland. *N Zeal Med J* 106:524–526.

McKenna MJ. 1992. Differences in vitamin D status between countries in young adults and the elderly. *Am J Med* 93:69–77.

McKnight-Hanes MC, Leverett DH, Adair SM, Sheilds CP. 1988. Fluoride content of infant formulas: Soy-based formulas as a potential factor in dental fluorosis. *Pediatr Dent* 10:189–194.

Meier DE, Luckey MM, Wallenstein S, Clemens TL, Orwoll ES, Waslien CI. 1991. Calcium, vitamin D, and parathyroid hormone status in young white and black women: Association with racial differences in bone mass. *J Clin Endocrinol Metab* 72:703–710.

Melton LJ III, Chrischilles EA, Cooper C, Lane AW, Riggs, BL. 1992. Perspective. How many women have osteoporosis? *J Bone Miner Res* 7:1005–1010.

Melton LJ III, Atkinson EJ, O'Fallon WM, Wahner HW, Riggs BL. 1993a. Long-term fracture prediction by bone mineral assessed at different skeletal sites. *J Bone Miner Res* 8:1227–1233.

Melton LJ III, Bryant SC, Wahner HW, O'Fallon WM, Malkasian GD, Judd HL, Riggs BL. 1993b. Influence of breastfeeding and other reproductive factors on bone mass later in life. *Osteopor Int* 3:76–83.

Merke J, Klaus G, Hugel U, Waldherr R, Ritz E. 1986. No 1,25-dihydroxyvitamin D_3 receptors on osteoclasts of calcium-deficient chicken despite demonstrable receptors on circulating monocytes. *J Clin Invest* 77:312–314.

Mertz W, Tsui JC, Judd JT, Reiser S, Hallfrisch J, Morris ER, Steele PD, Lashley E. 1991. What are people really eating? The relation between energy intake derived from estimated diet records and intake determined to maintain body weight. *Am J Clin Nutr* 54:291–295.

Mertz W, Abernathy CO, Olin SS. 1994. *Risk Assessment of Essential Elements.* Washington, DC: ILSI Press.

Meulmeester JF, vandenBerg H, Wedel M, Boshuis PG, Hulshof KF, Luyken R. 1990. Vitamin D status, parathyroid hormone and sunlight in Turkish, Moroccan and Caucasian children in The Netherlands. *Eur J Clin Nutr* 44:461–470.

Meyer F, White E. 1993. Alcohol and nutrients in relation to colon cancer in middle-aged adults. *Am J Epidemiol* 138:225–236.

Miller JZ, Smith DL, Flora L, Slemenda C, Jiang X, Johnston CC Jr. 1988. Calcium absorption from calcium carbonate and a new form of calcium (CCM) in healthy male and female adolescents. *Am J Clin Nutr* 48:1291–1294.

Mimouni FB. 1996. The ion-selective magnesium electrode: A new tool for clinicians and investigators. *J Am College Nutr* 15:4–5.

Mimouni F, Tsang RC, Hertzberg VS, Miodovnik M. 1986. Polycythemia hypomagnesemia and hypocalcemia infants of diabetic mothers. *Am J Dis Child* 140:798–800.

Mimouni F, Campaigne B, Neylan M, Tsang RC. 1993. Bone mineralization in the first year of life in infants fed human milk, cow-milk formula, or soy-based formula. *J Pediatr* 122:348–354.

Moncrief MW, Chance GW. 1969. Nephrotoxic effect of vitamin D therapy in vitamin D refractory rickets. *Arch Dis Child* 44:571–579.

Montalto MB, Benson JD. 1986. Nutrient intakes of older infants: Effect of different milk feedings. *J Am Coll Nutr* 5:331–341.

Mordes JP, Wacker WEC. 1978. Excessive magnesium. *Pharmacol Rev* 29:273–300.

Moser PB, Issa CF, Reynolds RD. 1983. Dietary magnesium intake and the concentration of magnesium in plasma and erythrocytes of postpartum women. *J Am Coll Nutr* 2:387–396.

Moser PB, Reynolds RD, Acharya S, Howard MP, Andon MB. 1988. Calcium and magnesium dietary intakes and plasma and milk concentrations of Nepalese lactating women. *Am J Clin Nutr* 47:735–739.

Moss AJ, Levy AS, Kim I, Park YK. 1989. *Use of Vitamin and Mineral Supplements in the United States: Current Users, Types of Products, and Nutrients.* Advance data from vital and health statistics, No. 174. Hyattsville, MD: National Center for Health Statistics.

Motoyama T, Sano H, Fukuzaki H. 1989. Oral magnesium supplementation in patients with essential hypertention. *Hypertension* 13:227–232.

Mountokalakis TD. 1987. Effects of aging, chronic disease, and multiple supplements on magnesium requirements. *Magnesium* 6:5–11.

Moya M, Cortes E, Ballester MI, Vento M, Juste M. 1992. Short-term polycose substitution for lactose reduces calcium absorption in healthy term babies. *J Pediatr Gastroenterol Nutr* 14:57–61.

Muhler JC. 1970. Ingestion from foods. In: Adler P, ed. *Fluorides and Human Health.* Monograph series no. 59. Geneva: World Health Organization. Pp. 32–40.

Muldowney WP, Mazbar SA. 1996. Rolaids-yogurt syndrome: A 1990s version of milk-alkali syndrome. *Am J Kidney Dis* 27:270–272.

Murphy SP, Calloway DH. 1986. Nutrient intakes of women in NHANES II, emphasizing trace minerals, fiber, and phytate. *J Am Diet Assoc* 86:1366–1372.

Naccache H, Simard PL, Trahan L, Demers M, Lapointe C, Brodeur JM. 1990. Variability in the ingestion of toothpaste by preschool children. *Caries Res* 24:359–363.

Naccache H, Simard PL, Trahan L, Brodeur JM, Demers M, Lachapelle D, Bernard PM. 1992. Factors affecting the ingestion of fluoride dentifrice by children. *J Pub Hlth Dent* 52:222–226.

Nadler JL, Malayan S, Luong H, Shaw S, Natarajan RD, Rude RK. 1992. Intracellular free magnesium deficiency plays a key role in increased platelet reactivity in type II diabetes mellitus. *Diabetes Care* 15:835–841.

Nadler JL, Buchanan T, Natarajan R, Antonipillai I, Bergman R, Rude RK. 1993. Magnesium deficiency produces insulin resistance and increased thromboxane synthesis. *Hypertension* 21:1024–1029.

Nagubandi S, Kumar R, Londowski JM, Corradino RA, Tietz PS. 1980. Role of vitamin D glucosiduronate in calcium homeostasis. *J Clin Invest* 66:1274–1280.

Nagy L, Tarnok F, Past T, Mozsik GY, Deak G, Tapsonyi Z, Fendler K, Javor T. 1988. Human tolerability and pharmacodynamic study of TISACID tablet in duodenal ulcer patients. A prospective, randomized, self-controlled clinico-pharmocological study. *Acta Medica Hung* 45:231–246.

Nakamura T, Turner CH, Yoshikawa T, Slemenda CW, Peacock M, Burr DB, Mizuno Y, Orimo H, Ouchi Y, Johnston CC Jr. 1994. Do variations in hip geometry explain differences in hip fracture risk between Japanese and white Americans? *J Bone Miner Res* 9:1071–1076.

Nakao H. 1988. Nutritional significance of human milk vitamin D in neonatal period. *Kobe J Med Sci* 34:121–128.

Narang NK, Gupta RC, Jain MK. 1984. Role of vitamin D in pulmonary tuberculosis. *J Assoc Physicians India* 32:185–188.

National Council for Nutrition (Conseil National de la Nutrition). 1994. *Recommandations nutritionelles pour la Belgique.* Bruxelles, Belgium: Ministère des Affairs Socialis de la Santé Publique et de l'Environnement.

National Food Administration. 1989. *Swedish Nutrition Recommendations, 2nd edition.* Uppsala, Sweden: National Food Administration.

Need AG, Morris HA, Horowitz M, Nordin C. 1993. Effects of skin thickness, age, body fat, and sunlight on serum 25-hydroxyvitamin D. *Am J Clin Nutr* 58:882–885.

Neri LC, Johansen HL. 1978. Water hardness and cardiovascular mortality. *Ann NY Acad Sci* 304:203–219.

Neri LC, Johansen HL, Hewitt D, Marier J, Langner N. 1985. Magnesium and certain other elements and cardiovascular disease. *Sci Total Environ* 42:49–75.

Netherlands Food and Nutrition Council. 1992. *Report on the Age Limit to be Adopted in Connection with "Guidelines for a Healthy Diet."* The Hague: Netherlands Food and Nutrition Council.

Neville MC, Keller, R, Seacat J, Lutes V, Neifert M, Casey C, Allen J, Archer P. 1988. Studies in human lactation: Milk volumes in lactating women during the onset of lactation and full lactation. *Am J Clin Nutr* 48:1375–1386.

Newmark K, Nugent P. 1993. Milk-alkali syndrome: A consequence of chronic antacid abuse. *Postgrad Med* 93:149–156.

Ng K, St John A, Bruce DG. 1994. Secondary hyperparathyroidism, vitamin D deficiency and hip fracture: Importance of sampling times after fracture. *Bone Miner* 25:103–109.

Niekamp RA, Baer JT. 1995. In-season dietary adequacy of trained male cross-country runners. *Int J Sport Nutr* 5:45–55.

Nielsen FH. 1990. Studies on the relationship between boron and magnesium which possibly affects the formation and maintenance of bones. *Magnes Trace Elem* 9:61–69.

Nielsen FH, Hunt CD, Mullen LM, Hunt JR. 1987. Effect of dietary boron on mineral, estrogen, and testosterone metabolism in postmenopausal women. *FASEB J* 1:394–397.

Nieves JW, Golden AL, Siris E, Kelsey JL, Lindsay R. 1995. Teenage and current calcium intake are related to bone mineral density of the hip and forearm in women aged 30–39 years. *Am J Epidemiol* 141:342–351.

NIH (National Institutes of Health). 1994. *Optimal Calcium Intake.* NIH Consensus Statement 12:4. Bethesda, MD: NIH.

NIN (National Institute of Nutrition). 1995. Dairy products in the Canadian diet. NIN Review No. 24. Ontario, Canada: NIN.

Nordin BEC. 1976. *Calcium, Phosphate and Magnesium Metabolism.* Edinburgh: Churchill Livingstone.

Nordin BEC. 1989. Phosphorus. *J Food Nutr* 45:62–75.

Nordin BEC, Polley KJ. 1987. Metabolic consequences of the menopause. A cross-sectional, longitudinal, and intervention study on 557 normal postmenopausal women. *Calcif Tissue Int* 41:S1–S59.

Nose O, Iida Y, Kai H, Harada T, Ogawa M, Yabuuchi H. 1979. Breath hydrogen test for detecting lactose malabsorption in infants and children: Prevalence of lactose malabsorption in Japanese children and adults. *Arch Dis Child* 54:436–440.

NRC (National Research Council). 1980. *Recommended Dietary Allowances, 9th Edition.* Committee on Dietary Allowances, Food and Nutrition Board. Washington, DC: National Academy Press.

NRC (National Research Council). 1982. *Diet, Nutrition, and Cancer.* Report of the Committee on Diet, Nutrition, and Cancer, Assembly of Life Sciences. Washington, DC: National Academy Press.

NRC (National Research Council). 1983. *Risk Assessment in the Federal Government: Managing the Process.* Washington, DC: National Academy Press.

NRC (National Research Council). 1986. *Nutrient Adequacy. Assessment Using Food Consumption Surveys.* Washington, DC: National Academy Press.

NRC (National Research Council). 1989a. *Recommended Dietary Allowances: 10th Edition.* Report of the Subcommittee on the Tenth Edition of the RDAs, Food and Nutrition Board, and the Commission on Life Sciences. Washington, DC: National Academy Press.

NRC (National Research Council). 1989b. *Diet and Health: Implications for Reducing Chronic Disease Risk.* Report of the Committee on Diet and Health, Food and Nutrition Board, Commission on Life Sciences. Washington, DC: National Academy Press.

NRC (National Research Council) 1993. *Health Effects of Ingested Fluoride.* Subcommittee on Health Effects of Ingested Fluoride. Washington, DC: National Academy Press.

NRC (National Research Council). 1994. *Science and Judgment in Risk Assessment.* Committee on Risk Assessment of Hazardous Air Pollutants. Board on Environmental Studies and Toxicology. Washington, DC: National Academy Press.

NRC (National Research Council). 1995. *Nutrient Requirements of Laboratory Animals.* Committee on Animal Nutrition, Board on Agriculture. Washington, DC: National Academy Press.

Nusser SM, Carriquiry AL, Dodd KW, Fuller WA. 1996. A semiparametric transformation approach to estimating usual daily intake distributions. *J Am Stat Assoc* 91:1440–1449.

O'Brien KO, Abrams SA, Stuff JE, Liang LK, Welch TR. 1996. Variables related to urinary calcium excretion in young girls. *J Pediatr Gastroenterol Nutr* 23:8–12.

O'Dowd KJ, Clemens TL, Kelsey JL, Lindsay R. 1993. Exogenous calciferol (vitamin D) and vitamin D endocrine status among elderly nursing home residents in the New York City area. *J Am Geriatr Soc* 41:414–421.

Ohlson MA, Brewer WD, Jackson L, Swanson PP, Roberts PH, Mangel M, Leverton RM, Chaloupka M, Gram MR, Reynolds MS, Lutz R. 1952. Intakes and retentions of nitrogen, calcium and phosphorus by 136 women between 30 and 85 years of age. *Fed Proc* 11:775–783.

Oliveri MB, Ladizesky M, Mautalen CA, Alonso A, Martinez L. 1993. Seasonal variations of 25 hydroxyvitamin D and parathyroid hormone in Ushuaia (Argentina), the southernmost city in the world. *Bone Miner* 20:99–108.

Ooms ME, Roos JC, Bezemer PD, VanDerVijgh WJ, Bouter LM, Lips P. 1995. Prevention of bone loss by vitamin D supplementation in elderly women: A randomized double-blind trial. *J Clin Endocrinol Metab* 80:1052–1058.

Ophaug RH, Singer L, Harland BF. 1980a. Estimated fluoride intake of 6-month-old infants in four dietary regions of the United States. *Am J Clin Nutr* 33:324–327.

Ophaug RH, Singer L, Harland BF. 1980b. Estimated fluoride intake of average two-year-old children in four dietary regions of the United States. *J Dent Res* 59:777–781.

Ophaug RH, Singer L, Harland BF. 1985. Dietary fluoride intake of 6-month and 2-year-old children in four dietary regions of the United States. *Am J Clin Nutr* 42:701–707.

Orimo H, Ouchi Y. 1990. The role of calcium and magnesium in the development of atherosclerosis. Experimental and clinical evidence. *Ann NY Acad Sci* 598:444–457.

Orwoll ES. 1982. The milk-alkali syndrome: Current concepts. *Ann Intern Med* 97:242–248.

Orwoll ES, Oviatt SK, McClung MR, Deftos LJ, Sexton G. 1990. The rate of bone mineral loss in normal men and the effects of calcium and cholecalciferol supplementation. *Ann Intern Med* 112:29–34.

Osis D, Kramer L, Wiatrowski E, Spencer H. 1974. Dietary fluoride intake in man. *J Nutr* 104:1313–1318.

Osteoporosis Society of Canada. 1993. Consensus on calcium nutrition. Official position of the Osteoporosis Society of Canada. *Nutr Quart* 18:62–69.

Osuji OO, Leake JL, Chipman ML, Nikiforuk G, Locker D, Levine N. 1988. Risk factors for dental fluorosis in a fluoridated community. *J Dent Res* 67:1488–1492.

OTA (Office of Technology Assessment). 1993. *Researching Health Risks.* Washington, DC: Office of Technology Assessment.

Outhouse J, Kinsman G, Sheldon D, Tworney I, Smith J. 1939. The calcium requirements of five pre-school girls. *J Nutr* 17:199–211.

Outhouse J, Breiter H, Rutherford E, Dwight J, Mills R, Armstrong W. 1941. The calcium requirement of man: Balance studies on seven adults. *J Nutr* 21:565–575.

Paganini-Hill A, Chao A, Ross RK, Henderson BE. 1991. Exercise and other factors in the prevention of hip fracture: The Leisure World Study. *Epidemiology* 2:16–25.

Pak CY. 1988. Medical management of nephrolithiasis in Dallas: Update 1987. *J Urol* 140:461–467.

Pak CY, Sakhaee K, Rubin CD, Zerwekh JE. 1997. Sustained-release sodium fluoride in the management of established menopausal osteoporosis. *Am J Med Sci* 313:23–32.

Pang DT, Phillips CL, Bawden JW. 1992. Fluoride intake from beverage consumption in a sample of North Carolina children. *J Dent Res* 71:1382–1388.

Paolisso G, Passariello N, Pizza G, Marrazzo G, Giunta R, Sgambato S, Varricchio M, D'Onofrio F. 1989. Dietary magnesium supplements improve B-cell response to glucose and arginine in elderly non-insulin-dependent diabetic subjects. *Acta Endocrinol Copenh* 121:16–20.

Paolisso G, Scheen A, D'Onofrio FD, Lefebvre P. 1990. Magnesium and glucose homeostasis. *Diabetologia* 33:511–514.

Paolisso G, Sgambato S, Gambardella A, Pizza G, Tesauro P, Varricchio M, D'Onofrio F. 1992. Daily magnesium supplements improve glucose handling in elderly subjects. *Am J Clin Nutr* 55:1161–1167.

Parfitt AM. 1977. Metacarpal cortical dimensions in hypoparathyroidism, primary hyperparathyroidism and chronic renal failure. *Calcif Tiss Res Suppl* 22:329–331.

Parfitt AM. 1988. Bone remodeling: Relationship to the amount and structure of bone, and the pathogenesis and prevention of fractures. In: Riggs BL, Melton LJ III eds. *Osteoporosis: Etiology, Diagnosis, and Management.* New York, NY: Raven Press.

Parfitt AM, Higgins BA, Nassim JR, Collins JA, Hilb A. 1964. Metabolic studies in patients with hypercalciuria. *Clin Sci* 27:463–482.

Parfitt AM, Chir B, Gallagher JC, Heaney RP, Johnston CC, Neer R, Whedon GD. 1982. Vitamin D and bone health in the elderly. *Am J Clin Nutr* 36:1014–1031.

Paunier L, Lacourt G, Pilloud P, Schlaeppi P, Sizonenko PC. 1978. 25-hydroxyvitamin D and calcium levels in maternal, cord and infant serum in relation to maternal vitamin D intake. *Helv Paediatr Acta* 33:95–103.

Peace H, Beattie JH. 1991. No effect of boron on bone mineral excretion and plasma sex steroid levels in healthy postmenopausal women. Monography, proceedings, roundtables, and discussions of the Seventh International Symposium on Trace Elements in Man and Animals, held May 20–25, 1990, in Dubrovnik, Croatia, Yugoslavia.

Peacock M. 1991. Calcium absorption efficiency and calcium requirements in children and adolescents. *Am J Clin Nutr* 54:261S–265S.

Pedersen AB, Bartholomew MJ, Dolence LA, Aljadir LP, Netteburg KL, Lloyd T. 1991. Menstrual differences due to vegetarian and nonvegetarian diets. *Am J Clin Nutr* 53:879–885.

Pendrys DG, Katz RV. 1989. Risk of enamel fluorosis associated with fluoride supplementation, infant formula, and fluoride dentifrice use. *Am J Epidemiol* 130:1199–1208.

Pendrys DG, Morse DE. 1990. Use of fluoride supplementation by children living in fluoridated communities. *J Dent Child* 57:343–347.

Pendrys DG, Stamm JW. 1990. Relationship of total fluoride intake to beneficial effects and enamel fluorosis. *J Dent Res* 69(Spec Iss):529–538.

Peng SK, Taylor CB. 1980. Editorial: Probable role of excesses of vitamin D in genesis of arteriosclerosis. *Arterial Wall* 6:63–68.

Peng SK, Taylor CB, Tham P, Mikkelson B. 1978. Role of mild excesses of vitamin D in arteriosclerosis. A study in squirrel monkeys. *Arterial Wall* 4:229.

Pennington JA. 1994. *Bowes and Church's Food Values of Portions Commonly Used.* Philadelphia, PA: JB Lippincott.

Pennington JA, Wilson DB. 1990. Daily intakes of nine nutritional elements: Analyzed vs. calculated values. *J Am Diet Assoc* 90:375–381.

Pennington JA, Young BE. 1991. Total diet study nutritional elements, 1982–1989. *J Am Diet Assoc* 91:179–183.

Perloff BP, Rizek RL, Haytowitz DB, Reid PR. 1990. Dietary intake methodology. II. USDA's Nutrient Data Base for Nationwide Dietary Intake Surveys. *J Nutr* 120:1530–1534.

Petley A, Macklin B, Renwick AG, Wilkin TJ. 1995. The pharmacokinetics of nicotinamide in humans and rodents. *Diabetes* 44:152–155.

Pett LB, Ogilvie GH. 1956. The Canadian Weight-Height Survey. *Hum Biol* 28:177–188.

Pettifor JM, Ross FP, Moodley G, Wang J, Marco G, Skjolde C. 1978a. Serum calcium, magnesium, phosphorus, alkaline phosphatase and 25-hydroxyvitamin D concentrations in children. *S Afr Med J* 53:751–754.

Pettifor JM, Ross P, Wang J, Moodley G, Couper-Smith J. 1978b. Rickets in children of rural origin in South Africa: Is low dietary calcium a factor? *J Pediatr* 92:320–324.

Pettifor JM, Bikle DD, Cavaleros M, Zachen D, Kamdar MC, Ross FP. 1995. Serum levels of free 1,25-dihydroxyvitamin D in vitamin D toxicity. *Ann Intern Med* 122:511–513.

Pietschmann P, Woloszczuk W, Pietschmann H. 1990. Increased serum osteocalcin levels in elderly females with vitamin D deficiency. *Exp Clin Endocrinol* 95:275–278.

Pillai S, Bikle DD, Elias PM. 1987. 1,25-Dihydroxyvitamin D production and receptor binding in human keratinocytes varies with differentiation. *J Biol Chem* 263:5390–5395.

Pitkin RM, Reynolds WA, Williams GA, Hargis GK. 1979. Calcium metabolism in normal pregnancy: A longitudinal study. *Am J Obstet Gynecol* 133:781–787.

Pittard WB III, Geddes KM, Sutherland SE, Miller MC, Hollis BW. 1990. Longitudinal changes in the bone mineral content of term and premature infants. *Am J Dis Child* 144:36–40.

Pluckebaum JM, Chavez N. 1994. Nutritional status of Northwest Indiana Hispanics in a congregate meal program. *J Nutr Elderly* 13:1–22.

PNUN (Standing Nordic Committee on Food). 1989. *Nordic Nutrition Recommendations,* 2nd Edition. Oslo: Nordic Council of Ministers.

Ponder SW, McCormick DP, Fawcett HD, Palmer JL, McKernan MG, Brouhard BH. 1990. Spinal bone mineral density in children aged 5.00 through 11.99 years. *Am J Dis Child* 144:1346–1348.

Ponz de Leon M, Roncucci L, Di Donato P, Tassi L, Smerieri O, Amorico MG, Malagoli G, De Maria D, Antonioli A, Chahin NJ. 1988. Pattern of epithelial cell proliferation in colorectal mucosa of normal subjects and of patients with adenomatous polyps or cancer of the large bowel. *Cancer Res* 48:4121–4126.

Portale AA, Booth BE, Halloran BP, Morris RC Jr. 1984. Effect of dietary phosphorus on circulating concentrations of 1,25-dihydroxyvitamin D and immunoreactive parathyroid hormone in children with moderate renal insufficiency. *J Clin Invest* 73:1580–1589.

Portale AA, Halloran BP, Murphy MM, Morris RC. 1986. Oral intake of phosphorus can determine the serum concentration of 1,25-dihydroxyvitamin D by determining its production rate in humans. *J Clin Invest* 77:7–12.

Portale AA, Halloran BP, Morris RC Jr. 1987. Dietary intake of phosphorus modulates the circadian rhythm in serum concentration of phosphorus. Implications for the renal production of 1,25-dihydroxyvitamin D. *J Clin Invest* 80:1147–1154.

Portale AA, Halloran BP, Morris RC Jr. 1989. Physiologic regulation of the serum concentration of 1,25-dihydroxyvitamin D by phosphorus in normal men. *J Clin Invest* 83:1494–1499.

Prentice A, Laskey MA, Shaw J, Cole TJ, Fraser DR. 1990. Bone mineral content of Gambian and British children aged 0–36 months. *Bone Miner* 10:211–214.

Prentice A, Jarjou LM, Cole TJ, Stirling DM, Dibba B, Fairweather-Tait S. 1995. Calcium requirements of lactating Gambian mothers: Effects of a calcium supplement on breast-milk calcium concentration, maternal bone mineral content, and urinary calcium excretion. *Am J Clin Nutr* 62:58–67.

Prichard JL. 1969. The prenatal and postnatal effects of fluoride supplements on West Australian school children, aged 6, 7 and 8, Perth, 1967. *Austral Dent J* 14:335–338.

Prince RL, Smith M, Dick IM, Price RI, Webb PG, Henderson NK, Harris MM. 1991. Prevention of postmenopausal osteoporosis. A comparative study of exercise, calcium supplementation, and hormone-replacement therapy. *N Engl J Med* 325:1189–1195.

Prince R, Devine A, Dick I, Criddle A, Kerr D, Kent N, Price R, Randell A. 1995. The effects of calcium supplementation (milk powder or tablets) and exercise on bone density in postmenopausal women. *J Bone Miner Res* 10:1068–1075.

Purdie DW, Aaron JE, Selby PL. 1988. Bone histology and mineral homeostasis in human pregnancy. *Br J Obstet Gynecol* 95:849–854.

Quamme GA. 1989. Control of magnesium transport in the thick ascending limb. *Am J Physiol* 256:F197–F210.

Quamme GA. 1993. Laboratory evlauation of magnesium status. Renal function and free intracellular magnesium concentration. *Clin Lab Med* 13:209–223.

Quamme GA, Dirks JH. 1986. The physiology of renal magnesium handling. *Renal Physiol* 9:257–269.

Raisz LG, Niemann I. 1969. Effect of phosphate, calcium and magnesium on bone resorption and hormonal responses in tissue culture. *Endocrinology* 85:446–452.

Rajalakshmi K, Srikantia SG. 1980. Copper, zinc, and magnesium content of breast milk of Indian women. *Am J Clin Nutr* 33:664–669.

Raman L, Rajalakshmi K, Krishnamachari KA, Sastry JG. 1978. Effect of calcium supplementation to undernourished mothers during pregnancy on the bone density of the neonates. *Am J Clin Nutr* 31:466–469.

Randall RE, Cohen D, Spray CC, Rossmeisl EC. 1964. Hypermagnesemia in renal failure. *Ann Intern Med* 61:73–88.

Rao DR, Bello H, Warren AP, Brown GE. 1994. Prevalence of lactose maldigestion. Influence and interaction of age, race, and sex. *Dig Dis Sci* 39:1519–1524.

Rasmussen HS, McNair P, Goransson L, Balslov S, Larsen OG, Aurup P. 1988. Magnesium deficiency in patients with ischemic heart disease with and without acute myocardial infarction uncovered by an intravenous loading test. *Arch Intern Med* 148:329–332.

Ray NF, Chan JK, Thamer M, Melton LJ III. 1997. Medical expenditures for the treatment of osteoporotic fractures in the United States in 1995: Report from the National Osteoporosis Foundation. *J Bone Miner Res* 12:24–35.

Reasner CA II, Dunn JF, Fetchick DA, Liel Y, Hollis BW, Epstein S, Shary J, Mundy GR, Bell NH. 1990. Alteration of vitamin D metabolism in Mexican-Americans. *J Bone Miner Res* 5:13–17.

Recker RR. 1985. Calcium absorption and aclorhydria. *N Engl J Med* 313:70–73.

Recker RR, Hassing GS, Lau JR, Saville PD. 1973. The hyperphosphatemic effect of disodium ethane-1-hydroxy-1, 1-diphosphonate (EHDP): Renal handling of phosphorus and the renal response to parathyroid hormone. *J Lab Clin Med* 81:258–266.

Recker RR, Davies KM, Hinders SM, Heaney RP, Stegman MR, Kimmel DB. 1992. Bone gain in young adult women. *J Am Med Assoc* 268:2403–2408.

Recker RR, Hinders S, Davies KM, Heaney RP, Stegman MR, Lappe JM, Kimmel DB. 1996. Correcting calcium nutritional deficiency prevents spine fractures in elderly women. *J Bone Miner Res* 11:1961–1966.

Reddy GS, Norman AW, Willis DM, Goltzman D, Guyda H, Solomon S, Philips DR, Bishop JE, Mayer E. 1983. Regulation of vitamin D metabolism in normal human pregnancy. *J Clin Endocrinol Metab* 56:363–370.

Reed A, Haugen M, Pachman LM, Langman CB. 1990. Abnormalities in serum osteocalcin values in children with chronic rheumatic diseases. *J Pediatr* 116:574–580.

Reed JA, Anderson JJ, Tylavsky FA, Gallagher PN Jr. 1994. Comperative changes in radial-bone density of elderly female lacto-ovovegetarians and omnivores. *Am J Clin Nutr* 59:1197S–1202S.

Reginster JY, Strause L, Deroisy R, Lecart MP, Saltman P, Franchimont P. 1989. Preliminary report of decreased serum magnesium in postmenopausal osteoporosis. *Magnesium* 8:106–109.

Reichel H, Koeffler HP, Norman AW. 1989. The role of vitamin D endocrine system in health and disease. *N Engl J Med* 320:980–991.

Reid IR, Ames RW, Evans MC, Gamble GD, Sharpe SJ. 1995. Long-term effects of calcium supplementation on bone loss and fractures in postmenopausal women: A randomized controlled trial. *Am J Med* 98:331–335.

Reinhart RA. 1988. Magnesium metabolism. A review with special reference to the relationship between intracellular content and serum levels. *Arch Intern Med* 148:2415–2420.

Reinhold JG, Fardadji B, Abadi P, Ismail-Beigi F. 1991. Decreased absorption of calcium, magnesium, zinc and phosphorus by humans due to increased fiber and phosphorus consumption as wheat bread. *Am J Clin Nutr* 49:204–206.

Resnick LM, Gupta RK, Laragh JH. 1984. Intracellular free magnesium in erythrocytes of essential hypertension: Relation to blood pressure and serum divalent cations. *Proc Natl Acad Sci USA* 81:6511–6515.

Resnick L, Gupta R, and Bhargava KK, Gruenspan H, Alderman MH, Laragh JH. 1991. Cellular ions in hypertension, diabetes and obesity: A nuclear magnetic resonance spectroscopic study. *Hypertension* 17:951–957.

Riancho JA, delArco C, Arteaga R, Herranz JL, Albajar M, Macias JG. 1989. Influence of solar irradiation on vitamin D levels in children on anticonvulsant drugs. *Acta Neurol Scand* 79:296–299.

Ricci JM, Hariharan S, Helfott A, Reed K, O'Sullivan MJ. 1991. Oral tocolysis with magnesium chloride: A randomized controlled prospective clinical trial. *Am J Obstet Gynecol* 165:603–610.

Richards A, Mosekilde L, Søgaard CH. 1994. Normal age-related changes in fluoride content of vertebral trabecular bone—relation to bone quality. *Bone* 15:21–26.

Riggs BL, Melton LJ III. 1995. The worldwide problem of osteoporosis: Insights afforded by epidemiology. *Bone* 17:505S–511S.

Riggs BL, O'Fallon WM, Muse J, O'Conner MK, Melton LJ III. 1996. Long-term effects of calcium supplementation on serum PTH, bone turnover, and bone loss in elderly women. *J Bone Miner Res* 11:S118.

Rigo J, Salle BL, Picaud JC, Putet G, Senterre J. 1995. Nutritional evaluation of protein hydrolysate formulas. *Eur J Clin Nutr* 49:S26–S38.

Riis B, Thomsen K, Christiansen C. 1987. Does calcium supplementation prevent postmenopausal bone loss? *N Engl J Med* 316:173–177.

Ritz E. 1982. Acute hypophosphatemia. *Kidney Int* 22:84–94.

Rizzoli R, Stoermann C, Ammann P, Bonjour J-P. 1994. Hypercalcemia and hyperosteolysis in vitamin D intoxication: Effects of clodronate therapy. *Bone* 15:193–198.

Robertson, WG. 1985. Dietary factors important in calcium stone formation. In: Schwille PO, Smith LH, Robertson WG, Vahlensieck W, eds. *Urolithiasis and Related Clinical Research.* New York: Plenum Press. Pp. 61–68.

Romani A, Marfella C, Scarpa A. 1993. Cell magnesium transport and homeostasis: Role of intracellular compartments. *Miner Electrolyte Metab* 19:282–289.

Roncucci L, Scalmati A, Ponz de Leon M. 1991. Pattern of cell kinetics in colorectal mucosa of patients with different types of adenomatous polyps of the large bowel. *Cancer* 68:873–878.

Ronis DL, Lang WP, Farghaly MM, Passow E. 1993. Tooth brushing, flossing, and preventive dental visits by Detroit-area residents in relation to demographic and socioeconomic factors. *J Pub Hlth Dent* 53:138–145.

Rosado JL, Lopez P, Morales M, Munoz E, Allen LH. 1992. Bioavailability of energy, nitrogen, fat, zinc, iron and calcium from rural and urban Mexican diets. *Br J Nutr* 68:45–58.

Rowe JW, Minaker KL, Pallotta JA, Flier JS. 1983. Characterization of the insulin resistance of aging. *J Clin Invest* 71:1581–1587.

Rubenowitz E, Axelsson G, Rylander R. 1996. Magnesium in drinking water and death from acute myocardial infarction. *Am J Epidemiol* 143:456–462.

Rubin H. 1975. Central role for magnesium in coordinate control of metabolism and growth in animal cells. *Proc Natl Acad Sci USA* 72:3551–3555.

Rude RK. 1993. Magnesium metabolism and deficiency. *Endocrinol Metab Clin North Am* 22:377–395.

Rude RK, Olerich M. 1996. Magnesium deficiency: Possible role in osteoporosis associated with gluten-sensitive enteropathy. *Osteopor Int* 6:453–461.

Rude RK, Singer FR. 1980. Magnesium deficiency and excess. *Ann Rev Med* 32:245–259.

Rude RK, Oldham SB, Singer FR. 1976. Functional hypoparathyroidism and parathyroid hormone end-organ resistance in human magnesium deficiency. *Clin Endocrinol* 5:209–224.

Rude RK, Bethune JE, Singer FR. 1980. Renal tubular maximum for magnesium in normal, hyperparathyroid and hypoparathyroid man. *J Clin Endocrinol Metab* 51:1425–1431.

Rude RK, Manoogian C, Ehrlich L, DeRusso P, Ryzen E, Nadler J. 1989. Mechanisms of blood pressure regulation by magnesium in man. *Magnesium* 8:266–273.

Rude RK, Stephen A, Nadler J. 1991. Determination of red blood cell intracellular free magnesium by nuclear magnetic resonance as an assessment of magnesium depletion. *Magnes Trace Elem* 10:117–121.

Rudloff S, Lonnerdal B. 1990. Calcium retention from milk-based infant formulas, whey-hydrolysate formula, and human milk in weanling rhesus monkeys. *Am J Dis Child* 144:360–363.

Rudnicki M, Frolich A, Rasmussen WF, McNair P. 1991. The effect of magnesium on maternal blood pressure in pregnancy-induced hypertension. A randomized double-blind placebo-controlled trial. *Acta Obstet Gynecol Scand* 70:445–450.

Ruiz JC, Mandel C, Garabedian M. 1995. Influence of spontaneous calcium intake and physical exercise on the vertebral and femoral bone mineral density of children and adolescents. *J Bone Miner Res* 10:675–682.

Russell AL. 1949. Dental effects of exposure to fluoride-bearing Dakota sandstone waters at various ages and for various lengths of time. II. Patterns of dental caries inhibition as related to exposure span, to elapsed time since exposure, and to periods of calcification and eruption. *J Dent Res* 28:600–612.

Russell AL, Elvove E. 1951. Domestic water and dental caries. VII. A study of the fluoride-dental caries relationship in an adult population. *Pub Hlth Rep* 66:1389–1401.

Ryan MP. 1987. Diuretics and potassium/magnesium depletion. Directions for treatment. *Am J Med* 82:38–47.

Ryzen E, Elbaum N, Singer FR, Rude RK. 1985. Parenteral magnesium tolerance testing in the evaluation of magnesium deficiency. *Magnesium* 4:137–147.

Ryzen E, Elkayam U, Rude RK. 1986. Low blood mononuclear cell magnesium in intensive cardiac care unit patients. *Am Heart J* 111:475–480.

Sacks FM, Brown LE, Appel L, Borhani NO, Evans D, Whelton P. 1995. Combinations of potassium, calcium, and magnesium supplements in hypertension. *Hypertension* 26:950–956.

Sakhaee K, Baker S, Zerwekh J, Poindexter J, Garcia-Hernandez PA, Pak CY. 1994. Limited risk of kidney stone formation during long-term calcium citrate supplementation in nonstone forming subjects. *J Urol* 152:324–327.

Salama F, Whitford GM, Barenie JT. 1989. Fluoride retention by children from toothbrushing. *J Dent Res* 68(Spec Issue):335.

Salle BL, Delvin E, Glorieux F, David L. 1990. Human neonatal hypocalcemia. *Biol Neonate* 58:S22–S31.

Sandberg AS, Larsen T, Sandstrom B. 1993. High dietary calcium level decreases colonic phytate degradation in pigs fed a rapeseed diet. *J Nutr* 123:559–566.

Sanders TA, Purves R. 1981. An anthropometric and dietary assessment of the nutritional status of vegan preschool children. *J Human Nutr* 35:349–357.

Sandler RB, Slemenda CW, LaPorte RE, Cauley JA, Schramm MM, Barresi ML, Kriska AM. 1985. Postmenopausal bone density and milk consumption in childhood and adolescence. *Am J Clin Nutr* 42:270–274.

Saunders D, Sillery J, Chapman R. 1988. Effect of calcium carbonate and aluminum hydroxide on human intestinal function. *Dig Dis Sci* 33:409–412.

Schanler RJ, Garza C, Smith EO. 1985. Fortified mothers' milk for very low birth weight infants: Results of macromineral balance studies. *J Pediatr* 107:767–774.

Schendel DE, Berg CJ, Yeargin-Allsopp M, Boyle CA, Decoufle P. 1996. Prenatal magnesium sulfate exposure and the risk for cerebral palsy or mental retardation among very low-birth-weight children aged 3 to 5 years. *J Am Med Assoc* 276:1805–1810.

Schiffl H, Binswanger U. 1982. Renal handling of fluoride in healthy man. *Renal Physiol* 5:192–196.

Schiller L, Santa Ana C, Sheikh M, Emmett M, Fordtran J. 1989. Effect of the time of administration of calcium acetate on phosphorus binding. *N Engl J Med* 320:1110–1113.

Schlesinger ES, Overton DE, Riverhead LI, Chase HC, Cantwell KT. 1956. Newburgh-Kingston caries-fluorine study XIII. Pediatric findings after ten years. *J Am Dent Assoc* 52:296–306.

Schlesinger L, Arevalo M, Arredondo S, Diaz M, Lonnerdal B, Stekel A. 1992. Effect of a zinc-fortified formula on immunocompetence and growth of malnourished infants. *Am J Clin Nutr* 56:491–498.

Schmidt LE, Arfken CL, Heins JM. 1994. Evaluation of nutrient intake in subjects with non-insulin-dependent diabetes mellitus. *J Am Diet Assoc* 94:773–774.

Schmidt-Gayk H, Goossen J, Lendle F, Seidel D. 1977. Serum 25-hydroxycalciferol in myocardial infarction. *Atherosclerosis* 26:55–58.

Schneider EL, Guralnik JM. 1990. The aging of America. Impact on health care costs. *J Am Med Assoc* 263:2335–2340.

Schofield FA, and Morrell E. 1960. Calcium, phosphorus and magnesium. *Fed Proc* 19:1014–1016.

Schuman CA, Jones HW III. 1985. The "milk-alkali" syndrome: Two case reports with discussion of pathogenesis. *Quart J Med (New Series)* 55:119–126.

Schutzmannsky G. 1971. Fluoride tablet application in pregnant females. *Dtsch Stomatol* 21:122–129.

Schwartz E, Chokas WV, Panariello VA. 1964. Metabolic balance studies of high calcium intake in osteoporosis. *Am J Med* 36:233–249.

Schwartz GG, Hulka BS. 1990. Is vitamin D deficiency a risk factor for prostate cancer? *Anticancer Res* 10:1307–1312.

Schwartz R, Walker G, Linz MD, MacKellar I. 1973. Metabolic responses of adolescent boys to two levels of dietary magnesium and protein. I. Magnesium and nitrogen retention. *Am J Clin Nutr* 26:510–518.

Schwartz R, Spencer H, Welsh JJ. 1984. Magnesium absorption in human subjects from leafy vegetables, intrinsically labeled with stable ^{26}Mg. *Am J Clin Nutr* 39:571–576.

Schwartz R, Apgar BJ, Wien EM. 1986. Apparent absorption and retention of Ca, Cu, Mg, Mn, and Zn from a diet containing bran. *Am J Clin Nutr* 43:444–455.

Schwartzman MS, Franck WA. 1987. Vitamin D toxicity complicating the treatment of senile, postmenopausal, and glucocorticoid-induced osteoporosis: Four case reports and a critical commentary on the use of vitamin D in these disorders. *Am J Med* 82:224–229.

Sebastian A, Harris ST, Ottaway JH, Todd KM, Morris RC Jr. 1994. Improved mineral balance and skeletal metabolism in postmenopausal women treated with potassium bicarbonate. *N Engl J Med* 330:1776–1781.

Sebert JL, Garabedian M, Chauvenet M, Maamer M, Agbomson F, Brazier M. 1995. Evaluation of a new solid formulation of calcium and vitamin D in institutionalized elderly subjects: A randomized comparative trial versus separate administration of both constituents. *Rev Rhum* 62:288–294.

Seelig MS. 1981. Magnesium requirements in human nutrition. *Magnes Bull* 3(suppl):26–47.

Seelig MS. 1993. Interrelationship of magnesium and estrogen in cardiovascular and bone disorders, eclampsia, migraine and premenstrual syndrome. *J Am Coll Nutr* 12:442–458.

Seelig MS, Elin RJ. 1996. Is there a place for magnesium in the treatment of acute myocardial infarction? *Am Heart J* 132:471–477.

Seki K, Makimura N, Mitsui C, Hirata J, Nagata I. 1991. Calcium-regulating hormones and osteocalcin levels during pregnancy: A longtitudinal study. *Am J Obstet Gynecol* 164:1248–1252.

Selby PL. 1994. Calcium requirement—A reappraisal of the methods used in its determination and their application to patients with osteoporosis. *Am J Clin Nutr* 60:944–948.

Selby PL, Davies M, Marks JS, Mawer EB. 1995. Vitamin D intoxication causes hypercalcemia by increased bone resorption which responds to pamidronate. *Clin Endocrinol* 43:531–536.

Sentipal JM, Wardlaw GM, Mahan J, Matkovic V. 1991. Influence of calcium intake and growth indexes on vertebral bone mineral density in young females. *Am J Clin Nutr* 54:425–428.

Seydoux J, Girardin E, Paunier L, Beguin F. 1992. Serum and intracellular magnesium during normal pregnancy and in patients with pre-eclampsia. *Br J Obstet Gynecol* 99:207–211.

Shapses SA, Robins SP, Schwartz EI, Chowdhury H. 1995. Short-term changes in calcium but not protein intake alter the rate of bone resorption in healthy subjects as assessed by urinary pyridinium cross-link excretion. *J Nutr* 125:2814–2821.

Sharma OP. 1996. Vitamin D, calcium, and sarcoidosis. *Chest* 109:535–539.

Shen YW, Taves DR. 1974. Fluoride concentrations in the human placenta and maternal and cord blood. *Am J Obstet Gynecol* 119:205–207.

Sherman HC, Hawley E. 1922. Calcium and phosphorus metabolism in childhood. *J Biol Chem* 52:375–399.

Shils ME. 1969. Experimental human magnesium depletion. *Medicine* 46:61–85.

Shils ME. 1994. Magnesium. In: Shils ME, Olson JA, Shike M, eds. *Modern Nutrition in Health and Disease.* Philadelphia, PA: Lea & Febiger. Pp. 164–184.

Shils ME, Rude RK. 1996. Deliberations and evaluations of the approaches, endpoints and paradigms for magnesium dietary recommendations. *J Nutr* 126:2398S–2403S.

Sibai BM, Villar MA, Bray E. 1989. Magnesium supplementation during pregnancy: A double-blind randomized controlled clinical trial. *Am J Obstet Gynecol* 161:115–119.

Siener R, Hesse A. 1995. Influence of a mixed and a vegetarian diet on urinary magnesium excretion and concentration. *Br J Nutr* 73:783–790.

Silverberg SJ, Shane E, Clemens TL, Dempster DW, Segre GV, Lindsay R, Bilezidian JP. 1986. The effect of oral phosphate administration on major indices of skeletal metabolism in normal subjects. *J Bone Miner Res* 1:383–388.

Silvis SE, Paragas PD Jr. 1972. Paresthesias, weakness, seizures, and hypophosphatemia in patients receiving hyperalimentation. *Gastroenterology* 62:513–520.

Simard PL, Lachapelle C, Trahan L, Naccache H, Demers M, Broduer JM. 1989. The ingestion of fluoride dentifrice by young children. *J Dent Child* 56:177–181.

Simard PL, Naccache H, Lachapelle D, Brodeur JM. 1991. Ingestion of fluoride from dentifrices by children aged 12 to 24 months. *Clin Pediatr Phila* 30:614–617.

Simmer K, Khanum S, Carlsson L, Thompson RP. 1988. Nutritional rehabilitation in Bangladesh—the importance of zinc. *Am J Clin Nutr* 47:1036–1040.

Singer L, Ophaug R. 1979. Total fluoride intake of infants. *Pediatrics* 63:460–466.

Singer L, Ophaug RH, Harland BF. 1980. Fluoride intakes of young male adults in the United States. *Am J Clin Nutr* 33:328–332.

Singer L, Ophaug RH, Harland BF. 1985. Dietary fluoride intake of 15–19-year-old male adults residing in the United States. *J Dent Res* 64:1302–1305.

Singh A, Jolly SS. 1970. Chronic toxic effects on the skeletal system. In: *Fluorides and Human Health.* Geneva: World Health Organization. Pp 238–249.

Skajaa K, Dorup I, Sandstrom BM. 1991. Magnesium intake and status and pregnancy outcome in a Danish population. *Br J Obstet Gynecol* 98:919–928.

Slattery ML, Sorenson AW, Ford MH. 1988. Dietary calcium intake as a mitigating factor in colon cancer. *Am J Epidemiol* 128:504–514.

Slemenda CW, Reister TK, Hui SL, Miller JZ, Christian JC, Johnston CC Jr. 1994. Influences on skeletal mineralization in children and adolescents: Evidence for varying effects of sexual maturation and physical activity. *J Pediatr* 125:201–207.

Slemenda CW, Peacock M, Hui S, Zhou L, Johnston CC Jr. 1997. Reduced rates of skeletal remodeling are associated with increased bone mineral density during the development of peak skeletal mass. *J Bone Miner Res* 12:676–682.

Slesinski MJ, Subar AF, Kahle LL. 1996. Dietary intake of fat, fiber, and other nutrients is related to the use of vitamin and mineral supplements in the United States: The 1992 National Health Interview Survey. *J Nutr* 126:3001–3008.

Smilkstein MJ, Smolinske SC, Kulig KW, Rumack, BH. 1988. Severe hypermagnesemia due to multiple-dose cathartic therapy. *West J Med* 148:208–211.

Smith EL, Gilligan C, Smith PE, Sempos CT. 1989. Calcium supplementation and bone loss in middle-aged women. *Am J Clin Nutr* 50:833–842.

Smith KT, Heaney RP, Flora L, Hinders SM. 1987. Calcium absorption from a new calcium delivery system (CCM). *Calcif Tissue Int* 41:351–352.

Smith R, Dent CE. 1969. Vitamin D requirements in adults. Clinical and metabolic studies on seven patients with nutritional osteomalacia. *Bibl Nutr Dieta* 13:44–45.

Snedeker SM, Smith SA, Greger JL. 1982. Effect of dietary calcium and phosphorus levels on the utilization of iron, copper, and zinc by adult males. *J Nutr* 112:136–143.

Sojka JE, Wastney ME, Abrams S, Froese S, Martin BR, Weaver CM. 1997. Magnesium kinetics in adolescent girls determined using stable isotopes: Effects of high and low calcium intakes. *Am J Physiol* 273:R170–R175.

Sojka JE, Weaver CM. 1995. Magnesium supplementation and osteoporosis. *Nutr Rev* 53:71–74.

Sokoll LJ, Dawson-Hughes B. 1992. Calcium supplementation and plasma ferritin concentrations in premenopausal women. *Am J Clin Nutr* 56:1045–1048.

Sorva A, Risteli J, Risteli L, Valimaki M, Tilvis R. 1991. Effects of vitamin D and calcium on markers of bone metabolism in geriatric patients with low serum 25-hydroxyvitamin D levels. *Calcif Tissue Int* 49:S88–S89.

Southgate DAT, Widdowson EM, Smits BJ, Cooke WT, Walker CHM, Mathers NP. 1969. Absorption and excretion of calcium and fat by young infants. *Lancet* 1:487–489.

Sowers M, Wallace RB, Lemke JH. 1985. Correlates of forearm bone mass among women during maximal bone mineralization. *Prev Med* 14:585–596.

Sowers M, Wallace RB, Lemke JH. 1986. The relationship of bone mass and fracture history to fluoride and calcium intake: A study of three communities. *Am J Clin Nutr* 44:889–898.

Sowers M, Clark MK, Jannausch ML, Wallace RB. 1991. A prospective study of bone mineral content and fracture in communities with differential fluoride exposure. *Am J Epidemiol* 133:649–660.

Sowers M, Corton G, Shapiro B, Jannausch ML, Crutchfield M, Smith ML, Randolph JF, Hollis B. 1993. Changes in bone density with lactation. *J Am Med Assoc* 269:3130–3135.

Sowers M, Randolph J, Shapiro B, Jannaush M. 1995a. A prospective study of bone density and pregnancy after an extended period of lactation with bone loss. *Obstet Gynecol* 85:285–289.

Sowers M, Eyre D, Hollis BW, Randloph JF, Shapiro B, Jannausch ML, Crutchfield M. 1995b. Biochemical markers of bone turnover in lactating and nonlactating postpartum women. *J Clin Endocrinol Metab.* 80:2210–2216.

Spak CJ, Ekstrand J, Zylberstein D. 1982. Bioavailability of fluoride added by baby formula and milk. *Caries Res* 16:249–256.

Spak CJ, Hardell LI, De Chateau P. 1983. Fluoride in human milk. *Acta Paediatr Scand* 72:699–701.

Spatling L, Spatling G. 1988. Magnesium supplementation in pregnancy. A double blind study. *Br J Obstet Gynecol* 95:120–125.

Specker BL. 1996. Evidence for an interaction between calcium intake and physical activity on changes in bone mineral density. *J Bone Miner Res* 11:1539–1544.

Specker BL, Tsang RC. 1987. Cyclical serum 25-hydroxyvitamin D concentrations paralleling sunshine exposure in exclusively breast-fed infants. *J Pediatr* 110:744–747.

Specker BL, Tsang RC, Hollis BW. 1985a. Effect of race and diet on human-milk vitamin D and 25-hydroxyvitamin D. *Am J Dis Child* 139:1134–1137.

Specker BL, Valanis B, Hertzberg V, Edwards N, Tsang RC. 1985b. Sunshine exposure and serum 25-hydroxyvitamin D concentrations in exclusively breast-fed infants. *J Pediatr* 107:372–376.

Specker BL, Lichtenstein P, Mimouni F, Gormley C, Tsang RC. 1986. Calcium-regulating hormones and minerals from birth to 18 months of age: A cross-sectional study. II. Effects of sex, race, age, season, and diet on serum minerals, parathyroid hormone, and calcitonin. *Pediatrics* 77:891–896.

Specker BL, Tsang RC, Ho ML, Miller D. 1987. Effect of vegetarian diet on serum 1,25-dihydroxyvitamin D concentrations during lactation. *Obstet Gynecol* 70:870–874.

Specker BL, Tsang RC, Ho ML. 1991a. Changes in calcium homeostasis over the first year postpartum: Effect of lactation and weaning. *Obstet Gynecol* 78:56–62.

Specker BL, Tsang RC, Ho ML, Landi TM, Gratton TL. 1991b. Low serum calcium and high parathyroid hormone levels in neonates fed "humanized" cow's milk-based formula. *Am J Dis Child* 145:941–945.

Specker BL, Ho ML, Oestreich A, Yin TA, Shui QM, Chen XC, Tsang RC. 1992. Prospective study of vitamin D supplementation and rickets in China. *J Pediatr* 120:733–739.

Specker BL, Vieira NE, O'Brien KO, Ho ML, Heubi JE, Abrams SA, Yergey AL. 1994. Calcium kinetics in lactating women with low and high calcium intakes. *Am J Clin Nutr* 59:593–599.

Specker BL, Beck A, Kalkwarf H, Ho M. 1997. Randomized trial of varying mineral intake on total body bone mineral accretion during the first year of life. *Pediatrics* 99:e12.

Spencer H, Menczel J, Lewin I, Samachson J. 1965. Effect of high phosphorus intake on calcium and phosphorus metabolism in man. *J Nutr* 86:125–132.

Spencer H, Lewin I, Fowler J, Samachson J. 1969. Influence of dietary calcium intake on Ca^{47} absorption in man. *Am J Med* 46:197–205.

Spencer H, Kramer L, Osis D, Norris C. 1978a. Effect of phosphorus on the absorption of calcium and on the calcium balance in man. *J Nutr* 108:447–457.

Spencer H, Lesniak M, Gatza CA, Kramer L, Norris C, Coffey J. 1978b. Magnesium-calcium interrelationships in man. *Trace Substances Environ Hlth* 12:241–247.

Spencer H, Kramer L, Lesniak M, DeBartolo M, Norris C, Osis D. 1984. Calcium requirements in humans. Report of original data and a review. *Clin Orthop Relat Res* 184:270–280.

Spencer H, Fuller H, Norris C, Williams D. 1994. Effect of magnesium on the intestinal absorption of calcium in man. *J Am Coll Nutr* 13:485–492.

Spenser H, Osis D, Lender M. 1981. Studies of fluoride metabolism in man. A review and report of original data. *Sci Total Environ* 17:1–12.

Stamp TCB, Haddad JG, Twigg CA. 1977. Comparison of oral 25-hydroxycholecalciferol, vitamin D, and ultraviolet light as determinants of circulating 25-hydroxyvitamin D. *Lancet* 1:1341–1343.

Stanbury SW. 1971. The phosphate ion in chronic renal failure. In: Hioco DJ, ed. *Phosphate et Metabolisme Phosphocalcique.* Paris: Sandoz Laboratories.

Stapleton FB. 1994. Hematuria associated with hypercalciuria and hyperuricosuria: A practical approach. *Pediatr Nephrol* 8:756–761.

Stearns G. 1968. Early studies of vitamin D requirement during growth. *Am J Pub Hlth* 58:2027–2035.

Steenbock H, Black A. 1924. The reduction of growth-promoting and calcifying properties in a ration by exposure to ultraviolet light. *J Biol Chem* 61:408–422.

Steichen JJ, Tsang RC. 1987. Bone mineralization and growth in term infants fed soy-based or cow milk-based formula. *J Pediatr* 110:687–692.

Stein JH, Smith WO, Ginn HE. 1966. Hypophosphatemia in acute alcoholism. *Am J Med Sci* 252:78–83.

Stendig-Lindberg G, Tepper R, Leichter I. 1993. Trabecular bone density in a two year controlled trial of peroral magnesium in osteoporosis. *Magnes Res* 6:155–163.

Stephen KW, McCall DR, Tullis JI. 1987. Caries prevalence in northern Scotland before, and 5 years after, water defluoridation. *Br Dent J* 163:324–326.

Stevenson CA, Watson AR. 1957. Fluoride osteosclerosis. *Am J Roentg Rad Ther Nucl Med* 78:13–18.

Stumpf WE, Sar M, Reid FA, Tanakay Y, DeLuca HF. 1979. Target cells for 1,25-dihydroxyvitamin D$_3$ in intestinal tract, stomach, kidney, skin, pituitary, and parathyroid. *Science* 206:1188-1190.

Suarez FL, Savaiano DA, Levitt MD. 1995. A comparison of symptoms after the consumption of milk or lactose-hydrolyzed milk by people with self-reported severe lactose intolerance. *N Engl J Med* 333:1–4.

Svenningsen NW, Lindquist B. 1974. Postnatal development of renal hydrogen ion excretion capacity in relation to age and protein intake. *Acta Paediatr Scand* 63:721–731.

Switzer RL. 1971. Regulation and mechanism of phosphoribosylpyrophosphate synthetase. III. Kinetic studies of the reaction mechanism. *J Biol Chem* 246:2447–2458.

Tanner JT, Smith J, Defibaugh P, Angyal G, Villalobos M, Bueno MP, McGarrahan ET, Wehr HM, Muniz JF, Hollis BW. 1988. Survey of vitamin content of fortified milk. *J Assoc Off Anal Chem* 71: 607–610.

Tanner JM. 1990. *Growth at Adolescence.* Oxford: Oxford University Press.

Tatevossian A. 1990. Fluoride in dental plaque and its effects. *J Dent Res* 69(Spec Iss): 645–652.

Taves DR. 1978. Fluoridation and mortality due to heart disease. *Nature* 272:361–362.

Taves DR. 1983. Dietary intake of fluoride ashed (total fluoride) v. unashed (inorganic fluoride) analysis of individual foods. *Br J Nutr* 49:295–301.

Taves DR, Neuman WF. 1964. Factors controlling calcification in vitro: Fluoride and magnesium. *Arch Biochem Biophys* 108:390–397.

Taylor AF, Norman ME. 1984. Vitamin D metabolite levels in normal children. *Pediatr Res* 18: 886–890.

Taylor CB, Hass GM, Ho KJ, Liu LB. 1972. Risk factors in the pathogenesis of arteriosclerotic heart disease and generalized atherosclerosis. *Ann Clin Lab Sci* 2:239.

Teegarden D, Proulx WR, Martin BR, Zhao J, McCabe GP, Lyle RM, Peacock M, Slemenda C, Johnston CC, Weaver CM. 1995. Peak bone mass in young women. *J Bone Miner Res* 10:711–715.

Ten Cate JM. 1990. In vitro studies on the effects of fluoride on de- and remineralization. *J Dent Res* 69(Spec Iss):614–619.

Terblanche S, Noakes TD, Dennis SC, Marais D, Eckert M. 1992. Failure of magnesium supplementation to influence marathon running performance or recovery in magnesium-replete subjects. *Int J Sport Nutr* 2:154–164.

Tesar R, Notelovitz M, Shim E, Kauwell G, Brown J. 1992. Axial and peripheral bone density and nutrient intakes of postmenopausal vegetarian and omnivorous women. *Am J Clin Nutr* 56:699–704.

Thatcher HS, Rock L. 1928. Clinical notes, suggestions and new instruments. *J Am Med Assoc* 91:1185–1186.

Theintz G, Buchs B, Rizzoli R, Slosman D, Clavien H, Sizonenko PC, Bonjour JP. 1992. Longitudinal monitoring of bone mass accumulation in healthy adolescents: Evidence for a marked reduction after 16 years of age at the levels of lumbar spine and femoral neck in female subjects. *J Clin Endocrinol Metab* 75:1060–1065.

Thompson FE, Byers T. 1994. Dietary assessment resource manual. *J Nutr* 124:2245S–2317S.

Thys-Jacobs S, Ceccarelli S, Bierman A, Weisman H, Cohen M-A, Alvir J. 1989. Calcium supplementation in premenstrual syndrome: A randomized crossover trial. *J Gen Intern Med* 4:183–189.

Tillman DM, Semple PF. 1988. Calcium and magnesium in essential hypertension. *Clin Sci* 75:395–402.

Touitou Y, Godard JP, Ferment O, Chastang C, Proust J, Bogdan A, Auzeby A, Touitou C. 1987. Prevalence of magnesium and potassium deficiencies in the elderly. *Clin Chem* 33:518–523.

Travis SF, Sugerman HJ, Ruberg RL, Dudrick SJ, Delivoria-Papadopoulos M, Miller L, Oski FA. 1971. Alterations of red cell glycolytic intermediates and oxygen transport as a consequence of hypophosphatemia in patients receiving intravenous hyperalimentation. *N Engl J Med* 285:763–768.

Tremaine WJ, Newcomer AD, Riggs BL, McGill DB. 1986. Calcium absorption from milk in lactase-deficient and lactase-sufficient adults. *Dig Dis Sci* 31:376–378.

Tsang RC, Strub R, Brown DR, Steichen J, Hartman C, Chen IW. 1976. Hypomagnesemia in infants of diabetic mothers: Perinatal studies. *J Pediatr* 89:115–119.

Tucker K. 1996. The use of epidemiological approaches and meta-analysis to determine mineral element requirements. *J Nutr* 126:2365S–2372S.

Tucker K, Kiel DP, Hannan MT, Felson DT. 1995. Magnesium intake is associated with bone-mineral density (BMD) in elderly women. *J Bone Miner Res* 10:S466.

Tylavsky FA, Anderson JJ. 1988. Dietary factors in bone health of elderly lactoovovegetarian and omnivorous women. *Am J Clin Nutr* 48:842–849.

Urakabe S, Nakata K, Ando A, Orita Y, Abe Y. 1975. Hypokalemia and metabolic acidosis from overuse of magnesium oxide. *Jpn Circ J* 39:1135–1137.

USDA (US Department of Agriculture). 1985. *Nationwide Food Consumption Survey. Continuing Survey of Food Intakes of Individuals.* Women 19–50 years and their children 1–5 years, 1 day, 1985. Report No. 85-1. Hyattsville, MD: Nutrition Monitoring Division, Human Nutrition Information Service, USDA.

USDA (US Department of Agriculture). 1991. *Provisional Table on the Vitamin D Content of Foods.* Hyattsville, MD: Nutrient Data Research Branch, USDA.

USDA (US Department of Agriculture), Center for Nutrition Policy and Promotion. 1997. *Nutrient Content of the U.S. Food Supply, 1909–1994.* Washington DC: Center for Nutrition Policy and Promotion, USDA.

USPHS (US Public Health Service). 1991. *Ad Hoc Subcommittee on Fluoride: Review of Fluoride Benefits and Risks.* Bethesda, MD: Department of Health and Human Services.

Venkataraman PS, Tsang RC, Greer FR, Noguchi A, Laskarzewski P, Steichen JJ. 1985. Late infantile tetany and secondary hyperparathyroidism in infants fed humanized cow milk formula. Longitudinal follow-up. *Am J Dis Child* 139:664–668.

Vicchio D, Yergey A, O'Brien K, Allen L, Ray R, Holick MF. 1993. Quantification and kinetics of 25-hydroxyvitamin D_3 by isotope dilution liquid chromatography/thermospray mass spectrometry. *Biol Mass Spectrom* 22:53–58.

Vik T, Try K, Thelle DS, Forde OH. 1979. Tromso heart study: Vitamin D metabolism and myocardial infarction. *Br Med J* 2:176.

Villar J, Repke JT. 1990. Calcium supplementation during pregnancy may reduce preterm delivery in high-risk populations. *Am J Obstet Gynecol* 163:1124–1131.

Villareal DT, Civitelli R, Chines A, Avioli LV. 1991. Subclinical vitamin D deficiency in postmenopausal women with low vertebral bone mass. *J Clin Endocrinol Metab* 72: 628–634.

Wacker WE, Parisi AF. 1968. Magnesium metabolism. *N Engl J Med* 45:658–663, 712–717, 772–776.

Wagener DK, Novrjah P, Horowitz AM. 1995. *Trends in Childhood Use of Dental Care Products Containing Fluoride: United States, 1983–1989.* Advance data from Vital Health Statistics of the Center for Disease Control. National Center for Health Statistics #219; Nov. 20, 1992. Hyattsville, MD: National Center for Health Statistics.

Walker AR, Richardson B, Walker F. 1972. The influence of numerous pregnancies and lactations on bone dimensions in South African Bantu and Caucasian mothers. *Clin Sci* 42:189–196.

Walker RM, Linkswiler HM. 1972. Calcium retention in the adult human male as affected by protein intake. *J Nutr* 102:1297–1302.

Wallach S, Verch RL. 1986. Tissue magnesium in spontaneously hypertensive rats. *Magnesium* 5:33–38.

Wang CC, Kern R, Kaucher M. 1930. Minimum requirement of calcium and phosphorus in children. *Am J Dis Child* 39:768–773.

Wardlaw GM, Pike AM. 1986. The effect of lactation on peak adult shaft and ultradistal forearm bone mass in women. *Am J Clin Nutr* 44:283–286.

Wasnich R, Yano K, Vogel J. 1983. Postmenopausal bone loss at multiple skeletal sites: Relationship to estrogen use. *J Chron Dis* 36:781–790.

Wastney ME, Ng J, Smith D, Martin BR, Peacock M, Weaver CM. 1996. Differences in calcium kinetics between adolescent girls and young women. *Am J Physiol* 271:R208–R216.

Waterhouse C, Taves D, Munzer A. 1980. Serum inorganic fluoride: Changes related to previous fluoride intake, renal function and bone resorption. *Clin Sci* 58:145–152.

Weaver CM. 1994. Age-related calcium requirements due to changes in absorption and utilization. *J Nutr* 124:1418S–1425S.

Weaver CM, Martin BR, Plawecki KL, Peacock M, Wood OB, Smith DL, Wastney ME. 1995. Differences in calcium metabolism between adolescent and adult females. *Am J Clin Nutr* 61:577–581.

Webb AR, Kline L, Holick MF. 1988. Influence of season and latitude on the cutaneous synthesis of vitamin D_3: Exposure to winter sunlight in Boston and Edmonton will not promote vitamin D_3 synthesis in human skin. *J Clin Endocrinol Metab* 67:373–378.

Webb AR, De Costa BR, Holick MF. 1989. Sunlight regulates the cutaneous production of vitamin D_3 by causing its photodegradation. *J Clin Endocrinol Metab* 68:882–887.

Webb AR, Pilbeam C, Hanafin N, Holick MF. 1990. An evaluation of the relative contributions of exposure to sunlight and of diet to the circulating concentrations of 25-hydroxyvitamin D in an elderly nursing home population in Boston. *Am J Clin Nutr* 51:1075–1081.

Wei SH, Hattab FN, Mellberg JR. 1989. Concentration of fluoride and selected other elements in teas. *Nutrition* 5:237–240.

Weinsier RL, Krumdieck CL. 1981. Death resulting from overzealous total parenteral nutrition: The refeeding syndrome revisited. *Am J Clin Nutr* 34:393–399.

Weisman Y, Harell A, Edelstein S, Spirer Z, Golander A. 1979. 1,25-dihydroxyvitamin D_3 and 24,25-dihydroxyvitamin D_3 in vitro synthesis by human decidua and placenta. *Nature* 281:317–319.

Weissberg N, Schwartz G, Shemesh O, Brooks BA, Algur N, Eylath U, Abraham AS. 1992. Serum and mononuclear cell potassium, magnesium, sodium and calcium in pregnancy and labour and their relation to uterine muscle contraction. *Magnes Res* 5:173–177.

Wester PO, Dyckner T. 1980. Diuretic treatment and magnesium losses. *Acta Med Scand* 647:145–152.

Whitford GM. 1994. Effects of plasma fluoride and dietary calcium concentrations on GI absorption and secretion of fluoride in the rat. *Calcif Tissue Int* 54:421–425.

Whitford GM. 1996. The metabolism and toxicity of fluoride. In Myers HM, ed. *Monographs in Oral Science, 2nd Revised Edition.* Basel, Switzerland: Karger.

Whitford GM, Allmann DW, Shahed AR. 1987. Topical fluorides: Effects on physiologic and biochemical processes. *J Dent Res* 66:1072–1078.

Whiting SJ, Pluhator MM. 1992. Comparison of in vitro and in vivo tests for determination of availability of calcium from calcium carbonate tablets. *J Am Coll Nutr* 11:553–560.

Whiting SJ, Wood RJ. 1997. Adverse effects of high-calcium diets in humans. *Nutr Rev* 55:1–9.

WHO (World Health Organization). 1984. *Fluorine and Fluorides.* Environmental Health Criteria 36. Geneva: World Health Organization. Pp. 77–79.

WHO (World Health Organization). 1987. *Principles for the Safety Assessment of Food Additives and Contaminants in Food.* Environmental Health Criteria 70. Geneva: World Health Organization.

WHO (World Health Organization). 1994. *Assessment of Fracture Risk and its Application to Screening for Postmenopausal Osteoporosis.* Technical Report Series 843. Geneva: World Health Organization.

WHO (World Health Organization). 1996. *Trace Elements in Human Nutrition and Health.* Prepared in collaboration with the Food and Agriculture Organization of the United Nations and the International Atomic Energy Agency. Geneva: World Health Organization.

Wickham CA, Walsh K, Cooper C, Barker DJ, Margetts BM, Morris J, Bruce SA. 1989. Dietary calcium, physical activity, and risk of hip fracture: A prospective study. *Br Med J* 299:889–892.

Widdowson EM. 1965. Absorption and excretion of fat, nitrogen, and minerals from "filled" milks by babies one week old. *Lancet* 2:1099–1105.

Widdowson EM, Dickerson JWT. 1964. The chemical composition of the body. In: Comar CL, Bronner F, eds. *Mineral Metabolism: An Advanced Treatise, Vol. II. The Elements, Part A.* New York: Academic Press.

Widdowson EM, McCance RA, Spray CM. 1951. The chemical composition of the human body. *Clin Sci* 10:113–125.

Widman L, Wester PO, Stegmayr BK, Wirell M. 1993. The dose-dependent reduction in blood pressure through administration of magnesium. A double blind placebo controlled cross-over study. *Am J Hypertens* 6:41–45.

Wiktorsson AM, Martinsson T, Zimmerman M. 1992. Caries prevalence among adults in communities with optimal and low water fluoride concentrations. *Community Dent Oral Epidemiol* 20:359–363.

Wilkinson R. 1976. Absorption of calcium, phosphorus, and magnesium. In: Nordin BEC, ed. *Calcium, Phosphate and Magnesium Metabolism.* Edinburgh: Churchill Livingstone. Pp. 36–112.

Willett W. 1990. *Nutritional Epidemiology.* New York, NY: Oxford University Press.

Willett WC, Sampson L, eds. 1997. Dietary assessment methods. *Am J Clin Nutr* 65:1097S–1368S.

Williams JE, Zwemer JD. 1990. Community water fluoride levels, preschool dietary patterns, and the occurrence of fluoride dental opacities. *J Pub Hlth Dent* 50:276–281.

Williams ML, Rose CS, Morrow G, Sloan SE, Barness LA. 1970. Calcium and fat absorption in neonatal period. *Am J Clin Nutr* 23:1322–1330.

Wilson SG, Retallack RW, Kent JC, Worth GK, Gutteridge DH. 1990. Serum free 1,25-dihydroxyvitamin D and the free 1,25-dihydroxyvitamin D index during a longitudinal study of human pregnancy and lactation. *Clin Endocrinol* 32:613–622.

Wise A, Gilburt DJ. 1982. Phytate hydrolysis by germfree and conventional rats. *Appl Environ Microbiol* 43:753–756.

Wisker E, Nagel R, Tanudjaja TK, Feldheim W. 1991. Calcium, magnesium, zinc, and iron balances in young women: Effects of a low-phytate barley-fiber concentrate. *Am J Clin Nutr* 54:553–559.

Witteman JC, Willett WC, Stampfer MJ, Colditz GA, Sacks FM, Speizer FE, Rosner B, Hennekens CH. 1989. A prospective study of nutritional factors and hypertension among U.S. women. *Circulation* 80:1320–1327.

Witteman JC, Grobbee DE, Derkx FH, Bouillon R, de Bruijn AM, Hofman A. 1994. Reduction of blood pressure with oral magnesium supplementation in women with mild to moderate hypertension. *Am J Clin Nutr* 60:129–135.

Wong NL, Quamme GA, Dirks JH. 1986. Effects of acid-base disturbances on renal handling of magnesium in the dog. *Clin Sci* 70:277–284.

Wood RJ, Zheng JJ. 1990. Milk consumption and zinc retention in postmenopausal women. *J Nutr* 120:398–403.

Wood RJ, Sitrin MD, Rosenberg IH. 1988. Effect of phosphorus on endogenous calcium losses during total parenteral nutrition. *Am J Clin Nutr* 48:632–636.

Woods KL, Fletcher S. 1994. Long-term outcome after intravenous magnesium sulphate in suspected acute myocardial infarction: The second Leicester Intravenous Magnesium Intervention Trial (LIMIT-2). *Lancet* 343:816–819.

Workshop Reports. 1992. *J Dent Res* 71:1218–1227.

Yamagata Z, Miyamura T, Iijima S, Asaka A, Sasaki M, Kato J, Koizumi K. 1994. Vitamin D receptor gene polymorphism and bone mineral density in healthy Japanese women. *Lancet* 344:1027.

Yamamoto ME, Applegate WB, Klag MJ, Borhani NO, Cohen JD, Kirchner KA, Lakatos E, Sacks FM, Taylor JO, Hennekens CH. 1995. Lack of blood pressure effect with calcium and magnesium supplementation in adults with high-normal blood pressure. Results from Phase I of the Trials of Hypertension Prevention (TOHP). Trials of Hypertension Prevention (TOHP) Collaborative Research Group. *Ann Epidemiol* 5:96–107.

Yano K, Heilbrun LK, Wasnich RD, Hankin JH, Vogel JM. 1985. The relationship between diet and bone mineral content of multiple skeletal sites in elderly Japanese men and women living in Hawaii. *Am J Clin Nutr* 42:877–888.

Young GP, Thomas RJ, Bourne DW, Russell DM. 1985. Parenteral nutrition. *Med J Aust* 143:597–601.

Zeghoud F, Vervel C, Guillozo H, Walrant-Debray O, Boutignon H, Garabedian M. 1997. Subclinical vitamin D deficiency in neonates: Definition and response to vitamin D supplements. *Am J Clin Nutr* 65:771–778.

Zemel PC, Zemel MB, Urberg M, Douglas FL, Geiser R, Sower JR. 1990. Metabolic and hemodynamic effects of magnesium supplementation in patients with essential hypertension. *Am J Clin Nutr* 51:665–669.

Ziegler EE, Fomon SJ. 1983. Lactose enhances mineral absorption in infancy. *J Pediatr Gastroenterol Nutr* 2:228–294.

Zielhuis RL, van der Kreek FW. 1979. The use of a safety factor in setting health-based permissible levels for occupational exposure. *Int Arch Occup Environ Health* 42:191–201.

Zipkin I, Zucas SM, Lavender DR, Fullmer HM, Schiffmann E, Corcoran BA. 1970. Fluoride and calcification of rat aorta. *Calcif Tissue Res* 6:173–182.

A

Origin and Framework of the Development of Dietary Reference Intakes

This report is the first in a series of publications resulting from the comprehensive effort being undertaken by the Food and Nutrition Board's (FNB) Standing Committee on the Scientific Evaluation of Dietary Reference Intakes (DRI Committee) and its panels and subcommittees.

ORIGIN

This initiative began in June 1993, when the FNB organized a symposium and public hearing entitled "Should the Recommended Dietary Allowances Be Revised?" Shortly thereafter, to continue its collaboration with the larger nutrition community on the future of the Recommended Dietary Allowances (RDAs), the FNB took two major steps: (1) it prepared, published, and disseminated the concept paper "How Should the Recommended Dietary Allowances Be Revised?" (IOM, 1994), which invited comments regarding the proposed concept, and (2) it held several symposia at nutrition-focused professional meetings to discuss the FNB's tentative plans and to receive responses to this initial concept paper.

The five general conclusions presented in the 1994 concept paper are as follows:

1. Sufficient new information has accumulated to support a reassessment of RDAs.
2. Where sufficient data for efficacy and safety exist, reduction in the risk of chronic degenerative disease is a concept that should be included in the formulation of future recommendations.

3. Upper levels of intake should be established where data exist regarding risk of toxicity.

4. Components of food of possible benefit to health, although not meeting the traditional concept of a nutrient, should be reviewed, and if adequate data exist, reference intakes should be established.

5. Serious consideration must be given to developing a new format for presenting future recommendations.

Subsequent to the symposium and release of the concept paper, the FNB held workshops at which invited experts discussed many issues related to the development of nutrient-based reference values, and FNB members have continued to provide updates and engage in discussions at professional meetings. In addition, the FNB gave attention to the international uses of the earlier RDAs and the expectation that the scientific review of nutrient requirements should be similar for comparable populations.

Concurrently, Health Canada and Canadian scientists were reviewing the need for revision of the *Recommended Nutrient Intakes* (RNIs) (Health Canada, 1990). Consensus following a symposium for Canadian scientists cosponsored by the Canadian National Institute of Nutrition and Health Canada in April 1995 was that the Canadian government should pursue the extent to which involvement with the developing FNB process would be of benefit to both Canada and the United States in terms of leading toward harmonization.

Based on extensive input and deliberations, the FNB initiated action to provide a framework for the development and possible international harmonization of nutrient-based recommendations that would serve, where warranted, for all of North America. To this end, in December 1995, the FNB began a close collaboration with the government of Canada and took action to establish the DRI Committee. It is hoped that representatives from Mexico will join in future deliberations.

RATIONALE FOR THE FRAMEWORK

The 1993 symposium and subsequent activities have provided substantial evidence that a comprehensive, coordinated approach to developing DRIs is needed for diet planning, nutritional assessment, and nutrition policy development. The current framework is based on the following four assumptions:

1. Since the publication of the tenth edition of *Recommended Dietary Allowances* (NRC, 1989a) in the United States and *Canadian Recommended Nutrient Intakes* (Health Canada, 1990), there has been a significant expansion and evolution of the research base in relation to a move toward defining functional endpoints that are relevant to the understanding of nutrient requirements and food constituents and their relationship to a number of aspects of human health.

2. These advances allow the refinement of the conceptual framework for defining nutrient requirements quantitatively and a clearer determination of the legitimate uses of nutrient requirement estimates and their derivatives in the interpretation and use of dietary intake data. Such uses might broadly be categorized according to whether they are (a) *prescriptive or planning* applications, where suitable levels of nutrient intake by individuals and/or population groups are established, and (b) *diagnostic or assessment* applications, where determinations are made about the likely nutritional adequacy of the observed intake when considered in relation to appropriate nutrient requirement data. Major differences in the types of information required about nutrient needs and relevant nutrient intake data are fundamental to appropriately focusing on the individual or on a defined population group (Beaton, 1994).

3. Neither the RDAs nor the Canadian RNIs have been applied appropriately in many settings. The availability of only a single type of reference value in the face of various needs has led to inappropriate applications. Moreover, inconsistent methods and criteria for deriving certain RDAs and RNIs and insufficient documentation of approaches and criteria have also contributed to inappropriate applications.

4. In these times of extensive international collaboration, agricultural and food exchange, and global nutrition-related health problems, harmonization of nutrient-based dietary standards between Canada and the United States is viewed as a first step, with the expectation that Mexico will be able to join in the near future. Such harmonization within the North American continent would further global development of similar efforts. Although the same general approaches have been used by most countries in developing recommended nutrient intakes (e.g., RDAs in the United States, RNIs in Canada, and Dietary Reference Values [DRVs] in Great Britain), and physiological requirements for nutrients are expected to be similar across healthy population groups, many of the quantitative values that have emerged from the different national expert groups are quite divergent, largely reflecting differences in the interpretation and use of scientific data and often based on different food

habits and indigenous diets. A mechanism is needed to determine the commonality of the bases on which recommendations are made and to use scientific data to indicate differences in requirements among apparently similar population groups in different geographic locations.

DESCRIPTION OF THE FRAMEWORK

In 1995, the DRI Committee was appointed to oversee and conduct this project. To accomplish this task over a period of 5 years, the DRI Committee devised a plan that involves the work of seven or more expert related nutrient group panels and two overarching subcommittees (Figure A-1). The process described below is expected to be used for subsequent panels, which will interact with an additional Subcommittee on the Uses and Interpretation of the DRIs.

The related nutrient group panels, composed of experts on those nutrients, are responsible for (1) reviewing the scientific literature concerning specific nutrients under study for each stage of the lifespan, (2) considering the roles of nutrients in decreasing risk of chronic and other diseases and conditions, and (3) interpreting the current data on intakes in North American population groups. The panels are charged with analyzing the literature, evaluating possible criteria or indicators of adequacy, and providing substantive rationales for their choices of each criterion. Using the criterion or criteria chosen for each stage of the lifespan, the panels estimate the average requirement for each nutrient or food component reviewed, assuming that adequate data are available. As the panel members review data on requirements, they also interact with two subcommittees regarding their group of nutrients. The Subcommittee on Upper Reference Levels is charged with reviewing possible risk assessment models for estimating levels of nutrients that may increase risk of toxicity or adverse effects and then assisting the panel to apply the model to each nutrient or food component reviewed. Similarly, a Subcommittee on the Uses and Interpretation of the DRIs is proposed to assist the panels and DRI Committee in the development of practical information and guidance using the many DRIs appropriately. Based on interaction with and from information provided by the panels and subcommittees, the DRI Committee determined the DRI values to be included in the report.

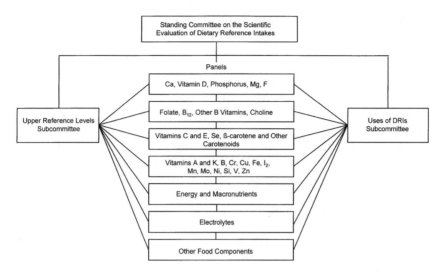

FIGURE A-1   Dietary Reference Intakes.

CHARGE TO THE PANEL ON CALCIUM AND RELATED NUTRIENTS AND SUBCOMMITTEE ON UPPER REFERENCE LEVELS

The National Institutes of Health's National Heart, Lung and Blood Institute, the U.S. Food and Drug Administration, and the U.S. Department of Agriculture's Agricultural Research Service requested that the Institute of Medicine review and develop dietary reference intakes for calcium, phosphorus, magnesium, vitamin D, and fluoride. In part, this nutrient group was given priority because of the high prevalence of osteoporosis among the growing population of people over 50 years of age, in addition to possible links of these nutrients to the development of risk factors for stroke and cardiovascular disease. Additionally, the need to establish upper levels of intake, which although not evaluated as having any benefit to the individual, would also not result in increased risk, was an important component of the task.

In April 1996, the DRI Committee of the FNB established the Panel on Calcium and Related Nutrients and the Subcommittee on Upper Reference Levels. The panel was charged with the following:

• Review the literature and interpret the depth of current knowledge of calcium, phosphorus, magnesium, vitamin D, and fluoride requirements for each stage of the lifespan.

• Analyze the literature coupled with information available from large epidemiological studies to determine dietary intakes of calcium, phosphorus, magnesium, vitamin D, and fluoride in the U.S. and Canadian populations and the potential for such intakes to be associated with decreased risk of chronic disease.

• Review the other components in foods that affect the utilization of calcium and related nutrients in human diets, including bioavailability from nonfood sources.

• Evaluate comparable standards from other countries and multinational groups for whom recommended nutrient ranges have been developed and consider the applicability of the recommended nutrient range for use in North America.

• Develop dietary reference intake values for calcium, phosphorus, magnesium, vitamin D, and fluoride, where adequate data are available, for each stage of the lifespan including people older than 50 years.

• Identify research needed to improve knowledge of calcium, phosphorus, magnesium, vitamin D, and fluoride requirements.

The Subcommittee on Upper Reference Levels was charged with the following:

• Develop a model to estimate the maximum level of nutrient intake that would pose a low risk of adverse effects.

• Apply the model to calcium, phosphorus, magnesium, vitamin D, and fluoride to develop Tolerable Upper Intake Levels.

B

Acknowledgments

The Panel on Calcium and Related Nutrients, the Subcommittee on Upper Reference Levels of Nutrients, the Standing Committee on the Scientific Evaluation of Dietary Reference Intakes, and the Food and Nutrition Board staff are grateful for the time and effort of the many contributors to the report and the workshops and meetings leading up to the report. Through openly sharing their considerable expertise and different outlooks, these individuals and organizations brought clarity and focus to the challenging task of setting calcium, phosphorus, magnesium, vitamin D, and fluoride requirements for humans. The list below mentions those individuals who we worked closely with, but many others also deserve our heartfelt thanks. Those individuals, whose names we do not know, made important contributions to the report by offering suggestions and opinions at the many professional meetings and workshops the committee members attended. The panel, subcommittee, and committee members, as well as the FNB staff thank the following named (as well as unnamed) individuals and organizations:

INDIVIDUALS

Richard Allison
Burton Altura
Harvey Anderson
John Anderson
Sue Anderson
Mark B. Andon
Laura Baird

Lewis A. Barness
George Beaton
Norman Bell
Bernice Berg
Douglas Buck
Albert W. Burgstahler
David Burmaster

Elsworth Buskirk
Doris Calloway
Mona Calvo
Alicia Carriquiry
Florian Cerkelwski
Kevin Cockell
Olwen Collins

Richard J. Deckelbaum
Hector DeLuca
Annette Dickinson
Kevin Dodd
Michael Dourson
Harold Draper
Jacqueline Dupont
Ronald J. Elin
Mark Epstein
Nancy Ernst
Richard Foulkes
Susan Fourt
Kay Franz
David Gaylor
Sheila Gibson
Michael Glade
George Glasser
Jay Goodman
Peter Greenwald
Janet Greger
Raj K. Gupta
Jean Pierre Habicht
Charles Halsted
Alfred Harper
Suzanne Harris
John Hathcock
Daniel Hatton
J.G.A.J. Hautvast
Mark Hegsted
James Heimbach
Charles Hennekens

Steven Heymsfield
Mark Horwitt
Lyn Howard
Curtiss Hunt
Howard Jacobson
Maureen Jones
Ruth Kavo
Carl Keen
Eileen Kennedy
Chor San Khoo
Anita Knight
Raymond Koteras
David Kritchevsky
John Lee
Sidney Lees
Orville Levander
Richard Levine
Christine Lewis
Bonnie Liebman
Fimo Lifshitz
David Lineback
Alberta Long
Anne Looker
Marjolaine Mailhot
Bernadette Marriott
Paul Mason
Alexander Mauskop
George McCabe
Donald McCormick
Linda Meyers
Gregory Miller
Curtis Morris

Alanna Moshfegh
Jerry Nadler
Malden Nesheim
Forrest Nielsen
Jeri Nieves
Charles Pak
Joyce Pekula
Roy Pitkin
Daniel Raiten
John Repke
Lawrence Resnick
Richard Rivlin
Robert Russell
L. Saldanho
Brittmarie Sandström
Mildred Seelig
Christopher Sempos
Jay Shapiro
Arleen B. Tate
Richard Troiano
John Vanderveen
William Waddell
Julie Walko
Roger Whitehead
Susan J. Whiting
John Wilson
Richard Wood
Jacqueline Wright
Elizabeth Yetley
Steven Zeisel
Stanley H. Zlotkin

ORGANIZATIONS

American Dental Association
American Institute of Nutrition
American Medical Association
American Society for Bone Mineral Research
Canadian Paediatric Society
Council for Responsible Nutrition
Dietary Reference Intakes Steering Committee
Federation of American Scientists for Experimental Biology
Health Canada
Institute of Food Technologists
Interagency Human Nutrition Research Council
Life Sciences Research Organization
National Dairy Council
National Osteoporosis Foundation
Osteoporosis Society of Canada
Researchers Against Deadly Water

C
Options for Dealing with Uncertainties

Methods for dealing with uncertainties in scientific data are generally understood by working scientists and require no special discussion here, except to point out that such uncertainties should be explicitly acknowledged and taken into account whenever a risk assessment is undertaken. More subtle and difficult problems are created by uncertainties associated with some of the inferences that need to be made in the absence of directly applicable data; much confusion and inconsistency can result if they are not recognized and dealt with in advance of undertaking a risk assessment.

The most significant inference uncertainties arise in risk assessments whenever attempts are made to answer the following questions (NRC, 1994):

• What set(s) of hazard and dose-response data (for a given substance) should be used to characterize risk in the population of interest?

• If animal data are to be used for risk characterization, which endpoints for adverse effects should be considered?

• If animal data are to be used for risk characterization, what measure of dose (e.g., dose per unit body weight, body surface, dietary intake) should be used for scaling between animals and humans?

• What is the expected variability in dose response between animals and humans?

• If human data are to be used for risk characterization, which adverse effects should be used?

- What is the expected variability in dose response among members of the human population?
- How should data from subchronic exposure studies be used to estimate chronic effects?
- How should problems of differences in route of exposure within and between species be dealt with?
- How should the threshold dose be estimated for the human population?
- If a threshold in the dose-response relationship seems unlikely, how should a low-dose risk be modeled?
- What model should be chosen to represent the distribution of exposures in the population of interest, when data relating to exposures are limited?
- When interspecies extrapolations are required, what should be assumed about relative rates of absorption from the gastrointestinal tract of animals and of humans?
- For which percentiles on the distribution of population exposures should risks be characterized?

Depending on the nutrient under review, at least partial, empirically based answers to some of these questions may be available, but in no case is scientific information likely to be sufficient to provide a highly certain answer; in many cases there will be no relevant data for the nutrient in question.

It should be recognized that, for several of these questions, certain inferences have been widespread for long periods of time, and thus, it may seem unnecessary to raise these uncertainties anew. When several sets of animal toxicology data are available, for example, and data are insufficient to identify the set (i.e., species, strain, adverse effects endpoint) that "best" predicts human response, it has become traditional to select that set in which toxic responses occur at lowest dose ("most sensitive"). In the absence of definitive empirical data applicable to a specific case, it is generally assumed that there will not be more than a 10-fold variation in response among members of the human population. In the absence of absorption data, it is generally assumed that humans will absorb the chemical at the same rate as the animal species used to model human risk. In the absence of complete understanding of biological mechanisms, it is generally assumed that, except possibly for certain carcinogens, a threshold dose must be exceeded before toxicity is expressed. These types of long-standing assumptions, which are necessary to complete a risk assessment, are recognized by risk assessors as attempts to deal with uncertainties in knowledge (NRC, 1994).

A past National Research Council (NRC) report (1983) recommended the adoption of the concepts and definitions that have been discussed in this paper. The NRC committee recognized that throughout a risk assessment, data and basic knowledge will be lacking and that risk assessors will be faced with several scientifically plausible options (called "inference options" by the NRC) for dealing with questions such as those presented above. For example, several scientifically supportable options for dose-scaling across species and for high-to-low dose extrapolation, but no ready means to identify those that are clearly best supported. The NRC committee recommended that regulatory agencies in the United States identify the needed "inference options" in risk-assessment and specify, through written risk assessment guidelines, the specific options that will be used for all assessments. Agencies in the United States have identified the specific models to be used to fill gaps in data and knowledge; these have come to be called *default options* (EPA, 1986).

The use of defaults to fill knowledge and data gaps in risk assessment has the advantage of ensuring *consistency* in approach (the same defaults are used for each assessment) and for minimizing or eliminating case-by-case manipulations of the conduct of risk assessment to meet predetermined risk management objectives. The major disadvantage of the use of defaults is the potential for displacement of scientific judgment by excessively rigid guidelines. A remedy for this disadvantage was also suggested by the NRC committee: risk assessors should be allowed to replace defaults with alternative factors in specific cases of chemicals for which relevant scientific data were available to support alternatives. The risk assessors' obligation in such cases is to provide explicit justification for any such departure. Guidelines for risk assessment issued by the U.S. Environmental Protection Agency, for example, specifically allow for such departures (EPA, 1986).

The use of preselected defaults is not the only way to deal with model uncertainties. Another option is to allow risk assessors complete freedom to pursue whatever approaches they judge applicable in specific cases. Because many of the uncertainties cannot be resolved scientifically, case-by-case judgments without some guidance on how to deal with them will lead to difficulties in achieving scientific consensus, and the results of the assessment may not be credible.

Another option for dealing with uncertainties is to allow risk assessors to develop a range of estimates, based on application of both defaults and alternative inferences that, in specific cases, have some degree of scientific support. Indeed, appropriate analysis of uncertainties would seem to require such a presentation of risk results. Although presenting a number of plausible risk estimates has clear advantages in that it would seem to reflect more faithfully the true state of scientific understanding, there are no well-established criteria for using such complex results in risk management.

The various approaches to dealing with uncertainties inherent to risk assessment, and discussed in the foregoing sections, are summarized in Table C-1.

As will be seen in the chapters on each nutrient, specific default assumptions for assessing nutrient risks have not been recommended. Rather, the approach calls for case-by-case judgments, with the recommendation that the basis for the choices made be explicitly stated. Some general guidelines for making these choices will, however, be offered.

TABLE C-1 Approaches for Dealing with Uncertainties in a Risk-Assessment Program

Program Model	Advantages	Disadvantages
Case-by-case judgments by experts	Flexibility High potential to maximize use of most relevant scientific information bearing on specific issues	Potential for inconsistent treatment of different issues Difficulty in achieving consensus Need to agree on defaults
Written guidelines specifying defaults for data and model uncertainties (with allowance for departures in specific cases)	Consistent treatment of different issues Maximize transparency of process Allow resolution of scientific disagreements by resort to defaults	May be difficult to justify departure, or to achieve consensus among scientists that departures are justified in specific cases Danger that uncertainties will be overlooked
Assessors asked to present full array of estimates, using all scientifically plausible models	Maximize use of scientific information Reasonably reliable portrayal of true state of scientific understanding	Highly complex characterization of risk, with no easy way to discriminate among estimates Size of required effort may not be commensurate with utility of the outcome

D

1994 CSFII Adjusted Data for Calcium, Phosphorus, and Magnesium

Tables D-1 through D-3 are the 1994 CSFII data adjusted for day-to-day variation (Nusser et al., 1996) for calcium, phosphorus, and magnesium.

TABLE D-1 Daily Calcium Intake (mg): Mean, standard error of the mean, selected percentiles, and associated standard errors for usual intake

Sex/Age Category	n	Mean	Percentile	
			1st	5th
0-6 mo	69	460.6	110	191
SE		33.3	36.3	43.5
7-12 mo	45	725.8	243	351
SE		78.6	58.9	61.6
1-3 y	702	792.5	287	399
SE		16.8	14.4	13.8
4-8 y	666	838.1	339	455
SE		25.0	21.4	21.3
M 9-13 y	180	1025	358	499
SE		50.2	28.4	33.4
M 14-18 y	191	1169	409	554
SE		55.7	24.3	25.0
M 19-30 y	328	1013	355	484
SE		35.4	21.2	24.2
M 31-50 y	627	912.6	313	429
SE		32.0	15.8	21.7
M 51-70 y	490	747.7	265	362
SE		26.1	18.3	19.1
M >70 y	237	729.2	267	368
SE		30.5	17.9	22.8
F 9-13 y	200	918.5	361	486
SE		40.4	28.7	31.7
F 14-18 y	169	752.9	246	348
SE		38.7	28.9	32.9
F 19-30 y	302	647.2	214	300
SE		46.3	19.0	24.4
F 31-50 y	590	636.8	209	297
SE		15.4	10.5	13.7
F 51-70 y	510	599.4	215	294
SE		16.6	10.7	11.2
F >70 y	221	535.7	204	277
SE		22.6	13.8	13.9
8 y and under	1482	800.3	257	382
SE		17.3	19.6	18.4
M 9+ y	2053	924.5	312	431
SE		19.3	11.3	14.4
F 9+ y	1992	657.4	228	316
SE		9.9	9.4	9.6
F Pregnant[a]	33	1168	481	656
SE		90.4	86.7	80.8
F Lactating[a]	16	1053	619	794
SE		330.3	427	492
All Indiv (+P/L)	5576	796.5	239	349
SE		10.8	7.5	7.9

NOTE: n represents the actual unweighted sample size in each group. Estimates were obtained using C-SIDE v1.0 (C-SIDE courtesy of Iowa State University Statistical Laboratory). Standard errors (SE) were estimated via jacknife replication. Each standard error has 43 d.f.

10th	25th	50th	75th	90th	95th	99th
245	343	457	569	674	745	898
44.9	43.7	36.3	35.1	38.8	43.3	66.5
418	544	703	883	1062	1177	1410
63.7	69.4	79.7	95.6	117.0	135.0	179.0
468	599	766	957	1151	1276	1533
13.7	14.5	17.1	22.0	28.7	34.0	47.1
524	649	808	993	1190	1325	1618
21.4	22.2	24.7	29.2	36.7	43	58.9
587	756	980	1245	1520	1702	2084
36.7	42.9	50.7	60.2	72.7	83.5	113.0
647	834	1094	1422	1785	2039	2601
26.9	34.2	49.3	73.0	104.0	128.0	188.0
566	729	954	1232	1536	1746	2206
26	29.3	34.3	43.9	62.1	79.4	128
503	651	857	1112	1393	1588	2015
24.4	27.3	31.4	40.4	51.7	63.8	127.0
424	545	708	908	1122	1268	1581
19.8	21.6	25.3	31.9	41.6	49.7	71.1
430	548	702	880	1064	1185	1434
25.3	28.0	31.2	37.1	42.7	48.4	80.8
562	705	889	1100	1313	1452	1737
35.7	37.3	41.9	55.4	60.9	69.5	163.0
413	541	713	922	1144	1293	1611
35.1	38.8	42.3	45.3	50.1	56.3	79.8
355	464	612	792	985	1116	1397
28.0	35.2	44.9	56.6	69.2	77.9	97.2
353	461	606	779	961	1082	1337
14.4	12.7	13.8	23.2	32.0	40.1	83.2
344	441	571	727	891	1001	1234
11.6	12.7	15.5	21.5	30.7	38.1	56.7
322	407	517	644	774	860	1037
14.7	17.1	22.0	29.3	37.2	42.6	57.3
457	595	767	969	1183	1330	1652
17.7	17.3	17.8	19.8	24.4	29.1	43.4
507	658	865	1126	1416	1620	2077
15.9	16.3	19.0	25.8	32.4	49.6	150
372	480	625	800	985	1109	1372
9.5	9.5	9.8	11.8	16.2	20.2	30.7
758	939	1154	1382	1596	1729	1986
78.3	77.9	87.3	112.0	150.0	180.0	248.0
875	982	1050	1120	1233	1324	1519
513.0	460.0	304.0	214.0	237.0	313.0	547.0
418	555	742	977	1241	1429	1855
8.2	9.1	10.8	13.5	17.4	21.1	33.7

[a]These estimates are less reliable due to extremely small sample size.

TABLE D-2   Daily Phosphorus Intake (mg): Mean, standard error of the mean, selected percentiles, and associated standard errors for usual intake

| Sex/Age Category | n | Mean | Percentile | |
			1st	5th
0-6 mo	69	325	72	131
SE		26.2	37.3	38.8
7-12 mo	45	642	212	302
SE		70.9	45.1	47.0
1-3 y	702	943.9	416	552
SE		13.1	18.2	15.0
4-8 y	666	1088	537	677
SE		23.7	21.8	18.1
M 9-13 y	180	1407	589	771
SE		54.3	50.3	48.5
M 14-18 y	191	1642	767	956
SE		61.8	46.8	46.4
M 19-30 y	328	1659	809	1002
SE		51.9	38.3	39.9
M 31-50 y	627	1530	705	907
SE		36.7	32.0	34.5
M 51-70 y	490	1307	604	769
SE		39.5	30.4	31.0
M >70 y	237	1191	559	721
SE		30.3	37.0	34.7
F 9-13 y	200	1203	606	768
SE		44.1	44.9	43.7
F 14-18 y	169	1128	484	632
SE		45.1	47.7	61.9
F 19-30 y	302	1031	433	580
SE		63.1	29.1	31.9
F 31-50 y	590	1014	448	593
SE		20.1	22.2	21.1
F 51-70 y	510	986.5	468	599
SE		20.4	20.7	19.8
F >70 y	221	874.3	406	521
SE		27.7	26.9	26.0
8 y and under	1482	982.4	313	483
SE		15.8	22.2	20.3
M 9+ y	2053	1495	684	874
SE		24.2	17.8	18.3
F 9+ y	1992	1024	485	620
SE		13.0	15.1	12.8
F Pregnant[a]	33	1572	773	1012
SE		292.6	294.0	327.0
F Lactating[a]	16	1496	1113	1211
SE		309.1	313.0	348.0
All Indiv (+P/L)	5576	1222	445	620
SE		12.9	9.6	8.0

NOTE: n represents the actual unweighted sample size in each group. Estimates were obtained using C-SIDE v1.0 (C-SIDE courtesy of Iowa State University Statistical Laboratory). Standard errors (SE) were estimated via jackknife replication. Each standard error has 43 d.f.

10th	25th	50th	75th	90th	95th	99th
171	244	322	399	479	532	642
36.9	38.0	31.5	27.2	32.5	42.0	83.1
358	467	612	784	965	1086	1338
49.7	57.6	71.2	88.8	109.0	124.0	159.0
629	764	926	1104	1280	1396	1635
13.8	12.9	13.6	16.9	22.1	26.2	36.7
755	892	1059	1250	1455	1596	1910
17.6	18.3	21.4	28.5	40.1	49.8	75.0
882	1090	1359	1672	1993	2203	2640
48.1	49.3	53.9	62.8	76.4	88.1	119.0
1072	1292	1582	1927	2290	2534	3053
47.3	51.5	60.7	75.6	96.3	113.0	157.0
1119	1336	1613	1932	2258	2472	2917
42.0	46.8	51.3	64.1	83.7	101.0	159.0
1022	1229	1484	1780	2094	2312	2791
34.3	32.8	36.3	45.2	65.5	86.1	144.0
866	1047	1274	1531	1789	1956	2295
32.1	35.2	40.0	46.2	53.9	60.1	76.7
814	979	1176	1386	1587	1712	1957
33.8	32.8	32.5	33.7	38.1	43.0	57.4
856	1005	1178	1372	1579	1725	2052
44.0	44.4	45.3	49.3	57.1	64.5	88.6
722	888	1097	1335	1573	1727	2040
67.6	62.3	47.8	57.1	65.9	61.2	101.0
665	818	1005	1215	1429	1571	1871
35.4	50.1	70.7	78.2	81.2	87.6	123.0
674	818	990	1183	1382	1516	1802
20.2	18.4	18.5	24.5	36.2	46.0	70.8
674	806	966	1144	1325	1444	1693
20.1	19.6	20.1	25.9	33.4	38.5	55.3
588	710	859	1022	1181	1282	1482
25.9	26.3	28.3	32.2	38.1	42.9	55.2
581	750	953	1181	1419	1582	1935
18.5	14.3	15.6	18.8	27.8	36.2	57.4
985	1189	1445	1745	2063	2282	2761
19.0	20.7	23.8	28.7	36.2	43.2	64.3
697	834	1001	1188	1381	1510	1783
11.8	10.8	12.1	16.1	22.5	28.4	46.6
1137	1348	1581	1804	1996	2108	2314
345.0	356.0	348.0	308.0	232.0	182.0	245.0
1266	1365	1483	1613	1741	1822	1985
369.0	362.0	283.0	254.0	311.0	374.0	548.0
724	915	1164	1463	1790	2020	2544
8.8	10.2	12.1	16.6	22.3	27.2	43.6

[a]These estimates are less reliable due to extremely small sample size.

TABLE D-3 Daily Magnesium Intake (mg): Mean, standard error of the mean, selected percentiles, and associated standard errors for usual intake

Sex/Age Category	n	Mean	Percentile	
			1st	5th
0-6 mo	69	57.8	12	21
SE		5.9	4.7	5.2
7-12 mo	45	112.7	46	61
SE		10.4	6.7	6.9
1-3 y	702	183.4	80	106
SE		2.6	3.3	3.0
4-8 y	666	211.5	102	128
SE		4	4.0	3.2
M 9-13 y	180	271	106	140
SE		12.0	9.5	9.8
M 14-18 y	191	315.6	132	168
SE		12.0	6.7	7.4
M 19-30 y	328	343.1	144	185
SE		13.1	7.1	7.9
M 31-50 y	627	341.2	149	194
SE		8.6	8.0	7.0
M 51-70 y	490	304.9	130	169
SE		8.4	6.3	6.6
M >70 y	237	282.1	123	160
SE		7.5	6.1	6.3
F 9-13 y	200	229.5	111	142
SE		7.8	8.6	8.4
F 14-18 y	169	224.5	90	123
SE		9.0	9.4	10.5
F 19-30 y	302	210.6	89	118
SE		8.8	6.0	6.3
F 31-50 y	590	236.1	100	133
SE		4.5	5.5	5.5
F 51-70 y	510	238.5	110	141
SE		6.5	5.3	4.7
F >70 y	221	209.4	89	118
SE		6.7	6.9	6.5
8 y and under	1482	190.3	59	91
SE		2.7	4.2	3.5
M 9+ y	2053	323.6	135	177
SE		5.5	4.4	4.5
F 9+ y	1992	228.1	104	134
SE		2.7	3.0	2.5
F Pregnant[a]	33	292.5	144	187
SE		23.4	28.8	26.1
F Lactating[a]	16	316.8	218	244
SE		58.1	37.5	43.7
All Indiv (+P/L)	5576	263.9	90	128
SE		3.0	1.6	1.5

NOTE: *n* represents the actual unweighted sample size in each group. Estimates were obtained using C-SIDE v1.0 (C-SIDE courtesy of Iowa State University Statistical Laboratory). Standard errors (SE) were estimated via jackknife replication. Each standard error has 43 d.f.

10th	25th	50th	75th	90th	95th	99th
27	39	55	73	93	105	131
5.3	5.2	5.4	7.6	12.5	17.2	30
70	86	109	134	161	179	216
7.3	8.7	10.8	13.1	15.5	17.4	22.1
121	148	180	215	250	274	323
2.9	2.7	2.6	3.2	4.6	5.9	9.4
143	171	205	245	287	315	377
2.9	2.9	3.8	5.3	7.3	8.9	12.9
161	203	258	325	397	445	548
10.1	10.7	11.9	14.6	19.2	23.5	35.1
191	236	298	376	462	522	656
8.1	9.6	11.8	14.9	19.9	24.5	38.0
211	261	328	408	495	553	679
8.8	10.8	13.4	16.1	19.3	22.4	32.2
220	268	329	401	477	529	645
7.7	9.2	8.6	12.1	15.3	18.3	31.5
193	238	295	362	429	474	566
6.9	7.3	8.2	10	12.5	14.6	21.3
182	223	275	333	392	429	507
6.4	6.9	7.8	9.2	11.6	13.9	20.0
159	188	223	263	307	339	412
8.4	8.3	8.3	8.8	10.5	12.2	18.0
142	175	217	266	318	352	423
10.0	9.4	10.6	11.2	11.6	12.1	19.7
135	166	205	250	293	322	379
6.6	7.4	8.7	10.7	13.3	15.2	19.8
152	187	229	278	329	363	437
6.0	4.9	4.0	7.4	9.7	11.9	28.8
159	191	231	277	327	362	438
4.6	4.8	6.0	8.2	10.8	12.6	16.6
136	167	206	248	288	314	365
6.4	6.3	6.7	8.0	10.5	12.7	18.5
110	144	184	230	278	310	379
3.1	2.5	2.5	3.5	5.1	6.3	9.7
202	249	310	384	462	516	634
4.7	5.0	5.5	6.4	8.0	9.7	15.2
152	184	222	266	311	342	407
2.3	2.2	2.5	3.5	4.9	6.1	9.5
210	249	292	336	375	399	444
25.5	23.5	24.3	30.7	31.6	30.6	40.0
259	285	315	347	377	396	433
47.3	53.5	59.7	64.9	69.3	72.3	79.5
151	193	248	318	396	452	578
1.6	2.0	2.9	4.0	5.4	6.7	10.7

[a]These estimates are less reliable due to extremely small sample size.

E

Model for Estimating Calcium Intake for Desirable Calcium Retention

The model used for fitting the relationship between calcium intake and calcium retention is described by the equation: $Y = ae^L/(1 + e^L) + d$, where Y is retention and L is a linear function of intake (L = b + c [intake]; where b is the intercept and c is the slope of function) (Jackman et al., 1997). The model was used to determine an estimate of calcium intake required to achieve the selected value for *desirable* calcium retention.[1]

As described in the initial version of this report, when the application of this model to the data was proposed it was thought that it could predict the lowest value of the plateau intake of calcium at which mean percent *maximal* calcium retention would occur in a group of individuals. This was considered advantageous in that it estimated a relative measure (percent of an individual's maximum) rather than an absolute measure (a quantified pre-set level of retention) as errors often associated with balance studies would have negligible impact.

Subsequent to the release of the initial version of this report, statistical issues were raised related to the use of percent maximal retention in the way initially described in the prepublication report. The non-linear regression curves derived by applying the Jackson et

---

[1] It should be recognized that the model is most appropriate only over the ranges of intake from which it was derived, and the model as described does not estimate the range of intakes that would result in the desired level of retention.

al. model ($Y = ae^L/(1 + e^L)$) (1997) were asymptotic, thus never reaching 100 percent, but approaching that goal at higher levels of intake. In a strict statistical sense, 100 percent of an individual's maximal retention due to calcium intake could never be achieved, regardless of intake, if it was an asymptotic relationship. Biologically, this was not a logical conclusion, in that maximal retention, at least to the extent that it can be measured, is a finite number for each individual at a given point in time. The second statistical issue raised was the appropriateness of selecting the level of calcium intake at which the upper limit of the confidence interval for the nonlinear asymptotic regression curve first coincided with 100 percent maximal retention; although this could be defended statistically, it was of concern biologically. For some of the curves to which it was applied, this level of intake was associated with a mean percent maximal retention of 26 percent, which made it difficult to justify as a goal for the average intake of individuals.

Given these concerns, the DRI Committee, supporting the concept that maximizing calcium retention and decreasing calcium loss to the extent possible via calcium intake is of benefit to maintaining bone mineral content and subsequent risk of fracture, had the data recalculated using the Jackman et al. non-linear regression model (1997). In this revised approach, absolute retention (corrected for predicted sweat loss) was employed in place of the percent maximal retention as the value of Y, which was then solved for x, the intake of calcium. Thus, for each age group, a specified *desirable* level of retention was estimated for the purposes of quantifying an intake associated with the designated calcium retention. Where necessary, the desirable level was based on the same estimates for growth and absorption used in the factorial approach.

To derive the estimates of calcium intake using the Jackman et al. model to achieve this absolute measure of desirable calcium retention (or minimize calcium loss), a value for sweat loss was added to the estimate of retention needed since the balance studies used had not accounted for calcium loss in sweat. The derived estimates of calcium intake which would provide for desirable calcium retention were used as part of the basis for establishing an AI for each age group. Table 4-5 provides the specific values used for desirable calcium retention and sweat loss for each age group for which the model was utilized. The non-linear regression curves derived from this method follow (Figures E-1 through E-3). The 95 percent confidence intervals shown on the curves represent the goodness-of-fit of the regression lines.

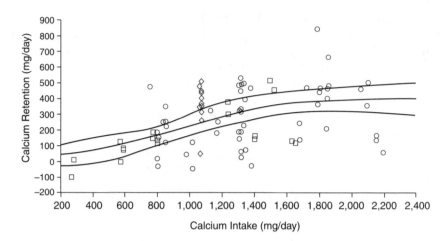

FIGURE E-1 Calcium retention as a function of intake in adolescents. The equation which describes the nonlinear regression model of Jackman et al. (1997) and applied as depicted in this figure to the balance study data of Jackman et al. (1997) as circles, Matkovic et al. (1990) as squares, and Greger et al. (1978) as diamonds is $Y = 436.90\ e^L / (1 + e^L)$, where $L = -2.96 + 0.0032$ (intake).

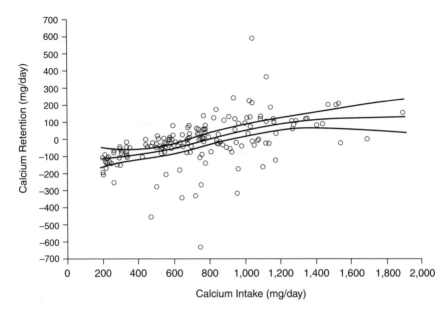

FIGURE E-2 Calcium retention as a function of intake in young adults aged 18–30 years as compiled by Matkovic and Heaney (1992). The equation which describes the nonlinear regression model of Jackman et al. (1997) and applied as depicted in this figure to the balance study data of Matkovic and Heaney (1992) is $Y = -133.79 + 290.16\, e^L/(1 + e^L)$, where $L = -3.15 + 0.0040$ (intake).

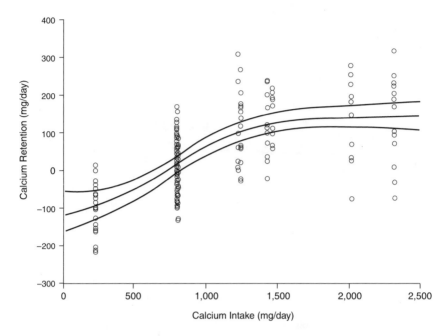

FIGURE E-3 Calcium retention as a function of intake in adult men from Spencer et al. (1984). The equation which describes the nonlinear regression model of Jackman et al. (1997) and applied as depicted in this figure to the balance study data of Spencer et al. (1984) is $Y = -130.73 + 274.93 \ e^L/(1 + e^L)$, where $L = -2.75 + 0.0036$ (intake).

F

Biographical Sketches of Committee, Subcommittee, Panel Members and Staff

STEPHANIE A. ATKINSON, Ph.D., R.D., is professor, Department of Pediatrics and associate member, Department of Biochemistry in the Faculty of Health Sciences, McMaster University in Hamilton, Ontario, Canada. She holds a clinical appointment as special professional staff at The Children's Hospital in Hamilton. Dr. Atkinson received her Ph.D. in nutritional sciences at the University of Toronto. The focus of her research has been on developmental aspects of bone in the pediatric population. Specifically, her research focuses on the impact of premature birth; nutrition; childhood diseases such as leukemia, asthma, and inflammatory bowel disease; and steroid therapy on bone metabolism and skeletal development in infants and children. Dr. Atkinson served as scientific chair of the 16th International Congress of Nutrition held in Montreal in 1997 and serves on the Board of Trustees of the National Institute of Nutrition in Canada. She is a member of the Canadian and American Societies for Nutritional Sciences, the American Society for Clinical Nutrition, the American Society for Bone and Mineral Research, and the Dietitians of Canada, and is a fellow of the American College of Nutrition.

STEVEN A. ABRAMS, M.D., is an associate professor of pediatrics at Baylor College of Medicine at the U.S. Department of Agriculture Center on Children's Nutrition Research. He received his B.S. in biology from the Massachusetts Institute of Technology and his M.D. from the Ohio State University College of Medicine. Dr.

Abrams' research centers on the assessment of mineral requirements in children using stable isotope techniques. He is a member of numerous professional associations including the American Society for Bone and Mineral Research, American Society for Clinical Nutrition, American Society for Nutritional Sciences, and Society for Pediatric Research, and is a fellow of the American Academy of Pediatrics.

LINDSAY H. ALLEN, Ph.D., R.D., is professor in the Department of Nutrition and a faculty member in the Program in International Nutrition at the University of California, Davis. She received her B.Sc. in nutrition and agriculture from the University of Nottingham, England, and her Ph.D. in nutrition from the University of California, Davis. Following post-graduate experience at the University of California, Berkeley, she joined the faculty at the University of Connecticut. Dr. Allen's research focuses on the causes, consequences, and prevention of micronutrient deficiencies (vitamin B_{12}, folic acid, iron, zinc, and riboflavin) in developing countries and on vitamin B_{12} deficiency in the elderly in the United States. She is an associate editor of the *Journal of Nutrition* and was awarded the Kellogg International Nutrition Prize in 1997. She is a member of the Food and Nutrition Board and the DRI Panel on Folate and Other B Vitamins and Choline. She previously served as chair of the Committee on International Nutrition, Institute of Medicine, National Academy of Sciences, and has authored over 120 publications.

BESS DAWSON-HUGHES, M.D., is a professor of medicine at Tufts University and chief of the Calcium and Bone Metabolism Laboratory at the Jean Mayer U.S. Department of Agriculture Human Nutrition Research Center on Aging at Tufts University. She directs the Metabolic Bone Disease Clinic at New England Medical Center. Dr. Dawson-Hughes received her B.A. in chemistry from Randolph-Macon Women's College and her M.D. from Tufts University School of Medicine. She is a member of the Board of Trustees of the National Osteoporosis Foundation and serves on the Councils of the American Society for Bone and Mineral Research and the American Society for Clinical Nutrition. Dr. Dawson-Hughes' research is directed at examining ways in which calcium, vitamin D, and other nutrients influence age-related loss of bone mass and risk of fragility fractures. She has published over 180 peer-reviewed journal articles, book chapters, abstracts, and reviews.

JOHANNA T. DWYER, D.Sc., R.D., is director of the Frances Stern Nutrition Center at New England Medical Center and professor in the Departments of Medicine and of Community Health at the Tufts Medical School and School of Nutrition Science and Policy in Boston. She is also a senior scientist at the Jean Mayer U.S. Department of Agriculture Human Nutrition Research Center on Aging at Tufts University. Dr. Dwyer's work centers on life-cycle related concerns such as the prevention of diet-related disease in children and adolescents, and maximization of quality of life and health in the elderly. She also has a long-standing interest in vegetarian and other alternative lifestyles. She is currently the editor of *Nutrition Today* and on the editorial board for *Family Economics and Nutrition Reviews.* She received her D.Sc. and M.Sc. from the Harvard School of Public Health, an M.S. from the University of Wisconsin, and received her undergraduate degree with distinction from Cornell University. She is a member of the Food and Nutrition Board, the Technical Advisory Committee of the Nutrition Screening Initiative, past president of the American Society for Nutritional Sciences, and a past president of the Society for Nutrition Education.

JOHN W. ERDMAN, JR., Ph.D., is professor of nutrition in food science and human nutrition and in internal medicine at the University of Illinois at Champaign-Urbana and director of the Division of Nutritional Sciences. Dr. Erdman received his B.S. and Ph.D. in food science at Rutgers University. His research interests include the effects of food processing on nutrient retention, the metabolic roles of vitamin A and beta carotene, and the bioavailability of minerals from foods. His research regarding soy protein has extended into studies on the impact of non-nutrient components of foods such as phytoestrogens on chronic disease. Dr. Erdman is currently vice-chair of the Food and Nutrition Board (FNB) and is a former member of the FNB's Committee on Opportunities in the Nutrition and Food Sciences and its Committee on the Nutrition Components of Food Labeling. He was also a member of the Subcommittee on the Bioavailability of Nutrients, Committee on Animal Nutrition, Board on Agriculture.

JOHN D. FERNSTROM, Ph.D., is professor of psychiatry, pharmacology, and behavioral neuroscience at the University of Pittsburgh School of Medicine and director, Basic Neuroendocrinology Program at the Western Psychiatric Institute and Clinic. He received his B.S. in biology and his Ph.D. in nutritional biochemistry from the Massachusetts Institute of Technology. He presently is a member of the National Advisory Council of the Monell Chemical Senses Center and of the American Society for Nutritional Sciences Council. He is a member of numerous professional societies, including the American Society for Clinical Nutrition, American Physiological Society, American Society for Pharmacology and Experimental Therapeutics, American Society for Neurochemistry, Society for Neuroscience, and Endocrine Society. Among other awards, Dr. Fernstrom received the Mead-Johnson Award from ASNS, a Research Scientist Award from the National Institute of Mental Health, a Wellcome Visiting Professorship in the Basic Medical Sciences, and an Alfred P. Sloan Fellowship in Neurochemistry. His current major research interest concerns the influence of the diet and drugs on the synthesis of neurotransmitters in the central and peripheral nervous systems.

SCOTT M. GRUNDY, M.D., Ph.D., is director of the Center for Human Nutrition and chairman of the Department of Clinical Nutrition at the University of Texas Southwestern Medical Center at Dallas. He received his M.D. from Baylor University Medical School and his Ph.D. from Rockefeller University. Dr. Grundy's major research area is in cholesterol and lipoprotein metabolism. He has published over 200 original papers and numerous solicited articles and book chapters. Dr. Grundy served as editor-in-chief of the *Journal of Lipid Research* for 5 years and is on the editorial boards of *American Journal of Physiology: Endocrinology and Metabolism, Arteriosclerosis,* and *Circulation.* He serves on numerous national and international committees including the Food and Nutrition Board and as chairman of the Cholesterol Education Program Adult Treatment Panel II for the National Institutes of Health. Dr. Grundy's numerous awards and honors include The Award of Merit from the American Heart Association, an honorary degree in medicine from the University of Helsinki, Finland, the Roger J. Williams Award in preventive nutrition, and the Bristol Myers Squibb/Mead Johnson Award for Distinguished Achievement in Nutrition Research. He was elected to the Institute of Medicine in 1995.

ROBERT P. HEANEY, M.D., is John A. Creighton University Professor and professor of medicine, Creighton University, Omaha, Nebraska. He received his B.S. and M.D. from Creighton. His principal professional interests have centered on human calcium and bone physiology and the education of health professionals. Dr. Heaney actively participates in research-related professional societies and serves as a consultant for scientific, academic, civic, and church-related organizations. He has served as chairman of the board of the Association of Academic Health Centers, and is a member of the Board of Directors of the National Osteoporosis Foundation. Dr. Heaney serves on the editorial boards of a number of scientific publications, is a past trustee of Loyola University of Chicago, and is a past member of the National Advisory Committee for the Pew Foundation Dental Project. He chaired the Scientific Advisory Panel on Osteoporosis of the U.S. Office of Technology Assessment. Dr. Heaney has spent over 40 years studying osteoporosis and human calcium physiology, and is an internationally recognized expert and lecturer in this field. He is the author of three books and has published over 300 original papers, chapters, monographs, and reviews. He has received numerous honors and awards, including the Kappa Delta Award of the American Academy of Orthopedic Surgeons; the Ohio State University Award for a continuing education program on osteoporosis; the Health Citizen of the Year Award from the Omaha Combined Health Agencies, in recognition of his community work while Creighton's vice president; and the Creighton University Alumni Achievement Citation. Dr. Heaney was awarded honorary membership in the American Dietetic Association, was elected fellow of the American Society for Nutritional Sciences, and in 1994 he received the Frederic C. Bartter Award of the American Society for Bone and Mineral Research.

CHARLES H. HENNEKENS, M.D., Dr.P.H., is Eugene Braunwald Professor of Medicine and professor of ambulatory care and prevention at Harvard Medical School, professor of epidemiology at Harvard School of Public Health, and chief of the Division of Preventive Medicine at Brigham and Women's Hospital. He received his M.D. from Cornell University Medical College and his M.P.H. and Dr.P.H. from the Harvard School of Public Health. Dr. Hennekens is president of the American Epidemiological Society, past president of the Society for Epidemiologic Research, and is a member of the Association of American Physicians. He has served as editor-in-chief of the *American Journal of Preventive Medicine* and founding editor-in-chief of the *Annals of Epidemiology*. Dr. Hennekens is a fellow of the American College of Preventive Medicine and the American College of Epidemiology, and is a member of the Food and Nutrition Board. His awards include the Bruce Award from the American College of Physicians, the Lilienfeld Award from American College of Epidemiology, and the 1996 American College of Nutrition Award. Dr. Hennekens is the principal or coprincipal investigator for several large, long-term observational studies and trials, including the Physician's Health Study and the Women's Health Study.

MICHAEL F. HOLICK, M.D., Ph.D., is professor of medicine, dermatology and physiology; chief of the Endocrinology, Nutrition and Diabetes Program; director for the General Clinical Research Center; and director of the Bone Health Care Clinic at Boston University Medical Center. He received his Ph.D. and M.D. from the University of Wisconsin. Dr. Holick has dedicated his career to understanding the biologic importance of vitamin D for human health. He determined how vitamin D is made in the skin during exposure to sunlight and established the importance of casual exposure to sunlight as a way for humans to obtain their vitamin D requirement. Dr. Holick pioneered the concept of using activated vitamin D for the treatment of psoriasis. He has received numerous awards for his innovative clinical and basic research activities. He serves on a number of editorial boards, has served as a consultant to NASA, and is a member of the NASA Life and Microgravity Sciences and Applications Advisory Committee.

JANET C. KING, Ph.D., R.D., is director of the U.S. Department of Agriculture Human Nutrition Research Center at the Presidio of San Francisco and professor in the Graduate School, University of California, Berkeley. Dr. King received a B.S. in dietetics from Iowa State University, a Ph.D. in nutrition from the University of California, Berkeley, and is a registered dietitian. She is a member of the American Society of Nutritional Sciences, American Society of Clinical Nutrition, American Dietetic Association, Society for Nutrition Education, and American Association for the Advancement of Science. Dr. King has served on the editorial board of the *Journal of Nutrition* and is associate editor of the *American Journal of Clinical Nutrition*. She is a past chair of the Food and Nutrition Board and has served on or chaired several of its committees. In 1994, Dr. King was elected to the Institute of Medicine. Other honors and awards include the Borden Award and Lederle Award from the American Society of Nutritional Sciences, Massee Lecturer in Human Nutrition from the University of North Dakota, Mary Shorb Lecturer from the University of Maryland, Lydia J. Roberts Award from the University of Chicago, International Prize in Modern Human Nutrition from the University of Lausanne, Switzerland, and University

Distinguished Professor in Nutrition from the University of California, Davis.

WALTER MERTZ, M.D., received his M.D. from the University of Mainz, Germany. He was an intern surgeon at the County Hospital, Hersfeld, and assistant resident at the Medical University Hospital, Frankfurt, Germany. He went to the National Institute of Health at Bethesda in 1953 where he worked on nutritional aspects of liver disease and on the glucose tolerance factor, later identified as the trace element chromium. Dr. Mertz continued his work on chromium in clinical studies at the Walter Reed Army Institute of Research as chief, Department of Biological Chemistry. He later joined the Human Nutrition Research Division, Agricultural Research Service, U.S. Department of Agriculture, as chief, Vitamin and Mineral Nutrition Laboratory. In 1972, he was appointed director of the Nutrition Institute, now the Beltsville Human Nutrition Research Center, a position he held until his retirement in 1993. Dr. Mertz is the author of more than 200 scientific publications.

RITA B. MESSING, Ph.D., received her Ph.D. in physiological psychology from Princeton University and did postdoctoral research in the Department of Nutrition and Food Science at the Massachusetts Institute of Technology in the Laboratory of Neuroendocrine Regulation. Dr. Messing has been in the Department of Pharmacology, University of Minnesota Medical School since 1981, and is currently an associate professor. Since 1990 her primary employment has been at the Minnesota Department of Health in environmental toxicology, where she supervises the Site Assessment and Consultation Unit, which conducts public health activities at hazardous waste sites and other sources of uncontrolled toxic releases. Dr. Messing has 70 publications in toxicology and risk assessment, neuropharmacology, psychobiology, and experimental psychology. She has taught at Rutgers University, Northeastern University, University of California at Irvine, and University of Minnesota, and had visiting appointments at Organon Pharmaceuticals in the Netherlands and the University of Paris.

SANFORD A. MILLER, Ph.D., is dean of the Graduate School of Biomedical Sciences and professor in the Departments of Biochemistry and Medicine at The University of Texas Health Science Center at San Antonio. He is the former director of the Center for Food Safety and Applied Nutrition at the Food and Drug Administration.

Previously, he was professor of nutritional biochemistry at the Massachusetts Institute of Technology. Dr. Miller has served on many national and international government and professional society advisory committees, including the Federation of American Societies for Experimental Biology Expert Committee on GRAS Substances, the National Advisory Environmental Health Sciences Council of the National Institutes of Health, the Food and Nutrition Board and its Food Forum, the Joint WHO/FAO Expert Advisory Panel on Food Safety (Chairman), and the Steering Committees of several WHO/FAO panels. He also served as chair of the Joint FAO/WHO Expert Consultation on the Application of Risk Analysis to Food Standards Issues. He is author or co-author of more than 200 original scientific publications. Dr. Miller received a B.S. in chemistry from the City College of New York, and a M.S. and Ph.D. from Rutgers University in physiology and biochemistry.

IAN C. MUNRO, Ph.D., is a leading authority on toxicology and has over 30 years experience in dealing with complex regulatory issues related to product safety. He has in excess of 150 scientific publications in the fields of toxicology and risk assessment. Dr. Munro formerly held senior positions at Health and Welfare Canada as director of the Bureau of Chemical Safety and director general of the Food Directorate, Health Protection Branch. He was responsible for research and standard setting activities related to microbial and chemical hazards in food and the nutritional quality of the Canadian food supply. He has contributed significantly to the development of risk assessment procedures in the field of public health, both nationally and internationally, through membership on various committees dealing with the regulatory aspects of risk assessment and risk management of public health hazards. Dr. Munro is a graduate of McGill University in biochemistry and nutrition and holds a Ph.D. from Queen's University in pharmacology and toxicology. He is a fellow of the Royal College of Pathologists, London. He also is a former director of the Canadian Centre for Toxicology at Guelph, Ontario.

SUZANNE P. MURPHY, Ph.D., R.D., is adjunct associate professor in the Department of Nutritional Sciences at the University of California, Berkeley, and director of the California Expanded Food and Nutrition Program at the University of California, Davis. She received her B.S. in mathematics from Temple University and her Ph.D. in nutrition from the University of California, Berkeley. Dr. Murphy's research interests include dietary assessment methodology, development of food composition databases, and nutritional epidemiology. She is a member of the National Nutrition Monitoring Advisory Council, and serves on the editorial boards for the *Journal of Nutrition, Journal of Food Composition and Analysis,* and *Family Economics and Nutrition Review.* Dr. Murphy is a member of numerous professional organizations including the American Dietetic Association, American Society for Nutritional Sciences, American Public Health Association, American Society for Clinical Nutrition, and Society for Nutrition Education. She has over 50 publications on dietary assessment methodology and has lectured nationally and internationally on this subject.

JOSEPH V. RODRICKS, Ph.D., is one of the founding principals of the ENVIRON Corporation, with internationally recognized expertise in assessing the risks to human health of exposure to toxic substances. He received his B.S. from the Massachusetts Institute of Technology and his Ph.D. in biochemistry from the University of Maryland. Dr. Rodricks is certified as a diplomate of the American Board of Toxicology. Before working as a consultant, he spent 15 years at the Food and Drug Administration (FDA). In his final 3 years at the FDA, he was Deputy Associate Commissioner for Science, with special responsibility for risk assessment. He was a member of the National Academy of Sciences (NAS) Board on Toxicology and Environmental Health Hazards, and has also served on or chaired ten other NAS Committees. Dr. Rodricks has more than 100 scientific publications on food safety and risk assessment and has lectured nationally and internationally on these subjects. He is the author of *Calculated Risks,* a non-technical introduction to toxicology and risk assessment.

IRWIN H. ROSENBERG, M.D., is an internationally recognized leader in nutrition science who serves as professor of physiology, medicine and nutrition at Tufts University School of Medicine and School of Nutrition, as well as director, Jean Mayer U.S. Department of Agriculture (USDA) Human Nutrition Research Center on Aging at Tufts University and dean for nutrition sciences, Tufts University. He is the first holder of the Jean Mayer Chair in Nutrition at Tufts. Prior to joining Tufts, Dr. Rosenberg held faculty positions at Harvard Medical School and the University of Chicago where he served as the first director of the Clinical Nutrition Research Center. As a clinical nutrition investigator, he has helped develop a nutritional focus within the field of gastroenterology with his primary research interest being in the area of folate metabolism. His research for the past decade has focused on nutrition and the aging process. Among his many honors are the Josiah Macy Faculty Award, Grace Goldsmith Award of the American College of Nutrition, Robert H. Herman Memorial Award of the American Society of Clinical Nutrition, Jonathan B. Rhoads Award of the American Society for Parenteral and Enteral Nutrition, and 1994 W.O. Atwater Memorial Lectureship of the USDA. Dr. Rosenberg was elected to the Institute of Medicine in 1994 and he received the Bristol Myers Squibb/ Mead Johnson Award for Distinguished Achievement in Nutrition Research in 1996.

ROBERT K. RUDE, M.D., is professor of medicine at the University of Southern California and director of the Endocrinology Research Laboratory and the University of Southern California/Orthopaedic Hospital Bone and Mineral Metabolism Clinic at the Orthopaedic Hospital. He received his B.S from the University of North Dakota and his M.D. from Northwestern University. Dr. Rude's research interests have been in the area of bone and mineral metabolism, with emphasis on the effect of magnesium depletion on calcium and bone homeostasis. Other areas of research include osteoporosis and hypercalcemia. He is a member of the American Federation for Clinical Research, Endocrine Society, American Society for Bone and Mineral Research, and American College of Nutrition. Dr. Rude has published close to 100 peer-reviewed journal articles and book chapters.

BONNY SPECKER, Ph.D., received her Ph.D. in epidemiology from the University of Cincinnati. Since that time she has been actively involved in calcium and vitamin D studies in infants and in lactating women. She was professor of pediatrics at the University of Cincinnati College of Medicine and Children's Hospital Medical Center, and recently accepted the position of director and chair of the Ethel Austin Martin Endowed Program in Human Nutrition at South Dakota State University where she is professor of nutrition and food sciences and adjunct professor of pediatrics at the University of South Dakota. Dr. Specker has over 80 peer-reviewed journal articles and book chapters. She is a member of the American Society for Bone and Mineral Research, Society for Pediatric Research, American Society of Nutritional Sciences, and American Society for Clinical Nutrition.

STEVE L. TAYLOR, Ph.D., serves as professor and head of the Department of Food Science and Technology and director of the Food Processing Center at the University of Nebraska. He also maintains an active research program in the area of food allergies through the Food Allergy Research and Resource Program at the University of Nebraska. He received his B.S. and M.S. in food science and technology from Oregon State University and his Ph.D. in biochemistry from the University of California, Davis. Dr. Taylor's primary research interests involve naturally occurring toxicants in foods, especially food allergens. His research involves the development of immunoassays for the detection of residues of allergenic foods contaminating other foods, the effect of processing on food allergens, and the assessment of the allergenicity of genetically engineered foods. Dr. Taylor has over 160 publications. He is a member of numerous professional associations including the Institute of Food Technologists, American Chemical Society, American Academy of Allergy, Asthma, and Immunology, and Society of Toxicology.

VERNON R. YOUNG, Ph.D., is a professor of nutritional biochemistry at the Massachusetts Institute of Technology and director of the Mass Spectrometry Facility, Shriners Burn Hospital, Boston. Dr. Young received a B.Sc. in agriculture from the University of Reading, United Kingdom and a Ph.D. in nutrition from the University of California, Davis. He later received a D.Sc. from the University of Reading for his research on various aspects of muscle and whole-body protein metabolism. Dr. Young has served as president of the American Society for Nutritional Sciences. He is a member of the Food and Nutrition Board, the American Society of Clinical Nutrition, and the Nutrition Society (UK). He has served on many editorial boards, including the *Journal of Nutrition* and *American Journal of Clinical Nutrition*. In 1990 Dr. Young was elected to the National Academy of Sciences and in 1993 to the Institute of Medicine. His research has focused mainly on human protein and amino acid metabolism and nutritional requirements. He is the recipient of numerous other awards including the Mead-Johnson Award and the Bordon Award from the ASNS, the McCollum Award from the American Society of Clinical Nutrition, the Rank Prize in Nutrition (UK), the Bristol-Myers Squibb/Mead Johnson Award for Excellence in Nutrition Research (US), and the Danone International Prize for Nutrition (France). He also received an M.D. (h.c.) from Uppsala University, Sweden.

ROBERT H. WASSERMAN, Ph.D., is James Law Professor of Physiology, College of Veterinary Medicine, Cornell University. He received his B.S. in microbiology and his Ph.D. in nutritional microbiology from Cornell University. Dr. Wasserman's research interest is the mechanisms and control of epithelial transport of mineral ions with emphasis given to the role of vitamin D on the intestinal absorption of calcium and phosphorus. He was elected to the National Academy of Sciences in 1980, chaired its Committee on the Scientific Basis of Meat and Poultry Inspection, and was a member of the Food and Nutrition Board. Dr. Wasserman has served on the editorial boards of *Proceedings of the Society for Experimental Biology and Medicine, The Cornell Veterinarian, Calcified Tissue International,* and *Journal of Nutrition.* Included among his numerous awards are the Mead Johnson Lectureship at Iowa State University, the Lichtwitz Prize of the Institut National de la Sante et de la Researche Medicale in Paris, the MERIT status award of the National Institutes of Health, the William F. Neuman Research Award from the American Society of Bone and Mineral Research, the Career Recognition Award from Vitamin D Workshop, Inc., and was elected a fellow of the American Institute of Nutrition.

CONNIE M. WEAVER, Ph.D., is professor and head of Foods and Nutrition at Purdue University. She received her B.S. and M.S. from Oregon State University and her Ph.D. from Florida State University, all in food science and human nutrition. She serves as president elect of the American Society for Nutritional Sciences, as scientific advisor to NASA and the International Life Sciences Institute, and on the editorial boards of the *Journal of Nutrition Biochemistry* and the *CRC Series in Contemporary Food Science.* Dr. Weaver's research focuses on mineral bioavailability and function.

GARY M. WHITFORD, Ph.D., D.M.D., is Regents' Professor in the Department of Oral Biology, Medical College of Georgia. He received his Ph.D. in toxicology from the University of Rochester and his D.M.D. from the Medical College of Georgia. Dr. Whitford received the H. Trendley Dean Distinguished Scientist Award from the International Association for Dental Research in 1986 and the ORCA-Rolex Award from the European Association for Caries Research in 1992. He is the author of over 100 publications, several chapters in various textbooks, and the monograph entitled the *Metabolism and Toxicity of Fluoride.*

FNB STAFF

ALICE L. KULIK, M.S.P.H., is a research associate with the Food and Nutrition Board (FNB). In addition to her work with the Panel on Calcium and Related Nutrients, she has worked on several other Institute of Medicine reports including those of the Panel on Folate, Other B Vitamins, and Choline and the Committee to Review the Department of Defense's Breast Cancer Research Program. Ms. Kulik received her B.A. in biology from Barnard College and her M.S.P.H. in epidemiology from the University of North Carolina School of Public Health. Prior to joining the FNB in 1996, Ms. Kulik was an assistant in the grants department of the Howard Hughes Medical Institute. She also worked as a biologist at the National Institute of Allergy and Infectious Diseases.

ELISABETH A. REESE, M.P.H., is a research associate with the Food and Nutrition Board (FNB). In addition to her work with the Subcommittee on Upper Reference Levels of Nutrients, Ms. Reese has worked on several Institute of Medicine and National Research Council reports including those of the Standing Committee on the Scientific Evaluation of Dietary Reference Intakes on calcium and related nutrients and folate and other B vitamins, and of the Committee to Ensure Safe Food from Production to Consumption. She also serves as president of the Society for Risk Analysis' Dose Response Specialty Group. Prior to joining the FNB in 1996, Ms. Reese was a staff scientist at an environmental consulting firm where she assessed and summarized the human health hazards of environmental chemicals and provided technical support for risk assessment projects. She earned a B.A. in chemistry and history from New York University, an M.P.H. in toxicology from the University of Michigan, and has since taken additional course work in epidemiology.

SANDRA A. SCHLICKER, Ph.D., is a senior program officer at the Food and Nutrition Board (FNB), and serves as the study director for the Subcommittee on Upper Reference Levels of Nutrients. Prior to joining the FNB, she was vice president of a Washington, D.C.-based consulting/research firm which focused on public policy issues in the fields of agriculture, health, and nutrition. Dr. Schlicker has served as a government relations representative, media spokes-person, and nutrition consultant to food manufacturers and trade associations. She is a licensed nutritionist and hold as B.S. in science and an M.S. and Ph.D. in food and nutrition from

The Pennsylvania State University. An active member of the American Dietetic Association, Dr. Schlicker has authored numerous nutrition articles in professional and consumer publications.

ALLISON A. YATES, Ph.D., R.D., is director of the Food and Nutrition Board (FNB), Institute of Medicine (IOM), and also serves as study director for the Standing Committee on the Scientific Evaluation of Dietary Reference Intakes. Dr. Yates received a B.S. in dietetics and an M.S. in public health (nutrition) from U.C.L.A., a Ph.D. in nutrition from the University of California, Berkeley, and is a registered dietitian. She is a member of the American Society for Nutrition Sciences, American Society of Clinical Nutrition, American Dietetic Association, Institute of Food Technologists, and the American Public Health Association. Dr. Yates served as a member of the FNB Committee on Military Nutrition Research prior to assuming her position at IOM in 1994. Most recently, Dr. Yates was professor of foods and nutrition and dean of the College of Health and Human Sciences at the University of Southern Mississippi.

Index

A

Achlorhydria, 74, 142
Adenylate cyclase, 191
Adequate Intakes (AIs), *see also* Calcium AIs;
    Fluoride, AIs; Vitamin D, AIs
  applicable population, 22
  criteria used to derive, 12-13
  defined, 4, 6, 24, 25, 48, 301, 315, 317
  derivation of, 4, 5-8, 32-33, 48-50, 317
  discrepancies between usual intakes and,
    324
  extrapolation from other age groups, 26
  gender and, 17, 34
  increasing consumption of nutrients, 10-
    12, 28, 323
  indicators used to set, 27, 40, 91, 261-
    263, 298-301
  RDAs compared, 5-8, 26
  replacement of, 25
  safety factors, 8
  uncertainty in, 317
  uses, 4, 5, 11, 28, 317
Adolescents, 9 through 18 years. *See also*
    Puberty
  ages 9 through 13 years, 34, 41, 99-106,
    169-173, 210-218, 268-269, 303; *see
    also* Puberty
  ages 14 through 18 years, 34, 99-106,
    169-173, 179, 180, 186-187, 210-218,
    219, 239, 240, 241, 303

Body Mass Index, 36
bone mass, 102, 104, 105
bone mineral content, 100, 101-102,
    103, 133-134
bone mineral density, 100, 102, 103,
    104-105
calcium , 41, 73, 75, 87, 99-106, 143, 144,
    215, 324, 396
fluoride, 295, 296, 303
indicators used to set AIs, 100-105
indicators used to set EARs, 169-172,
    210-212
lactation, 133-134, 179, 180, 241
magnesium, 194, 195, 206, 210-213, 214-
    215, 216-219, 240, 241, 244-246, 268
phosphorus, 154, 159, 165, 169-173, 177-
    178, 179, 180, 184-185, 186, 187-189,
    321
pregnancy, 114, 177-178, 239, 240, 276
RDAs, 172-173, 218, 219, 239
supplements, 96-97, 215
ULs, 141-142, 188, 244-246, 285, 310-311
vitamin D, 262, 268-269, 276, 277, 284-
    285, 286
weights and heights, reference, 35-36
Adults, 19 through 30 years
  Body Mass Index, 36, 37
  bone mass, peak, 34, 106-107
  calcium, 75-76, 87, 106-109, 111, 397
  derivation of DRIs for, 34-35

413

F

Factorial approach
  calcium, 6, 7, 48, 49, 102, 104, 105, 108, 109, 110-111
  phosphorus, 16, 40, 164-166, 168, 170, 172
Fetal
  calcium needs, 117
  growth retardation, 234, 235-237
  sensitivity to nutrients, 60, 303-304
Fiber. *See* Dietary fiber
Fluorhydroxyapatite, 288
Fluoride
  absorption, 289, 291, 313
  adolescents, 295, 296, 303
  adults, 289, 293, 296, 301, 303
  AIs, 8, 14, 19, 40, 50, 298-300, 301-306
  balance studies, 289, 300-301, 304
  bioavailability, 291
  and bone mineral content, 38, 288, 300, 307, 310
  and caffeine, 291, 294
  and calcification of tissues, 300, 307, 313
  and calcium, 288, 289, 290, 291
  children, 289, 290, 291-292, 293, 294-296, 298-299, 301, 303, 304, 305, 306, 308-309, 311-312
  and dental caries, 8, 14, 19, 50, 288-289, 290, 297-300, 301, 302, 313
  in dental products, 45, 291, 295-296, 300, 307, 311-312, 318
  derivation of DRI, 8, 40, 50
  in drinking water, 45, 291-292, 293, 295, 297-300, 301, 305, 307, 308, 310, 318
  and enamel fluorosis, 298-299, 300-302, 305-307, 308-309, 311-313, 318
  excretion, 289-290, 313
  factors affecting nutrient requirement, 291
  food sources, 291, 293-294
  gender differences, 19, 303
  and geographic differences, 298-300, 307-308
  in human milk, 19, 291, 292, 301, 302, 305, 306, 311
  indicators of nutrient requirements, 19, 40, 298-301
  infants, 290, 293, 295, 300, 301-302, 304, 305-306, 309, 311, 312
  intakes, 45, 291-296, 301, 306, 308

  interactions with food components, 291
  international comparisons, 298-300
  lactation and, 12, 19, 305-306
  life-stage group and, 19, 301-306
  menopausal status and, 300
  metabolism, 289-290, 305
  and osteoporosis, 288, 300, 307
  and osteosclerosis, 307, 308, 310
  phosphate, 290
  physiological role, 288-289
  pregnancy and, 12, 19, 303-305
  research recommendations, 14, 313
  skeletal fluorosis, 307-308, 310-311
  sources of, 45, 318
  special considerations, 305-306, 311
  supplements, 295, 298-299, 302, 304, 311-312
  sustained release form, 288
  toddlers, 293, 302-303, 309
  toothpastes, 291, 295-296, 300
  ULs, 13, 20, 68, 306-313, 318
  uncertainty factor, 68, 310
  young adults, 289
Food additives, 57, 154, 155, 180, 189
Food and Agriculture Organization, 22, 52, 319, 322
Food composition databases, 42-43
Food sources
  calcium, 45, 47, 81-82
  fluoride, 291, 293-294
  magnesium, 193, 196, 199-200
  phosphorus, 151-152, 155-156, 161, 173-174, 180, 181, 183-184, 189
  vitamin D, 256-257, 261-262, 268, 269, 270, 271, 283, 284, 285-286
Formulas, infant
  bioavailability of nutrients from, 32, 94-95, 96, 210
  calcium, 94-96, 141
  fluoride in, 291, 292, 293, 301-302, 306
  magnesium, 210
  phosphorus, 149, 152, 153, 155, 159, 161, 163, 183
  special considerations, 163, 210, 265
  vitamin D, 257, 262, 265, 266
Fortified foods, 4, 10-11, 12, 26, 28, 59, 143, 256, 261-262, 283, 284, 285-286, 318. *See also* Formulas, infant
Fracture. *See* Bone fracture
Fruits and vegetables, 82, 193, 196, 199-200, 229

M

and renal disease, 280
research recommendations, 14, 286-287
and rickets, 8, 50, 254, 257-258, 259,
    260, 263, 264-265, 277
risk characterization, 286
safety factor, 8, 50
serum, 260
and skeletal health, 257-258, 260-261,
    262-264
special considerations, 255, 265, 275,
    285
submariners, 270, 271
sun exposure and, 45, 50, 250, 252, 253-
    254, 255-256, 260, 262-276, 284, 285,
    286
sunscreen and, 14, 256, 261, 271, 286
supplements, 45-46, 255, 257, 262, 264,
    267, 268, 271-272, 274-277, 281-283,
    286, 318
toddlers, 266-268, 284-285
ULs, 13, 20, 68, 277-286, 318
uncertainty and uncertainty factors, 68,
    281, 282, 284
vegetarians, 267, 270
Vitamin E, 139
Vitamin K, 38-39, 60

W

Water. *See* Drinking water
Weight. *See* Reference weights and heights

Weight-bearing practices, 42, 68
Women. *See also* Gender differences;
    Lactation; Menopausal status;
    Pregnancy
amenorrheic, 76
balance studies, 220, 221, 225, 226
calcium, 72, 75, 109-110, 111-114, 135,
    143
fluoride, 301-306
indicators used to set AIs, 111-114
indicators used to set EARs, 221, 226
intakes of nutrients, 43-45
magnesium, 30, 220, 222-223, 225, 227,
    230-231, 233
phosphorus, 30, 31, 155, 316, 321, 322-
    323
vitamin D, 43-45, 256, 272, 273
World Health Organization, 22, 52, 83, 319,
    322

Y

Young adults. *See* Adults, 19 through 30
    years

Z

Zinc, 38, 59, 137, 140, 141, 142, 171, 180-
    181, 189, 214
Zinc oxide, 53